ESSENTIALS IN OPHTHALMOLOGY: Pediatric Ophthalmology, Neuro-Ophthalmology, Genetics

B. Lorenz · A.T. Moore (Eds.)

ESSENTIALS IN OPHTHALMOLOGY

G. K. Krieglstein · R. N. Weinreb
Series Editors

Glaucoma

Cataract and Refractive Surgery

Uveitis and Immunological Disorders

Vitreo-retinal Surgery

Medical Retina

Oculoplastics and Orbit

Pediatric Ophthalmology, Neuro-Ophthalmology, Genetics

Cornea and External Eye Disease

Editors B. Lorenz
A.T. Moore

Pediatric Ophthalmology, Neuro-Ophthalmology, Genetics

With 89 Figures, Mostly in Color, and 25 Tables

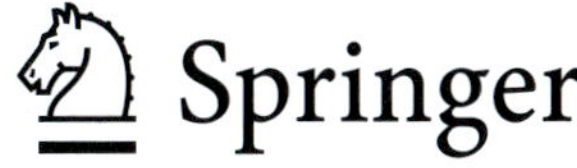

Series Editors

Guenter K. Krieglstein, MD
Professor and Chairman
Department of Ophthalmology
University of Cologne
Joseph-Stelzmann-Strasse 9
50931 Cologne
Germany

Robert N. Weinreb, MD
Professor and Director
Hamilton Glaucoma Center
Department of Ophthalmology – 0946
University of California at San Diego
9500 Gilman Drive
La Jolla, CA 92093-0946
USA

Volume Editors

Birgit Lorenz, MD
Professor of Ophthalmology
and Ophthalmic Genetics
Head of Department
Department of Paediatric Ophthalmology
Strabismology and Ophthalmogenetics
Klinikum, University of Regensburg
Franz Josef Strauss Allee 11
93053 Regensburg, Germany

Anthony T. Moore, MA, FRCS, FRCOphth
Division of Inherited Eye Disease
Institute of Ophthalmology
Moorfields Eye Hospital, City Road
London, EC1V 9EL, UK

ISBN-10 3-540-22594-3
Springer Berlin Heidelberg New York

ISBN-13 978-3-540-22594-2
Springer Berlin Heidelberg New York

ISSN 1612-3212

Library of Congress Control Number: 2005928345

Springer is a part of Springer Science + Business Media

springeronline.com

Cover picture "Cataract and Refractive Surgery" from Kampik A, Grehn F (eds) Augenärztliche Therapie. Georg Thieme Verlag Stuttgart, with permission.

Editor: Marion Philipp, Springer-Verlag Heidelberg, Germany
Desk editor: Martina Himberger, Springer-Verlag Heidelberg, Germany
Production: ProEdit GmbH, Elke Beul-Göhringer, Heidelberg, Germany
Cover design: Erich Kirchner, Heidelberg, Germany
Typesetting and reproduction of the figures: AM-productions GmbH, Wiesloch, Germany

Printed on acid-free paper
24/3151beu-göh 5 4 3 2 1 0

Foreword

Essentials in Ophthalmology is a new review series covering all of ophthalmology categorized in eight subspecialties. It will be published quarterly; thus each subspecialty will be reviewed biannually.

Given the multiplicity of medical publications already available, why is a new series needed? Consider that the half-life of medical knowledge is estimated to be around 5 years. Moreover, it can be as long as 8 years between the description of a medical innovation in a peer-reviewed scientific journal and publication in a medical textbook. A series that narrows this time span between journal and textbook would provide a more rapid and efficient transfer of medical knowledge into clinical practice, and enhance care of our patients.

For the series, each subspecialty volume comprises 10–20 chapters selected by two distinguished editors and written by internationally renowned specialists. The selection of these contributions is based more on recent and noteworthy advances in the subspecialty than on systematic completeness. Each article is structured in a standardized format and length, with citations for additional reading and an appropriate number of illustrations to enhance important points. Since every subspecialty volume is issued in a recurring sequence during the 2-year cycle, the reader has the opportunity to focus on the progress in a particular subspecialty or to be updated on the whole field. The clinical relevance of all material presented will be well established, so application to clinical practice can be made with confidence.

This new series will earn space on the bookshelves of those ophthalmologists who seek to maintain the timeliness and relevance of their clinical practice.

G. K. Krieglstein
R. N. Weinreb
Series Editors

Preface

In an era of increasing subspecialization pediatric ophthalmology stands out as the one area of ophthalmology where the generalist holds sway. The pediatric ophthalmologist must have a good working knowledge of general ophthalmology, have an understanding of visual development, visual electrophysiology and molecular genetics and be comfortable with dealing with children with a wide range of systemic disorders. It is a major challenge to keep up to date in all these areas. The aim of this monograph is to highlight recent advances in key fields of pediatric ophthalmology and inherited eye disease and to present this material in a concise readable format. The chapters encompass both pediatric ophthalmology and inherited eye disease; neuro-ophthalmology will be covered in detail in the next volume we edit.

Retinopathy of prematurity (ROP) has become more prevalent as advances in neonatal care have led to the survival of increasing numbers of very-low-birthweight preterm infants. This monograph includes reviews of current knowledge of the pathogenesis of ROP and screening and treatment protocols. There are also updates on the management of pediatric ocular tumors, infantile cataract and glaucoma, conditions which are best managed in specialized tertiary referral centers. One of the commonest eye problems in childhood is refractive error and amblyopia. This volume includes a review of current knowledge of the causes of myopia in experimental animal models and the implications for the understanding of the pathogenesis of myopia in man. There are also chapters on preschool vision screening and management of amblyopia.

Advances in molecular biology have led to improved understanding of the pathogenesis of inherited eye disease, and we have included chapters summarizing recent advances in understandings of the molecular genetic basis of early onset-retinal dystrophies and childhood retinal detachment. There is also a chapter highlighting the role of ocular electrophysiology in the investigation of visual loss in infancy. Finally, we cover two areas of pediatric ophthalmology where ophthalmologists work closely with their pediatric colleagues, firstly congenital infections affecting the eye and secondly the role of the ophthalmologist in assessing children with suspected non-accidental injury.

The individual chapters are written by leading authorities in their field. We are grateful to them for their excellent contributions and also to the publishers for their encouragement and support.

Birgit Lorenz
Anthony T. Moore

Contents

Chapter 1
Development of Ocular Refraction: Lessons from Animal Experiments
Frank Schaeffel, Howard C. Howland

1.1 Introduction ... 1
1.2 Overview on the Experimental Results in Animal Models ... 2
1.2.1 What Is the Evidence for Visual Control of Refractive Development and Axial Eye Growth? ... 2
1.2.2 Which Kind of Visual Stimulation Induces Refractive Errors in Animal Models? ... 2
1.2.3 What Is Known About the Retinal Image Processing That Leads to Refractive Errors? ... 4
1.2.4 How Long Must Defocus Persist to Induce Changes in Eye Growth? 5
1.2.5 What Is Known About the Tissue Responses and the Signaling Cascade from the Retina to the Sclera? ... 5
1.3 Can Animal Models Help to Improve the Management of Myopia in Children? ... 7
1.3.1 Undercorrection, Overcorrection, and Full Correction of Myopia ... 7
1.3.2 Reading Glasses ... 8
1.3.3 Contact Lenses Versus Spectacle Lenses ... 8
1.3.4 Illumination, Reading Distance, Computer Work Versus Reading Text in a Book ... 9
1.3.5 How Long Must the Near Work Be Performed to Induce Myopia? .. 10
1.3.6 Night Light, Blue Light ... 10
1.3.7 How Could Visual Acuity Improve Without Glasses? ... 12
1.3.8 Age Window for Intervention ... 13
1.3.9 Pharmacological Intervention for Myopia ... 13
1.3.10 Emmetropization in Hyperopia with and Without Optical Correction ... 13
1.4 Summary of Effects of Different Intervention Regimens on Myopia 15
References ... 15

Chapter 2
Preschool Vision Screening: Is It Worthwhile?
Josefin Ohlsson, Johan Sjöstrand

2.1 Introduction ... 19
2.1.1 Definition of Screening ... 19
2.1.2 Aims of Vision Screening ... 20
2.2 Preschool Vision Screening ... 20
2.2.1 Definition of Preschool Vision Screening ... 20
2.2.2 Target Conditions for Preschool Vision Screening ... 21
2.2.3 Natural History of Untreated Amblyopia ... 22
2.2.4 Whom to Screen? ... 22
2.3 Vision Screening Methodology ... 23
2.3.1 What Test to Use for Screening? ... 23
2.3.2 Visual Acuity ... 23
2.3.3 Stereo Tests ... 23
2.3.4 Orthoptic Assessment ... 24
2.3.5 Photorefractive Screening ... 24
2.3.6 Cost-Effectiveness of Different Tests ... 24
2.3.7 Who Should Perform the Screening? ... 24
2.3.8 At What Level Should Pass/ Fail Criteria Be Set? ... 24
2.4 When to Screen? ... 25
2.4.1 Treatment Outcome and Age ... 25

2.4.2 Testability and Age 26
2.4.3 Age at Vision Screening and Risk of New Cases or Rebounding Amblyopia 26
2.4.4 Age and Psychosocial Impact of Treatment 26
2.4.5 Current Recommendations on Suitable Age for Vision Screening 27
2.5 The Effect of Preschool Vision Screening 27
2.5.1 The Necessity of High Participation Rates 27
2.5.2 Evaluating the Effect of Preschool Vision Screening 29
2.6 What is the "Best Buy" for Vision Screening? 30
2.6.1 Early Versus Late Vision Screening 30
2.6.2 What Test Should Be Used? 31
2.6.3 What Age Is the "Best Buy" for Preschool Vision Screening? ... 31
2.7 Is Preschool Vision Screening Worthwhile? 32
2.7.1 The Risk of Losing the Nonamblyopic Eye 32
2.7.2 Is It Disabling to Be Amblyopic? ... 32
2.7.3 Cost-Effectiveness of Screening and Treatment for Amblyopia 33
2.8 Future Evidence Needed 34
References 34

Chapter 3
Modern Treatment of Amblyopia
Michael Clarke

3.1 Introduction 37
3.2 What Is Amblyopia? 37
3.3 Should Amblyopia Be Treated? 38
3.4 What Difference Does It Make When the Patient Is a Child? 39
3.5 Why Treat Amblyopia? 39
3.6 What Are Patient Perceptions of the Disability Due to Amblyopia? 41
3.7 Identification of Amblyopia 41
3.8 Treatment of Amblyopia 42
3.8.1 Evidence for Effectiveness of Amblyopia Treatment 43
3.8.2 Correction of Refractive Error 43
3.8.3 Patching 43
3.8.4 Atropine 45
3.8.5 Why Does Amblyopia Treatment Not Always Work? 46
3.9 New Developments 46
3.9.1 L-DOPA 46
3.9.2 Visual Stimulation 48
3.10 Translation into Practice 48
References 48

Chapter 4
Retinopathy of Prematurity: Molecular Mechanism of Disease
Lois E.H. Smith

4.1 Introduction 51
4.2 Pathogenesis: Two Phases of ROP .. 51
4.2.1 Phase I of ROP 52
4.2.2 Phase II of ROP 52
4.3 Mouse Model of ROP 52
4.4 Vascular Endothelial Growth Factor and Oxygen in ROP 52
4.4.1 VEGF and Phase II of ROP 53
4.4.2 VEGF and Phase I of ROP 53
4.5 Other Growth Factors Are Involved in ROP 54
4.5.1 IGF-1 Deficiency in the Preterm Infant 54
4.5.2 GH and IGF-1 in Phase II of ROP .. 55
4.5.3 IGF-1 and VEGF Interaction 55
4.5.4 Low Levels of IGF-I and Phase I of ROP 56
4.5.5 Clinical Studies: Low IGF-1 Is Associated with Degree of ROP ... 56
4.5.6 Low IGF-1 Is Associated with Decreased Vascular Density .. 56
4.5.7 IGF-1 and Brain Development 57
4.6 Conclusion: A Rationale for the Evolution of ROP.......... 57
References 58

Chapter 5
Screening for Retinopathy of Prematurity
Birgit Lorenz

5.1 Introduction 63
5.2 The Disease 64
5.2.1 Classification 65
5.2.2 Treatment Requiring ROP 65
5.2.3 Treatment of Acute ROP 69
5.3 Epidemiology of ROP 69
5.3.1 Risk Factors 70
5.3.2 Incidence of ROP 70
5.4 Screening Guidelines 72
5.5 Screening Methods 73

5.5.1 Conventional Screening 73
5.5.2 Digital Photography 75
5.5.3 Telemedicine 76
5.6 Conclusions 77
References 77

Chapter 6
Controversies in the Management of Infantile Cataract
Scott R. Lambert

6.1 Introduction 81
6.1.1 Epidemiology 81
6.2 Optimal Age for Infantile Cataract Surgery 82
6.2.1 Aphakic Glaucoma 83
6.2.2 Pupillary Membranes 83
6.2.3 Lens Reproliferation 84
6.2.4 General Anesthesia During the Neonatal Period 84
6.3 Visual Rehabilitation in Children with a Unilateral Congenital Cataract 84
6.3.1 Visual Rehabilitation in Children with Bilateral Congenital Cataracts 85
6.3.2 Contact Lenses 85
6.3.3 Intraocular Lenses 85
6.3.4 Surveys of North American Pediatric Ophthalmologists 87
6.4 Infant Aphakia Treatment Study ... 89
6.4.1 Eligibility Criteria 89
6.4.2 Surgical Procedure for Infants Randomized to Contact Lenses 89
6.4.3 Surgical Procedure for Infants Randomized to IOL 89
6.4.4 Type of IOL 90
6.4.5 IOL Power 90
6.5 Bilateral Simultaneous Surgery 91
6.5.1 Endophthalmitis 91
6.5.2 Visual Rehabilitation 92
References 92

Chapter 7
Management of Infantile Glaucoma
Thomas S. Dietlein, Guenter K. Krieglstein

7.1 Classification 95
7.2 Diagnostic Aspects 96
7.2.1 Clinical Background 96
7.2.2 Tonometry 97
7.2.3 Optic Disc Evaluation 97
7.2.4 Sonography 98
7.2.5 Corneal Morphology 98
7.2.6 Visual Field Testing 99
7.2.7 Objective Refraction 99
7.3 Medical Treatment 100
7.3.1 Miotics 100
7.3.2 Beta-Blockers 101
7.3.3 Carbonic Anhydrase Inhibitors 101
7.3.4 Prostaglandins 101
7.3.5 Alpha-2 Agonists 101
7.4 Surgical Therapy 101
7.4.1 Goniotomy 102
7.4.2 Trabeculotomy 102
7.4.3 Trabeculotomy Combined with Trabeculectomy 103
7.4.4 Trabeculectomy 103
7.4.5 Use of Antifibrotic Agents 104
7.4.6 Glaucoma Implants 104
7.4.7 Nonperforating Glaucoma Surgery 105
7.4.8 Cyclodialysis 105
7.4.9 Cyclodestructive Procedures 105
7.4.10 Surgical Iridectomy (Laser Iridotomy) 106
7.4.11 Special Aspects 106
7.5 Surgical Complications 106
7.5.1 Intraoperative Complications 106
7.5.2 Postoperative Complications 107
7.6 Prognosis 108
7.7 Concluding Remarks 108
References 108

Chapter 8
Pediatric Ocular Oncology
Carol L. Shields, Jerry A. Shields

8.1 General Considerations 111
8.1.1 Clinical Signs of Childhood Ocular Tumors 112
8.1.2 Diagnostic Approaches 112
8.1.3 Therapeutic Approaches 113
8.2 Eyelid Tumors 114
8.2.1 Capillary Hemangioma 114
8.2.2 Facial Nevus Flammeus 115
8.2.3 Kaposi's Sarcoma 115
8.2.4 Basal Cell Carcinoma 115
8.2.5 Melanocytic Nevus 116
8.2.6 Neurofibroma 116
8.2.7 Neurilemoma (Schwannoma) 116

8.3 Conjunctual Tumors 117
8.3.1 Dermoid 117
8.3.2 Epibulbar Osseous Choristoma 117
8.3.3 Complex Choristoma 117
8.3.4 Papilloma 117
8.3.5 Nevus 118
8.3.6 Congenital Ocular Melanocytosis .. 118
8.3.7 Pyogenic Granuloma 119
8.3.8 Kaposi's Sarcoma 119
8.4 Intraocular Tumors 119
8.4.1 Retinoblastoma 119
8.4.2 Retinal Capillary Hemangioma ... 121
8.4.3 Retinal Cavernous Hemangioma .. 121
8.4.4 Retinal Racemose Hemangioma ... 122
8.4.5 Astrocytic Hamartoma of Retina .. 122
8.4.6 Melanocytoma of the Optic Nerve 122
8.4.7 Intraocular Medulloepithelioma ... 123
8.4.8 Choroidal Hemangioma 123
8.4.9 Choroidal Osteoma 123
8.4.10 Uveal Nevus 124
8.4.11 Uveal Melanoma 124
8.4.12 Congenital Hypertrophy of Retinal Pigment Epithelium 125
8.4.13 Leukemia 126
8.5 Orbital Tumors 126
8.5.1 Dermoid Cyst 126
8.5.2 Teratoma 127
8.5.3 Capillary Hemangioma 127
8.5.4 Lymphangioma 127
8.5.5 Juvenile Pilocytic Astrocytoma 127
8.5.6 Rhabdomyosarcoma 128
8.5.7 Granulocytic Sarcoma (Chloroma) 128
8.5.8 Lymphoma 129
8.5.9 Langerhans Cell Histiocytosis 129
8.5.10 Metastatic Neuroblastoma 129
References 129

Chapter 9
Paediatric Electrophysiology: A Practical Approach
Graham E. Holder, Anthony G. Robson

9.1 Introduction 133
9.2 Electrophysiological Techniques ... 133
9.2.1 Electroretinography 133
9.2.2 Pattern Electroretinography 135
9.2.3 Cortical Visual Evoked Potentials .. 136
9.2.4 Electro-oculography 136
9.3 Investigation of Night Blindness ... 137
9.3.1 Retinitis Pigmentosa (Rod-Cone Dystrophy) 137
9.3.2 Congenital Stationary Night Blindness 140
9.3.3 Enhanced S-Cone Syndrome 142
9.4 Early Onset Nystagmus 143
9.4.1 Cone and Cone-Rod Dystrophy ... 143
9.4.2 Leber Congenital Amaurosis 145
9.4.3 Cone Dysfunction Syndromes 145
9.4.4 Albinism 145
9.4.5 Optic Nerve Hypoplasia 146
9.5 Visual Impairment in Multisystem Disorders 147
9.6 Investigation of Children Who Present with Unexplained Visual Acuity Loss 147
9.6.1 Macular Dystrophies 147
9.6.2 Optic Nerve Dysfunction 149
9.7 Unexplained Visual Loss in the Normal Child 151
9.7.1 Amblyopia 151
9.7.2 Nonorganic Visual Loss 151
9.8 Conclusions 152
References 152

Chapter 10
Clinical and Molecular Genetic Aspects of Leber's Congenital Amaurosis
Robert Henderson, Birgit Lorenz, Anthony T. Moore

10.1 Introduction 157
10.1.1 Clinical Findings 157
10.1.2 Differential Diagnosis 157
10.2 Molecular Genetics 158
10.2.1 GUCY-2D (LCA1 Locus) 160
10.2.2 RPE65 (LCA2) 160
10.2.3 CRX 162
10.2.4 AIPL1 (LCA4) 164
10.2.5 RPGRIP1 (LCA6) 165
10.2.6 TULP1 166
10.2.7 CRB1 167
10.2.8 RDH12 169
10.2.9 Other Loci 169
10.3 Heterozygous Carriers 170
10.4 Future Therapeutic Avenues 170
10.4.1 Gene Therapy 170
10.4.2 Retinal Transplantation and Stem Cell Therapy 171
10.4.3 Pharmacological Therapies 171
References 172

Chapter 11
Childhood Stationary Retinal Dysfunction Syndromes
Michel Michaelides, Anthony T. Moore

11.1 Introduction 179
11.2 Stationary Retinal Dysfunction Syndromes 182
11.2.1 Rod Dysfunction Syndromes (Stationary Night Blindness) 182
11.2.2 Cone Dysfunction Syndromes 184
11.3 Management of Stationary Retinal Dysfunction Syndromes 188
11.4 Conclusions 188
References 189

Chapter 12
Childhood Retinal Detachment
Arabella V. Poulson, Martin P. Snead

12.1 Introduction 191
12.2 Trauma 192
12.2.1 Blunt Ocular Trauma 192
12.2.2 Penetrating Ocular Trauma 193
12.3 Nontraumatic Retinal Dialysis..... 193
12.4 Familial Retinal Detachment 194
12.4.1 The Stickler Syndromes 194
12.4.2 Kniest Syndrome 197
12.4.3 Spondyloepiphyseal Dysplasia Congenita 197
12.4.4 Spondyloepimetaphyseal Dysplasia (Strudwick Type)................ 198
12.4.5 Vitreoretinopathy Associated with Phalangeal Epiphyseal Dysplasia 198
12.4.6 Dominant Rhegmatogenous Retinal Detachment 198
12.4.7 Marfan Syndrome 198
12.4.8 Ehlers-Danlos Syndrome 198
12.4.9 Wagner Vitreoretinopathy 199
12.4.10 X-Linked Retinoschisis........... 199
12.4.11 Familial Exudative Vitreoretinopathy 199
12.4.12 Norrie Disease 200
12.4.13 Incontinentia Pigmenti 200
12.5 Retinal Detachment Complicating Developmental Abnormalities..... 201
12.5.1 Congenital Cataract 201
12.5.2 Ocular Coloboma 201
12.5.3 Optic Disc Pits and Serous Macular Detachment .. 201
12.5.4 Retinopathy of Prematurity....... 202
12.6 Other 202
12.6.1 Inflammatory or Infectious 202
12.6.2 Exudative Retinal Detachment 202
12.7 Prophylaxis in Rhegmatogenous Retinal Detachment 203
References 203

Chapter 13
Eye Manifestations of Intrauterine Infections
Marilyn Baird Mets, Ashima Verma Kumar

13.1 Introduction 205
13.2 Toxoplasma gondii 205
13.2.1 Agent and Epidemiology 205
13.2.2 Diagnosis 205
13.2.3 Systemic Manifestations.......... 206
13.2.4 Eye Manifestations 206
13.2.5 Treatment 207
13.2.6 Prevention 207
13.3 Rubella Virus 207
13.3.1 Agent and Epidemiology 207
13.3.2 Transmission 207
13.3.3 Diagnosis 208
13.3.4 Systemic Manifestations.......... 208
13.3.5 Eye Manifestations 208
13.3.6 Treatment 209
13.3.7 Prevention 209
13.4 Cytomegalovirus 209
13.4.1 Agent and Epidemiology 209
13.4.2 Transmission 209
13.4.3 Diagnosis 209
13.4.4 Systemic Manifestations.......... 209
13.4.5 Eye Manifestations 209
13.4.6 Treatment 210
13.4.7 Prevention 210
13.5 Herpes Simplex Virus 210
13.5.1 Agent and Epidemiology 210
13.5.2 Transmission 210
13.5.3 Diagnosis 211
13.5.4 Systemic Manifestations.......... 211
13.5.5 Eye Manifestations 211
13.5.6 Treatment 211
13.5.7 Prevention 212

13.6 Lymphocytic Choriomeningitis Virus 212
13.6.1 Agent and Epidemiology 212
13.6.2 Transmission 212
13.6.3 Diagnosis 212
13.6.4 Systemic Manifestations 212
13.6.5 Eye Manifestations 213
13.6.6 Treatment 213
13.6.7 Prevention 213
13.7 Others 213
13.7.1 Treponema Pallidum 213
13.7.2 Varicella–Zoster Virus 213
13.7.3 Human Immunodeficiency Virus .. 214
13.7.4 Epstein–Barr Virus 214
13.8 West Nile Virus 214
13.8.1 Agent and Epidemiology 214
13.8.2 Transmission 214
13.8.3 Diagnosis 214
13.8.4 Systemic and Eye Manifestations .. 215
13.8.5 Treatment 215
13.8.6 Prevention 215
References 215

Chapter 14
Nonaccidental Injury. The Pediatric Ophthalmologist's Role
Alex V. Levin

14.1 Introduction 219
14.1.1 Basics 219
14.1.2 Reporting 219
14.1.3 Testifying 220
14.2 Physical Abuse 221
14.2.1 Blunt Trauma 221
14.2.2 Shaken Baby Syndrome 222
14.2.3 Munchausen Syndrome by Proxy (Factitious Illness by Proxy) 225
14.3 Sexual Abuse 226
14.4 Neglect and Noncompliance 227
14.5 Emotional Abuse 227
14.6 Conclusion 227
References 228

Subject Index 231

Contributors

Michael Clarke, MD
Reader in Ophthalmology
Claremont Wing Eye Department
Royal Victoria Infirmary
Newcastle upon Tyne NE1 4LP, UK

Thomas S. Dietlein, MD
Department of Ophthalmology
University of Cologne
Joseph-Stelzmann-Strasse 9, 50931 Cologne
Germany

Robert Henderson, BSc, MRCOphth
Honorary Research Fellow
IoO, Moorfields Eye Hospital
& Great Ormond Street Hospital
Institute of Ophthalmology
Dept. Molecular Genetics
11–43 Bath Street, London, EC1V 9EL, UK

Graham E. Holder, BSc, MSc, PhD
Consultant Electrophysiologist
Director of Electrophysiology
Moorfields Eye Hospital, City Road
London, EC1 V2PD, UK

Howard C. Howland, MS, PhD
Department of Neurobiology
and Behavior Cornell University
W-201 Mudd Hall
Ithaca, NY 14853, USA

Guenter K. Krieglstein, MD
Professor and Chairman
Department of Ophthalmology
University of Cologne
Joseph-Stelzmann-Strasse 9
50931 Cologne, Germany

Ashima Verma Kumar, MD
Division of Ophthalmology
2300 Children's Plaza Box 70
Chicago, IL 60614, USA

Scott R. Lambert, MD
Emory Eye Center
1365-B Clifton Road, N.E.
Atlanta, GA 30322, USA

Alex V. Levin, MD, MHSc, FAAP, FAAO, FRCSC
Staff Ophthalmologist
Department of Ophthalmology
M158, The Hospital for Sick Children
555 University Avenue
Toronto, Ontario, M5G 1X8, Canada

Birgit Lorenz, MD
Professor of Ophthalmology
and Ophthalmic Genetics
Head of Department
Department of Paediatric Ophthalmology
Strabismology and Ophthalmogenetics
Klinikum, University of Regensburg
Franz Josef Strauss Allee 11
93053 Regensburg, Germany

Marilyn Baird Mets, MD
Division of Ophthalmology
2300 Children's Plaza Box 70
Chicago, IL 60614, USA

Michel Michaelides,
BSc, MB, BS, MD, MRCOphth
Department of Molecular Genetics
Institute of Ophthalmology
11–43 Bath Street, London, EC1V 9EL, UK
Moorfields Eye Hospital, City Road
London, EC1V 2PD, UK

Anthony T. Moore, MA, FRCS, FRCOphth
Division of Inherited Eye Disease
Institute of Ophthalmology, UCL, London, UK
Moorfields Eye Hospital, City Road
London, EC1V 9EL, UK

Josefin Ohlsson, MD, PhD
Department of Clinical Neurophysiology
Göteborg University
Sahlgrenska University Hospital
41345 Göteborg, Sweden

Arabella V. Poulson, MB, BS, FRCOphth
Vitreoretinal Service, Box 41
Cambridge University Hospitals
NHS Foundation Trust
Addenbrooke's Hospital
Hills Road, Cambridge, CB2 2QQ, UK

Anthony G. Robson, BSc, MSc, PhD
Moorfields Eye Hospital, City Road
London, EC1V 2PD, UK

Frank Schaeffel, PhD
Professor and Head of the Section
of Neurobiology of the Eye
Dept. of Pathophysiology of Vision
and Neuroophthalmology
University Eye Hospital, Calwerstrasse 7/1
72076 Tübingen, Germany

Carol L. Shields, MD
Ocular Oncology Service, Wills Eye Hospital
900 Walnut Street, Philadelphia, PA 19107
USA

Jerry A. Shields, MD
Ocular Oncology Service, Wills Eye Hospital
900 Walnut Street, Philadelphia, PA 19107
USA

Johan Sjöstrand, MD, PhD
Department of Ophthalmology
Göteborg University, SU/Mölndal
431 80 Mölndal, Sweden

Lois E.H. Smith, MD, PhD
Department of Ophthalmology
Children's Hospital, Harvard Medical School
Boston, MA 02115, USA

Martin P. Snead, MD
Vitreoretinal Service, Box 41
Cambridge University Hospitals
NHS Foundation Trust
Addenbrooke's Hospital, Hills Road
Cambridge, CB2 2QQ, UK

1 Development of Ocular Refraction: Lessons from Animal Experiments

Frank Schaeffel, Howard C. Howland

Core Messages

- There is overwhelming evidence in both animal models and humans that refractive development and axial eye growth are under visual control
- The retina can analyze the sign and amount of defocus over time and control the growth of the underlying sclera
- Myopia is generally increasing in the industrialized world, in particular in the Far East
- Although genetic factors modulate the predisposition to become myopic, the high incidence of myopia in the industrialized world is likely to be due to environmental factors
- There are two major strategies to interfere with myopia development: (1) reducing "critical visual experience" (which is about to be defined). More individually adapted spectacle corrections may be a way since they can reduce progression of myopia by up to 50% in selected children. (2) inhibiting axial eye growth pharmacologically. Atropine is effective, but the mechanism of its action is not understood and its side effects preclude prolonged application

1.1 Introduction

The size of the organs in the body is continuously regulated to match their functional capacity as required (review: Wallman and Winawer [79]). There is, however, probably no other organ so precisely controlled in size as the eye: to achieve full visual acuity, its length must be matched to the optical focal length of cornea and lens with a tolerance of about a tenth of a millimeter (equivalent to 0.25 D). A normal-sighted (emmetropic) eye that increases in length by more than this amount will be slightly myopic and experience a detectable loss of visual acuity at far distances.

Until about 1975, it was thought that this match was achieved by tight genetic control of growth, even though this appeared an improbable (or improbably impressive) achievement. About this time, it was discovered that, in monkeys whose lids were monocularly fused to study the development of binocular neurons in the visual cortex, the deprived eyes became longer and myopic [84]. This observation stimulated research into myopia in animal models. The idea was that eye growth, and therefore also refractive development, might be under visual control which is accessible to experimental studies in which the visual experience is intentionally altered. It also revived an older discussion as to whether myopia is environmental or genetic.

Today, despite the results from animal models that demonstrate visually controlled eye growth, this discussion has not come to an end (e.g., [42]). Major studies in the United States concluded that "heritability was the most important factor" in myopia development and that only less than 20% can be modulated by visual experience (Orinda study [43]; twin studies, e.g., [18]). In contrast, a recent major review of the literature reaches the conclusion that the significant increase in the incidence of myopia in the last 40 years must be due to environmental factors [39].

By using animal models, a lot has been learned about the mechanisms of visual control of eye growth. However, the definition of the visual cues that make the eye grow longer in children is more difficult than expected. Nevertheless, the observations in animal models were often unexpected and gave rise to new theories and ideas about human myopia development. At least, a number of suggestions can be derived from the experimental results in animals. They will be described in this chapter but, first, the basic features of the mechanisms of visual control of eye growth in animal models will be summarized.

1.2 Overview on the Experimental Results in Animal Models

1.2.1 What Is the Evidence for Visual Control of Refractive Development and Axial Eye Growth?

It was first demonstrated in young chickens that fitting the animals with spectacle lenses that impose a defined amount of defocus on the retina made the eyes grow so that the imposed defocus was compensated [23, 56].

In the case of a negative lens, the plane of focus of the projected image is shifted, on average, behind the retina. It was found that axial length grew faster than normal, apparently to "catch the new focal plane." Cornea and lens did not show biometric or optical changes. The longer eye was then myopic without the negative lens in place but was about in focus with the lens. The compensation of a negative lens of 4 D took 3–4 days. In the case of a positive lens, axial eye growth was inhibited until the focal length of cornea and lens had sufficiently increased to produce hyperopia of the magnitude that was necessary to compensate for the lens power.

Developmental adaptation of refractive state by visual cues was first assumed to be a special feature of the bird eye. It was subsequently shown that young monkey eyes could also compensate for imposed defocus (Fig. 1.1) [21, 66]. Given that chicks and monkeys are phylogenetically not closely related, and that monkeys are much closer to humans than to chicks, it seems very likely that also the growing human eye can compensate for imposed defocus.

1.2.2 Which Kind of Visual Stimulation Induces Refractive Errors in Animal Models?

There are two different visual stimulations that interfere with axial eye growth: either globally degrading the retinal image sharpness and contrast, or imposing defined amounts of defocus.

1.2.2.1 Stimulation of Axial Eye Growth by Retinal Image Degradation

Lid fusion, as performed in the initial experiments [84], is an experimental manipulation with several effects: the retina no longer has access to spatial information (although it is not completely light-deprived), the mechanical pressure on the cornea is changed, and the metabolic conditions and temperature in the eye may be different. Although each of these factors could interfere with eye growth, it was found that the most important component was the deprivation of the retina of sharp vision and contrast. Accordingly, this type of myopia has been called form deprivation myopia (FDM) because form vision is no longer possible. In the meantime, it became clear that even a minor reduction of image sharpness and contrast may already stimulate axial eye growth: "deprivation myopia is a graded phenomenon" [67] and this has been shown in both chickens [3], and rhesus monkeys [67]. Therefore, the term "form deprivation myopia" may be an exaggerated description of the visual condition and could be replaced by "deprivation myopia" since this term makes no assumptions about the exact nature of the deprivation.

Deprivation myopia has been observed in almost all vertebrates that have been studied [79]. It is commonly induced by placing a frosted occluder in front of an eye for a period of several days or weeks. The speed by which deprivation myopia develops depends on the species

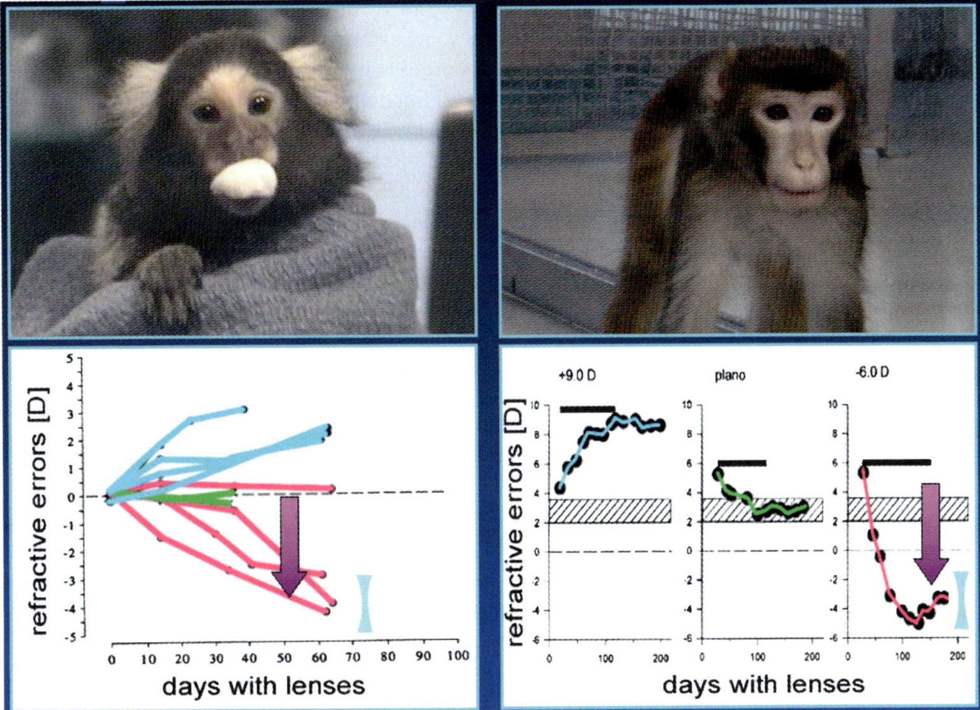

Fig. 1.1. If an emmetropic eye is wearing a negative lens, the focal plane is displaced behind the retina. Several animal models, including marmosets and rhesus monkeys, have shown that the eye develops compensatory axial elongation and myopia. With a positive lens, axial eye growth is inhibited, and a compensatory hyperopia develops (redrawn after [83], marmosets, *left*; [66], rhesus monkeys, *right*)

and the age of the animal [58]. In 1-day-old chickens, up to 20 D can be induced over 1 week of deprivation [77], but only 1 D at the age of 1 year [48]. Rhesus monkeys develop about 5 D on average during an 8-week deprivation period at the age of 30 weeks, but only 1 D at adolescence [68]. Deprivation myopia is strikingly variable among different individuals (range 0–11 D in rhesus monkeys, standard deviations about 5 D [67] (a similar standard deviation is typical also in the other animal models). Although the variability cannot be explained by differences in individual treatment of the animals, it is unclear whether the variability is due to genetic factors. Epigenetic variance could also account for it (R.W. Williams, personal communication, 2003) although it is striking that both eyes respond very similarly despite the lack of visual feedback [57].

Deprivation myopia can be induced in chickens after the optic nerve has been cut [76] and in local fundal areas if only part of the visual field is deprived [78]. Local degradation of the retinal image also produces local refractive error in tree shrews [63]. There are data in both chickens [35] and tree shrews [46] showing that deprivation myopia also can be induced after the ganglion cell action potentials are blocked by intravitreal application of tetrodotoxin, a natural sodium channel blocker. Taken together, the results show that image processing in the retina, excluding its spiking neurons, is sufficient to stimulate axial elongation.

1.2.2.2
Control of Eye Growth by Imposed Defocus

One of the most unexpected results of the chicken studies was that imposed defocus was compensated even if the connection of the eye to the brain was disrupted by cutting the optic nerve. Even though the baseline refraction of the eye without optic nerve moved to more hyperopia, suggesting general growth inhibition, negative lenses still caused axial elongation, and positive lenses growth inhibition on top of the new baseline refraction [86, 85]. These results suggest that the retina releases factors to control the growth of the underlying sclera. Furthermore, they show that the retina can make a distinction between positive and negative defocus. A retinal control of eye growth is further suggested by the observation that image defocus [6] is compensated in local fundal areas. Since accommodation requires an optic nerve and since accommodation shifts the focal plane, at least in humans and chickens, equally across the visual field, local compensation of refractive errors cannot be explained by a feedback loop that involves accommodation. Any potential effect of accommodation on axial eye growth must be indirect, by changing the focus of the retinal image.

Experiments with lenses after optic nerve section have not yet been conducted with monkeys. Therefore, it cannot be safely concluded that monkey eyes compensate imposed defocus based on a purely retinal mechanism. At least, it has already been shown [90] that the transcription factor Egr-1 in the monkey retina is regulated by the sign of imposed defocus, similar to the chicken [4, 12, 65].

1.2.3
What Is Known About the Retinal Image Processing That Leads to Refractive Errors?

Ignoring accommodation (which is, at least, apparently not necessary), to determine the sign of the refractive error of the eye, the retina could compare the focus for different viewing distances. However, additional information must be available on the dioptric distance of the viewing target. The other option is that the retina has a mechanism to measure the vergence of incoming rays instantaneously. Even though this idea seems hard to accept, experimental evidence is clearly in favor of this hypothesis.

Chickens that are individually kept in the center of a large drum so that they have only one viewing distance can compensate the power of lenses of either sign. In this case, lens powers were chosen so that the far point of the eyes was either behind or in front of the walls of the drum by the same dioptric amount of 12 D. In addition, accommodation was suppressed by cycloplegic agents. If the retina would only measure image sharpness and contract, all these treatments should have led to deprivation myopia. That hyperopia was induced despite massive image degradation, can only be explained by postulating that the retina can determine the sign of defocus [55]. It is quite impressive that the growth inhibition signal overwrites the deprivation-related signal for enhanced eye growth. Similar experiments have not yet been conducted with monkeys but, given the similarities among the results from different animal models, it is possible that also the mammalian retina can measure the sign of defocus.

Which image processing algorithms or which optical tricks the retina uses to measure vergence of rays is not clear. The most likely mechanisms are not used or, at least, not required (chromatic aberration, spherical aberration, astigmatism): Chickens compensate spectacle lenses equally well in white or monochromatic light [57]. They also compensate lenses at different illuminances and, hence, different pupil sizes and amounts of spherical aberration [38]. They compensate the spherical refractive errors even in the presence of extreme astigmatism [36]. Recent observations in chickens suggest that the sign of defocus detection is no longer possible if the chicks were exposed to the same visual experience under anesthetized conditions (M. Bitzer, personal communication, 2004).

Both chickens [7] and humans (e.g., [81]) can rapidly adapt to low image contrast. Since this adaptation is spatial frequency-specific, contrast adaptation can also partially compensate for the visual effects of defocus [37]. As a result, visual acuity can increase over time when defocus is maintained – a well-known experience of myopic subjects who take off their glasses. The increase in acuity is not based on refractive changes and there are no biometric changes in the eye [26]. It has also been shown that contrast adaptation is possible both at the retinal and cortical level [19]. A comparison of contrast adaptation levels at different spatial frequencies could be used as a measure of the amount of defocus over time [20]. Therefore, it has been speculated that more contrast adaptation at high spatial frequencies may indicate the presence of defocus, and that this could be a signal that could trigger axial eye growth [7]. It is clear, however, that contrast adaptation does not carry any information on the sign of defocus. Rather, it should be related to the retinal mechanisms that cause deprivation myopia.

1.2.4 How Long Must Defocus Persist to Induce Changes in Eye Growth?

The kinetics have been extensively studied by Winawer and Wallman [87] in chickens. Their finding that the temporal summation of defocus is highly nonlinear was not totally unexpected, as this was indicated by the experiments of Schmid and Wildsoet [64], who showed that the response of refraction to brief periods of normal vision in lens-reared chicks varied greatly with the sign of the lens. Winawer and Wallman found that multiple daily periods of defocus produce much larger changes in eye growth than one single period of the same total duration. If the single periods of lens treatment were shorter than 20 s, the lenses had no effect on eye growth. The most compelling result was, however, that the effects of positive and negative lenses did not cancel each other out: if negative lenses were worn all day, but were replaced with positive lenses for only 2 min, four times a day, the refractive state shifted still in the hyperopic direction [91]. Similarly, if monkeys wore negative lenses all day except for 1 h, the refraction remained in the range of normal animals [25]. These results suggest that the eye normally has a built-in protection against myopia development. It is also striking that the time constants for inhibition of deprivation or negative lens-induced myopia by interruption of treatment are very similar among different animal models [70]. A difference between chicks and monkeys was that interruption of negative lens wearing with positive lens wearing did not inhibit myopia more than interruption without lenses. However, the positive lenses used in the rhesus monkeys were +4.5 D and may have been too strong, given that the linear range of compensation is narrower in monkeys, compared to chickens.

1.2.5 What Is Known About the Tissue Responses and the Signaling Cascade from the Retina to the Sclera?

Once the retina has detected a consistent defocus, the release of yet unknown signaling molecules is altered, which changes the growth rate of the underlying sclera. The cellular candidates for the release of growth-controlling messengers are the amacrine cells, although this is not proven [12]. The signaling molecules reach the retinal pigment epithelium (RPE), where they bind to receptors to trigger the release of secondary messengers at the choroidal side of the RPE. It is less likely that they are transported through the tight junctions of the RPE to diffuse toward the sclera. Wallman et al. [80] were the first to observe in chickens that the choroid rapidly changes its thickness in such a way that the retina is moved closer to the focal plane (thinning when the image plane is behind the photoreceptor layer and thickening when it is in front). In chickens, this mechanism can effectively compensate for considerable amounts of refractive errors (up to 7 D), but in monkeys, where it has also been observed (marmoset: [44, 45]; rhesus monkey: [22]), it has only a minor effect in the range of a fraction of a diopter. Interestingly, the molecular signals for changes in choroidal thickness are different from those that regulate the growth of the sclera (summarized by Wallman and Winawer [79], p 455).

The biochemical nature of "the" retinal growth signal is not yet resolved. Several trans-

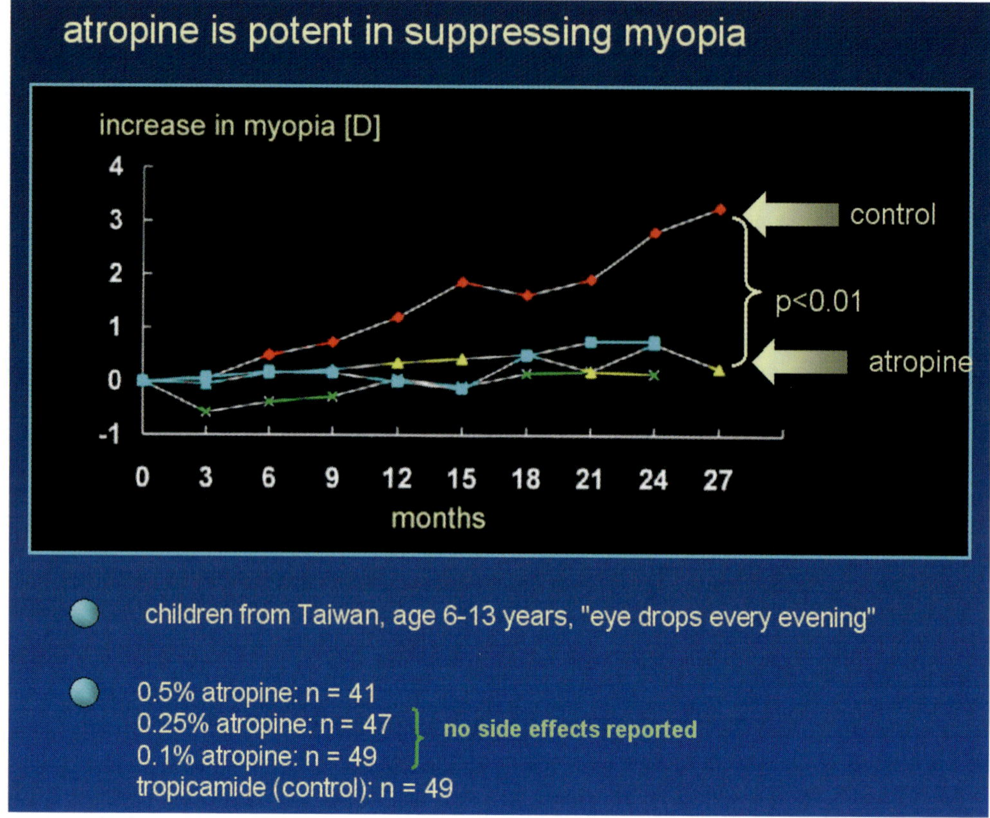

Fig. 1.2. Inhibition of myopia development in three groups of children in Taiwan, who received eye drops every evening with different concentrations of atropine. Note that all concentrations used inhibited myopia. In the case of 0.5% solution (*green crosses*), there was even an initial regression of myopia (redrawn after Shih et al. 1999 [62])

mitters seem to play a role. The major candidates are glucagon (which responds in correlation with the sign of defocus in chickens [11, 12]), dopamine (which responds only to image degradation but not the sign of defocus [47, 71]), potentially acetylcholine (because cholinergic receptor antagonists inhibit deprivation and lens-induced myopia [72]), but several other transmitters, neuromodulators, and growth factors have also been shown to play a role. In particular, the potential role of acetylcholine has been extensively studied. Although most muscarinic [31] and nicotinic [73] antagonists have an inhibitory effect on myopia development, there are many arguments that the inhibition is not based on specific binding of the antagonist to the respective receptors. The burning question of how cholinergic antagonists can inhibit axial eye growth in a variety of vertebrates (chick: [34, 72]; rhesus monkey: [74]; human: for example [62]; Fig. 1.2) remains unanswered.

In the case of atropine, currently still the most effective drug against myopia, at least five different target tissues have been identified (summarized by Wallman and Winawer [79]).

The sclera defines the shape and size of the globe and was therefore always at the center of interest in myopia research. In an attempt to identify targets for pharmacological intervention of myopia, its metabolism has been extensively studied in the recent years (summarized by Wallman and Winawer [79] and [33]). Atropine appears to have a direct inhibitory effect on scleral metabolism [30].

1.3 Can Animal Models Help to Improve the Management of Myopia in Children?

Several questions regarding the management of myopia in children and adolescents cannot be answered from available epidemiological studies. In these cases, the results from animal models may provide helpful suggestions. It should be kept in mind, however, that some children develop myopia even though they had the same visual environment as others, who do not develop myopia. Furthermore, children develop myopia without any treatment with lenses or deprivation, which is definitely a difference to experimental animals.

1.3.1 Undercorrection, Overcorrection, and Full Correction of Myopia

This question is closely related to the question whether the primate retina evaluates only global image sharpness or also the sign of imposed defocus, as previously observed in chickens (see Sect. 1.2.3). If the retina would only respond to the visual deprivation associated with defocus, undercorrection should induce deprivation myopia, with more eye growth (although a myopic or undercorrected eye is still in focus for close viewing distances). It is known that the mechanism for deprivation myopia is actually active in a human eye since ocular diseases that interfere with retinal image sharpness or contrast during childhood cause axial elongation and myopia (i.e., early unoperated cataracts, ptosis, and keratitis). It has not yet been proven that the primate retina can make the sign of defocus distinction to control eye growth in a bi-directional way although, at least, the transcription factor egr-1 in the primate retina has been found to respond to the sign of defocus, just as in chickens (see Sect. 1.2.2.2). If "sign of defocus sensitivity" is present, undercorrection should be beneficial.

Myopia has traditionally been slightly undercorrected with the weakest negative lens that permitted good acuity. However, there are almost no data in the literature to suggest that undercorrection may be beneficial, other than Tokoro and Kabe [75]. This study was not very well designed since treatments were mixed (atropine treatment and undercorrection by 1 D in ten children, compared to 13 fully corrected children). Nevertheless, it was confirmed by Goss [14] that the undercorrected group progressed more slowly (−0.54 D per year) compared to the fully corrected group (−0.75 D per year; $p<0.001$). More recently, a better designed study was conducted in Malaysia [5]. Full correction was given to 47 children (aged 9–13) and 47 children were intentionally undercorrected by 0.75 D. In this study, the fully corrected group progressed more slowly (−0.77 D per year) than the undercorrected group (−1.01 D per year; difference about 20 %, $p<0.01$). In both groups, the average progression of myopia was strikingly high. Although the second study should be more trustworthy, three additional points have to be kept in mind: (1) even with full correction at the time the glasses were prescribed, all children were undercorrected already after a few weeks due to the generally high myopia progression, (2) most myopic subjects have observed that their progression is restarted once new spectacles were prescribed, (3) that undercorrected eyes have a faster progression does not fit with what has been learned from animal models. Undercorrection should have a similar optical effect as wearing a positive lens and, accordingly, should generate a strong inhibitory signal for axial eye growth (see Sect. 1.2.3).

On the other hand, overcorrection would be comparable to wearing an additional negative lens and should stimulate myopia progression. Overcorrection by 1–2 D has been used in 4-year-old children as a potential therapy for intermittent exotropia [28]. However, myopia progression was not enhanced in the overcorrected group (on average about 2.5 D progression over the following 6 years).

Summary for the Clinician

- **In summary, at present, the results from animal models and the human studies are not complementary. It may be necessary to wait for the results of another study on the effects of undercorrection in children, preferably with another racial group, before the correction strategies are adopted**

1.3.2 Reading Glasses

The link between "near work" (such as reading and writing) and myopia has been extensively studied in the recent years ([54]; short summary in [39]), and there is little doubt that the correlation is, on average, highly significant. Although it is not clear what exactly the critical visual experience is, a current hypothesis is that reading imposes a slight defocus to the retina because subjects accommodate too little. In fact, most studies have found a "lag of accommodation" of around half a diopter at a 3-D reading distance [60]. The lag of accommodation places the focal plane behind the retina and could have a similar effect on eye growth as wearing a negative lens. Inspired by this idea, a number of studies have been conducted with reading glasses in children since they should reduce the lag. The first major study from Hong Kong [29] showed a clear beneficial effect of progressive addition lenses with +1.5 or +2.0 D addition, which reduced progression to about half of the progression with single vision lenses (–1.2 D in 2 years). The idea was also tested in a larger multicentric study in the United States, the Correction Of Myopia Evaluation Trial (COMET). This study also showed some beneficial effect of progressive addition lenses (on average, 14 % inhibition of the progression with single vision lenses of about 1 D in 2 years [16]). The authors considered the inhibitory effect as "clinically not significant". However, if the children were clustered according to their lag of accommodation and phorias, the inhibition could rise to almost 60 % in those children who were esophoric, had a large lag of accommodation (>0.43 D) and had less myopia at the beginning of the treatment (>–2.25 D) [17]. It is important also to recognize that the effects of the progressive addition lenses were generally more expressed when myopia was still low. A third major study from Hong Kong (the Hong Kong Lens Myopia Control Study [9]) found only a trend of a beneficial effect of progressive addition lenses, but the effect appeared significant when only children with low myopia were considered.

Summary for the Clinician

- **In summary, these studies demonstrate convincingly that refractive development is also controlled by visual experience in humans (not a trivial statement, after all). They further show that the treatment with reading glasses is worthwhile, at least in a subgroup of children**

1.3.3 Contact Lenses Versus Spectacle Lenses

There is some evidence in the literature that rigid gas permeable (RGP) contact lenses have a beneficial effect on myopia development [50]. A more recent study could not find a difference between contact lens wearers and spectacle wearers (–1.33 vs –1.28 D progression in 2 years [24]). In this study, 105 children aged 6–12 years wearing contact lenses were compared with 192 children wearing spectacles. Because this is a potentially important issue, another major study is underway (the CLAMP study, Contact Lens and Myopia Progression study). Why myopia should be inhibited with hard contact lenses, but not with soft ones is also an interesting question [13]. It is clear that hard contact lenses flatten the cornea for several days, and that this mimics a reduction of myopia. Therefore, vitreous chamber depth measurements are necessary to confirm that there was really growth inhibition.

The observation from animal models that refractive state is locally controlled, also in the peripheral retina (see Sects. 1.2.2.1 and 1.2.2.2), suggests another possible explanation: spectacle lenses could produce more hyperopic refractions in the peripheral retina than hard contact lenses and this could stimulate more eye growth. Until now, only very limited data have been published on the peripheral refraction of human eyes with hard contact lenses compared to spectacle lenses [61]. This study found that, on average, there was 0.43 D more hyperopia at 22° off-axis with spectacle lenses, compared to hard contact lenses (p=0.026). The question merits further studies in a larger sample.

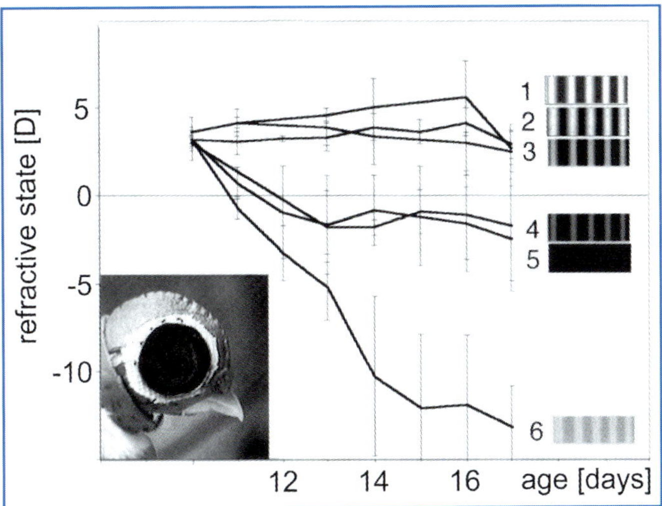

Fig. 1.3. Lowering the retinal image brightness in the chick eye by light neutral density filters has no effect on refractive development as long as the filters are weak (*1* no attenuation, *2* 0.5 log units, *3* 1.0 log units). If the filters are more dense (*4* 2.0 log units attenuation) some myopia develops, similar to when the filters are completely black (*5*). However, frosted diffusers that attenuate the light only a little (0.38 log units) cause much more myopia (*6*). This result suggests that low retinal image brightness interferes with eye growth. Furthermore, if the chicks are kept in low light (2.0 log units less than controls), even clear occluders cause some myopia, suggesting that eye growth becomes more sensitive to minor image degradation. Redrawn after [10]

Summary for the Clinician

- **The evidence for an inhibitory effect of hard contact lenses on myopia development is mixed. It is advisable to wait for the results of the CLAMP study**

1.3.4 Illumination, Reading Distance, Computer Work Versus Reading Text in a Book

It is surprising that there are only studies from chickens to determine whether ambient illuminance has an effect on myopia development. It was found that refractive errors imposed by spectacle lenses are similarly compensated over a wide range of illuminances (see Sect. 1.2.3). Therefore, these experiments provide no evidence that reading at low light may represent a risk factor. Only Feldkaemper et al. [10] have studied whether reduction of retinal image brightness by covering the eyes with neutral density filters can induce deprivation myopia. Refractive development was not altered if the filters attenuated the ambient light (illuminance 400 lux) by less than 2 log units. With darker filters, however, the refractions became more myopic, although not as myopic as with frosted eye occluders that degraded the retinal image, but attenuated light only by 0.38 log units. Furthermore, when the animals were placed in dim light (2.0 log units lower than controls) they did not become myopic without eye occluders but, even "clear" filters (denoted as "1" in Fig. 1.3), caused some myopia. These results suggest that eye growth becomes more sensitive to minor image degradation when the retinal image brightness is reduced (Fig. 1.3).

A possible reason why this could happen is that both retinal image brightness and retinal image contrast and sharpness reduce the release of dopamine in the retina [10], and dopamine release has been shown to have an inhibitory effect on eye growth [47]. Even though these observations are from chickens, they suggest that reading (which also represents a minor image degradation due to the lag of accommodation) might be more myopigenic at poor illumination.

One would expect that reading distance is also important because the lag of accommodation increases with decreasing target distance. Pärssinnen and Lyrra [49] studied 238 Finish school children at 10 years of age and found that myopia progression was higher in those children who read at 20 cm distance than in those reading at 30 cm distance. However, it should be kept in mind that this relationship need not be causal – it could be that children with higher myopia progression also have the habit of reading with shorter target distances.

There is no evidence that a computer screen has a different effect on myopia progression as a text printed on paper. It is likely, however, that extended work on the computer causes myopia due to the constantly short viewing distances. Several studies have come to this conclusion [41]. Given the extreme growth rates of the computer market in the Far East, it appears likely that the rapid increase in myopia in schoolchildren is, in fact, related to computers. Everybody who has children realizes how fascinating computer games are for them, compared to books. There is no doubt the "dose" of near work is greatly increased with computers.

Summary for the Clinician

- That reading at poor illumination increases the risk of myopia development is only suggested by experiments in chickens. Despite the lack of other evidence, it is still advisable to use appropriate illumination. Reading distance is a critical factor and reading should occur at sensible distances (i.e., 30 cm). There is no evidence that computer work is more myopigenic than reading a book at the same distance, but the computer is more attractive, increasing the "dose" of near work

1.3.5 How Long Must the Near Work Be Performed to Induce Myopia?

Initially, the amount of near work was quantified in "diopter hours" (amount of accommodation × duration in hours). However, there was an inherently low correlation between myopia progression and the amount of near work, as measured in diopter hours [43], although significant correlations were achieved because of the large numbers of samples already in the early studies (i.e., 793 children [88]). A large study on the relationship of near work and myopia in 1,005 school children in Singapore, 7–9 years old [54], showed that axial eye length was correlated to the myopia of the parents but also to the numbers of books that were read per week. There was a significant increase in myopia when two books were read vs when one book was read, but only in those children whose two parents were myopic. One possible explanation for the relatively low correlation between near work and myopia is that the exact behavioral pattern during reading may be important. It was already suggested by Winawer and Wallman [87] that diopter hour may not the best unit to predict myopia from near work.

Summary for the Clinician

- If the observations in animal models (see Sect. 1.2.4) are applicable to human myopia, interruption of reading for only short periods, and looking at a distance, should effectively inhibit the growth signal for the eye. More research is necessary in the monkey model and in children to find out whether temporary wearing of positive lenses could further strengthen this inhibitory signal for axial eye growth

1.3.6 Night Light, Blue Light

Based on the observation that the ocular growth rhythms are disturbed during development of deprivation myopia in chickens [82, 44], whether diurnal light rhythms might interfere with myopia development in children was tested. In the initial study [52], a high correlation between exposure to light during the night and myopia development was found. Later studies [15, 89] could not confirm this relationship and one possible explanation was that myopic parents had the lights on at night more frequently. The higher incidence of myopia in their children

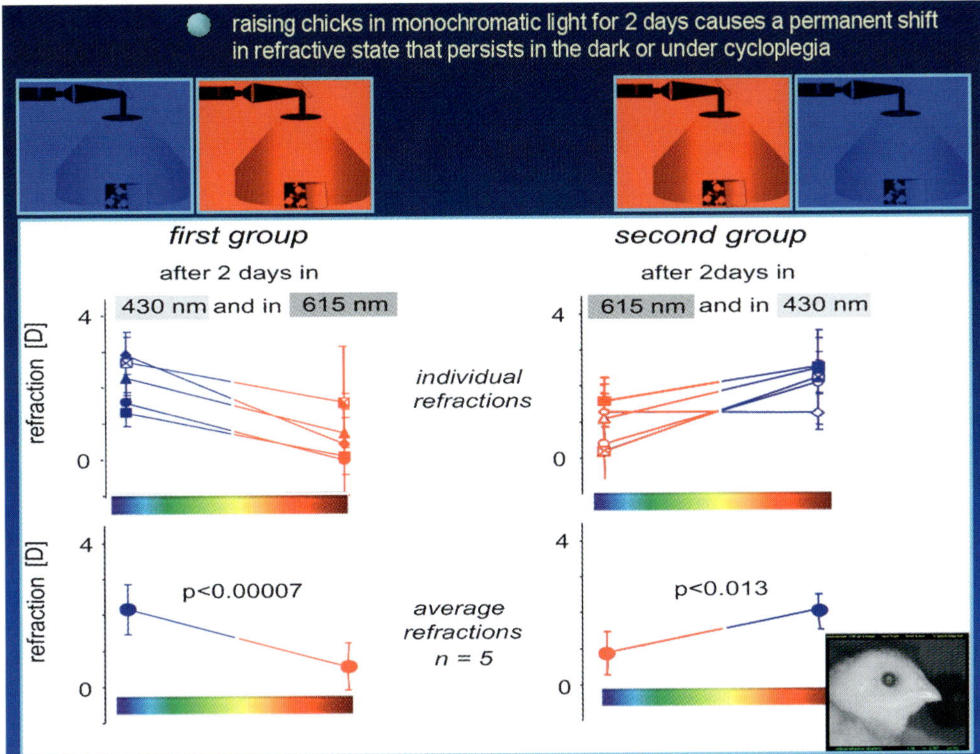

Fig. 1.4. Emmetropization responds to the chromatic shift in focus at different wavelengths. The chickens were raised first in quasi-monochromatic blue light, then refracted and then placed in quasi-monochromatic red light for 2 days. A shift in the myopic direction of about 1.1 D was observed, in line with the expected chromatic shift. A second group was first placed in the red and then in the blue, and the shift in refraction was in the other direction. All chickens were refracted in complete darkness and under cycloplegia, to avoid potentially confounding effects of a possible shift in tonic accommodation. Replotted after [59]

could then be explained by inheritance. Also, in monkeys, no effect of continuous light on emmetropization could be found [69]. Although chromatic aberration is not necessary for emmetropization (see Sect. 1.2.3), each of the three classes of cones can control accommodation independently (humans: [53, 27]; chickens: [59]). Because short wavelength light is focused closer to the cornea and lens, less accommodation is necessary to focus a near object onto the retina. Using this argument, Kroger and Binder [27] proposed that children should become less myopic if they read in blue light or from paper that reflects preferentially at short wavelengths. However, if accommodation already adjusts for the chromatic shift in focus, it is not clear how the retina can detect a different focus error signal, which would make the eye grow less in the blue. This question could only be resolved by an experiment: chickens were kept in red and in blue light for 2 days. To exclude that only the tonic accommodation level had shifted, they were refracted both in the dark or in white light under cycloplegia. There was a significant shift to more hyperopia (1.1 D) in the group that was raised in blue light (Fig. 1.4). In conclusion, the basic idea of Kroger and Binder [27] seemed to work in chickens, but it has not yet been tested in monkeys or humans.

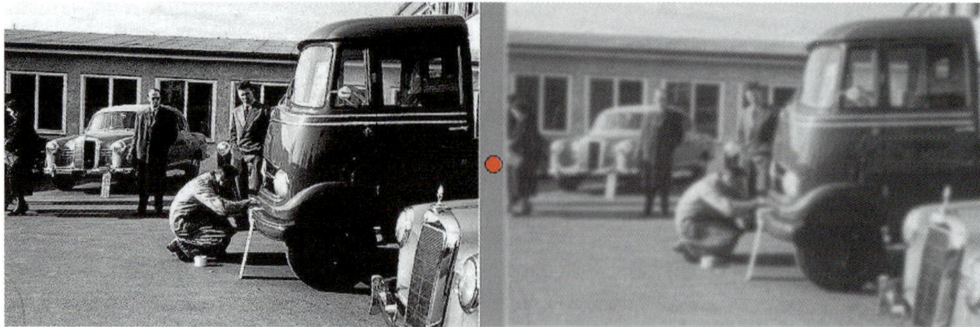

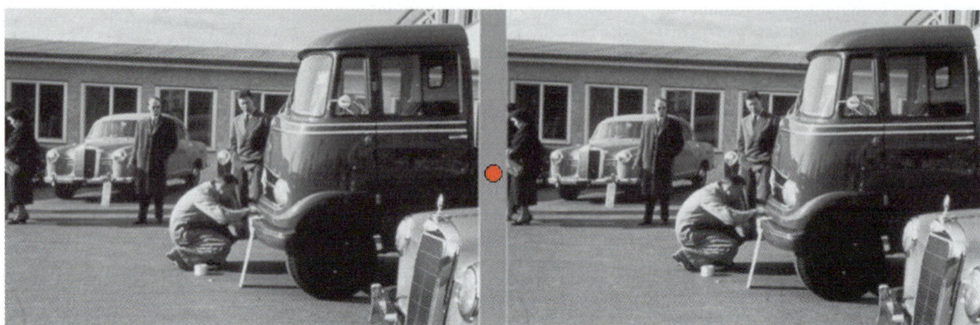

Fig. 1.5. Illustration of the effect of spatial frequency selective contrast adaptation on the impression of focus. First fixate the red spot in the *upper picture* for about 20 s. Then rapidly move your fixation to the red spot in the *lower picture*. For a short period of time, the picture on the *right* appears sharper and has more contrast, even though the left and right picture are identical (demonstration replotted with new sample pictures after Webster et al. [81])

Summary for the Clinician

- **Night light does not seem to be a risk factor as initially assumed. Reading in light of shorter wavelengths (i.e., around 430 nm) or from paper that reflects preferentially at short wavelengths could have a small inhibitory effect on myopia, although these conditions are difficult to create**

1.3.7 How Could Visual Acuity Improve Without Glasses?

Although for many years it has been known that contrast adaptation occurs in the visual system, it was discovered only recently that contrast adaptation can partially compensate for poor focus. This mechanism can also increase visual acuity without there being any optical changes in the eye. A compelling demonstration was published by Webster et al. [81]. If the subject views an image that has been low pass filtered or defocussed and has, accordingly, low contrast or complete absence of high spatial frequency components, the visual system increases its sensitivity at the respective spatial frequencies. As a result, the image appears sharper (Fig. 1.5).

On the other hand, if an image is viewed that has high contrast and high spatial frequency content, the visual system reduces its contrast sensitivity at the respective spatial frequencies. Since contrast adaptation has a fast and a slow component, extended exposure to defocus makes the image appear sharper [37]. Contrast adaptation has to be taken into account when an increase of visual acuity is claimed following eye training procedures. No biometrical and optical changes have been found in the eye, following vision training [26].

Summary for the Clinician

- **Visual acuity can somewhat be improved under prolonged defocus as a result of contrast adaptation. In contrast to occasional claims, there are no solid data showing a regression of myopia and a reduction of eye growth as a result of vision training**

1.3.8 Age Window for Intervention

Experiments in animal models have shown that myopia can be experimentally induced both in young and adolescent animals in which axial eye growth has already leveled off (Sect. 1.2.2.1). The older the animal, the less myopia develops and the longer treatment periods are necessary.

It has never been shown that an eye can be made shorter by treatment with positive lenses, once the final length had been reached (a minor decline in axial length was found, however, with high doses atropine, which was also accompanied by a shift in the hyperopic direction [8, 62]. Because the eye apparently cannot effectively be made shorter by visual feedback, there is also no recovery from induced myopia, once the animal has grown up (i.e., rhesus monkey: [51]).

In extrapolation to humans, one would expect that myopia can always be induced by changes in visual experience (i.e., a change in profession that includes a heavy load of near work), although with lower gain. This "adult onset myopia" has been described in the literature before [1, 32].

Summary for the Clinician

- **The older the eye, the less important the input of visual experience is. The most sensitive period is the phase with the fastest growth. However, myopia can still be induced in adult animals and humans**

1.3.9 Pharmacological Intervention for Myopia

Given that the effects of different optical corrections on myopia development are relatively small, except perhaps for a subgroup of children (see Sect. 1.3.2), and given that the visual experience in the industrialized world cannot be changed much, other treatment regimens are of interest. A drug such as atropine would be very attractive if it did not include the side effects of cycloplegia, photophobia, and if it did not lose its effects over a time period of 2–3 years. This could perhaps be prevented by less frequent application. However, there are no controlled studies yet to explore how often atropine must be applied to exert an inhibitory effect on axial eye growth. It is possible that application as eye drops every evening at high doses may be exaggerated. Nevertheless, atropine could be used as a model drug: once the mechanism by which it suppresses axial eye growth has been understood, a more specific target could be defined and a more selective drug developed. It is obvious that this area of research is particularly exciting.

Summary for the Clinician

- **Atropine applied as eye drops is the most potent inhibitor of axial eye elongation. However, the underlying mechanisms are not yet understood. Its side effects preclude extended application in children. Atropine could be used as a model to discover target tissues and mechanisms to develop more specific drugs. Other similar drugs are also effective, but less so**

1.3.10 Emmetropization in Hyperopia with and Without Optical Correction

Since emmetropization appears to be guided by the focus of the retinal image, the question arises whether optical correction of hyperopia in children could delay or exclude emmetropization to normal refractions. There are a number of studies on this topic: Mulvihill et al. [40] have shown that children with high hyperopia (approximately 6 D) are surprisingly stable in their refractions, whether they have been optically corrected or not. Apparently, the visual feedback to eye growth is inactive in high hyperopia. In line with this observation, another major study [2] has shown that there is little effect of

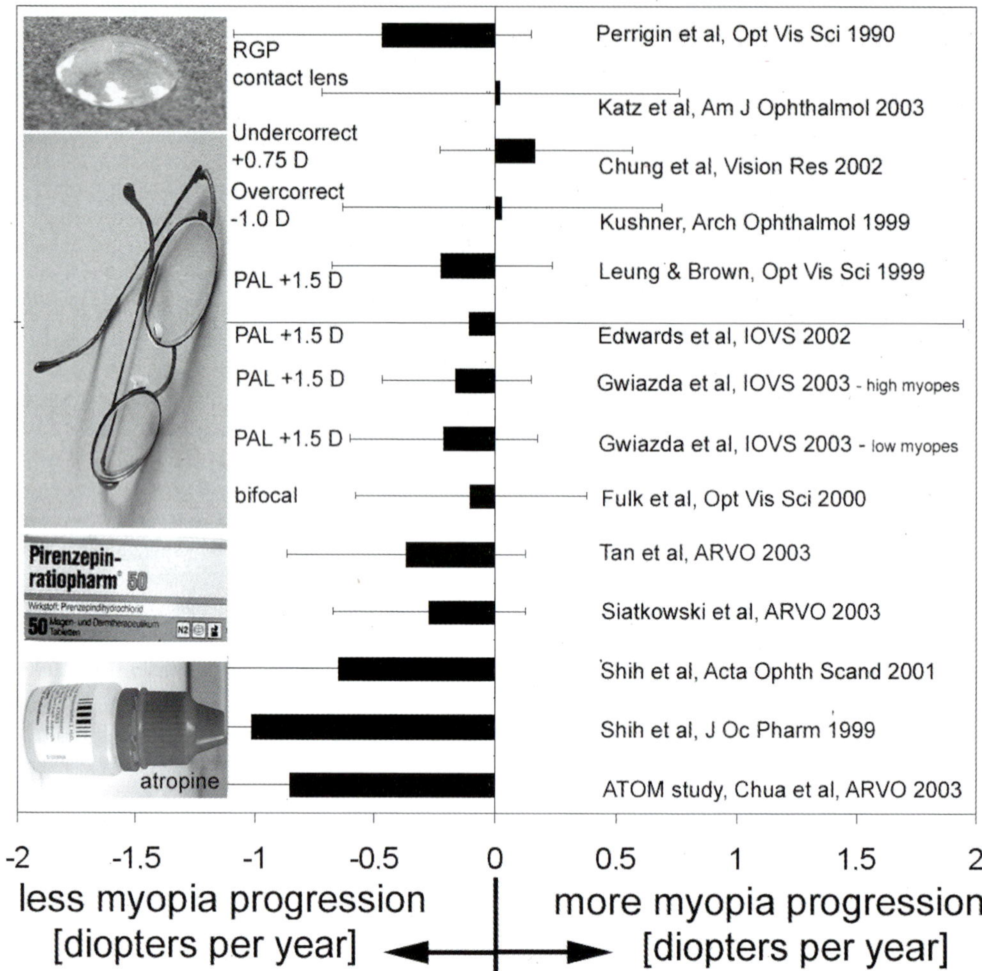

Fig. 1.6. Comparison of the effects of different treatment protocols on myopia progression in children. By far the most effective treatment was atropine, applied every evening by eye drops (complete inhibition of further progression). Pirenzepine was effective in the 1st year (about 50 % suppression). The different optical treatments reduced progression between 20 % and 40 %. Overcorrection had no significant effect. Undercorrection had a weak stimulatory effect. Data from hard contact lenses are variable and require further studies (CLAMP study underway). Note that the baseline progression may have varied in the different groups. Note further that atropine and pirenzepine treatment lost its effect in the 3rd year (data not shown, see text). (replotted after a slide shown by W.-H. Chua at the ARVO meeting, Ft. Lauderdale, 2004)

optical correction on the development of hyperopia in those children who were more than 3 D hyperopic. Children who were less hyperopic showed clear emmetropization, with the refractive changes per year negatively correlated with the amount of hyperopia in the beginning. In this group, refractive correction should have an effect, but it was not found in this study [2]. In conclusion, it seems as if the mechanism of emmetropization is ineffective or lacking in highly hyperopic children, and that full correction is probably the best treatment. In those children who are less than 3 D hyperopic, emmetropization could be slowed down by full correction although larger studies may be necessary to prove this assumption.

Summary for the Clinician

- Hyperopia seems to represent a failure of the emmetropization process since eye growth no longer responds to visual experience. Possibly for this reason, highly hyperopic children show no developmental change in refraction, neither with nor without spectacle correction. Children who are less than about 3 D hyperopic show emmetropization and may lose their hyperopia more slowly when fully corrected

1.4 Summary of Effects of Different Intervention Regimens on Myopia

There is little doubt that the pattern of focus on the retina determines the growth rate of the eye but it is difficult to control this variable precisely, due to effects of binocular input, uncontrolled fluctuations of accommodation, habits of preferred reading distance, contrast adaptation and blur sensitivity, and near work interruption patterns. It should be possible to develop individual optical corrections that are most appropriate to reduce myopia progression in a given individual that take these variables into account. Pharmacological intervention appears to be another promising means of treatment, although the best targets have not yet been defined. A summary of the effects of the different treatment attempts is shown in Fig. 1.6.

Summary for the Clinician

- Atropine treatment is the most powerful way to inhibit myopia. There is even a regression of myopia during the first months. Unfortunately, the system adapts to the treatment and atropine loses its effect in the 2nd or 3rd year. The other treatments described can only inhibit myopia development, by up the 50 %, but cannot stop it

References

1. Adams AJ (1987) Axial length elongation, not corneal curvature, as a basis of adult onset myopia. Am J Optom Physiol Opt 64:150–152
2. Atkinson J, Anker S, Bobier W, Braddick O, Durden K, Nardini M, Watson P (2000) Normal emmetropization in infants with spectacle correction for hyperopia. Invest Ophthalmol Vis 41: 3726–3731
3. Bartmann M, Schaeffel F (1994) A simple mechanism for emmetropization without cues from accommodation or colour. Vision Res 34:873–876
4. Bitzer M, Schaeffel F (2002) Defocus-induced changes in ZENK expression in the chicken retina. Invest Ophthalmol Vis Sci 43:246–252
5. Chung K, Mohidin N, O'Leary DJ (2002) Undercorrection of myopia enhances rather than inhibits myopia progression. Vision Res 42:2555–2559
6. Diether S, Schaeffel F (1997) Local changes in eye growth induced by imposed local refractive error despite active accommodation. Vision Res 37: 659–668
7. Diether S, Schaeffel F (1999) Long-term changes in retinal contrast sensitivity in chicks from frosted occluders and drugs: relations to myopia? Vision Res 39:2499–2510
8. Diether S, Schaeffel F, Fritsch C, Trendelenburg AU, Payor R, Lambrou G (2004) Contralateral inhibition of lens induced myopia in the chick by ipsilateral intravitreal atropine application: can a simple dilution model account for the effect? Invest Ophthalmol Vis Sci 45, #1238 (ARVO abstract)
9. Edwards MH, Li RW, Lam CS, Lew JK, Yu BS (2002) The Hong Kong progressive lens myopia control study: study design and main findings. Invest Ophthalmol Vis Sci 43:2852–2858
10. Feldkaemper M, Diether S, Kleine G, Schaeffel F (1999) Interactions of spatial and luminance information in the retina of chickens during myopia development. Exp Eye Res 68:105–115
11. Feldkaemper MP, Burkhardt E, Schaeffel F (2004) Localization and regulation of glucagon receptors in the chick eye and preproglucagon and glucagon receptor expression in the mouse eye. Exp Eye Res 79:321–329
12. Fischer AJ, McGuire JJ, Schaeffel F, Stell WK (1999) Light- and focus-dependent expression of the transcription factor ZENK in the chick retina. Nat Neurosci 2:706–712
13. Fulk GW, Cyert LA, Parker DE, West RW (2003) The effect of changing from glasses to soft contact lenses on myopia progression in adolescents. Ophthalmic Physiol Opt 23:71–77

14. Goss DA (1994) Effect of spectacle correction on the progression of myopia in children – a literature review. J Am Optom Assoc 65:117–128
15. Gwiazda J, Ong E, Held R, Thorn F (2000) Myopia and ambient night-time lighting. Nature 404:14
16. Gwiazda J, Hyman L, Hussein M, Everett D, Norton TT, Kurtz D, Leske MC, Manny R, Marsh-Tootle W, Scheiman M (2003) A randomized clinical trial of progressive addition lenses versus single vision lenses on the progression of myopia in children. Invest Ophthalmol Vis Sci 44:1492–1500
17. Gwiazda JE, Hyman L, Norton TT, Hussein ME, Marsh-Tootle W, Manny R, Wang Y, Everett D; COMET Group (2004) Accommodation and related risk factors associated with myopia progression and their interaction with treatment in COMET children. Invest Ophthalmol Vis Sci 45: 2143–2155
18. Hammond CJ, Snieder H, Gilbert CE, Spector TD (2001) Genes and environment in refractive error: the twin eye study. Invest Ophthalmol Vis Sci 42:1232–1236
19. Heinrich TS, Bach M (2001) Contrast adaptation in human retina and cortex. Invest Ophthalmol Vis Sci 42:2721–2727
20. Heinrich TS, Bach M (2002) Contrast adaptation in retinal and cortical evoked potentials: no adaptation to low spatial frequencies. Vis Neurosci 19:645–650
21. Hung LF, Crawford ML, Smith EL (1995) Spectacle lenses alter eye growth and the refractive status of young monkeys. Nat Med 1:761–765
22. Hung LF, Wallman J, Smith EL 3rd (2000) Vision-dependent changes in the choroidal thickness of macaque monkeys. Invest Ophthalmol Vis Sci 41:1259–1269
23. Irving EL, Sivak JG, Callender MG (1992) Refractive plasticity of the developing chick eye. Ophthalmic Physiol Opt 12:448–455
24. Katz J, Schein OD, Levy B, Cruiscullo T, Saw SM, Rajan U, Chan TK, Yew Khoo C, Chew SJ (2003) A randomized trial of rigid gas permeable contact lenses to reduce progression of children's myopia. Am J Ophthalmol 136:82–90
25. Kee CS, Hung LF, Qiao Y, Ramamirtham R, Winawer JA, Wallman J, Smith EL (2002) Temporal constraints on experimental emmetropization in infant monkeys. Invest Opthalmol Vis Sci 43 [Suppl], # 2925 (ARVO abstract)
26. Klan T (2000) A meta-analysis on the potency of visual training procedures to inhibit myopia development (in German). Verhaltenstherapie und Verhaltensmedizin 31:296–312
27. Kroger RH, Binder S (2000) Use of paper selectively absorbing long wavelengths to reduce the impact of educational near work on human refractive development. Br J Ophthalmol 84:890–893
28. Kushner BJ (1999) Does overcorrecting minus lens therapy for intermittent exotropia cause myopia? Arch Ophthalmol 117:638–642
29. Leung JT, Brown B (1999) Progression of myopia in Hong Kong Chinese schoolchildren is slowed by wearing progressive lenses. Optom Vis Sci 76:346–354
30. Lind GJ, Chew SJ, Marzani D, Wallman J (1998) Muscarinic acetylcholine receptor antagonists inhibit chick scleral chondrocytes. Invest Ophthalmol Vis Sci 39:2217–2231
31. Luft WA, Ming Y, Stell WK (2003) Variable effects of previously untested muscarinic receptor antagonists on experimental myopia. Invest Ophthalmol Vis Sci 44:1330–1338
32. McBrien NA, Adams DW (1997) A longitudinal investigation of adult-onset and adult-progression of myopia in an occupational group. Refractive and biometric findings. Invest Ophthalmol Vis Sci 38:321–333
33. McBrien NA, Gentle A (2003) Role of the sclera in the development and pathological complications of myopia. Prog Retin Eye Res 22:307–38
34. McBrien NA, Moghaddam HO, Reeder AP (1993) Atropine reduces experimental myopia and eye enlargement via a nonaccommodative mechanism. Invest Ophthalmol Vis Sci 34:205–215
35. McBrien NA, Moghaddam HO, Cottriall CL, Leech EM, Cornell LM (1995) The effects of blockade of retinal cell action potentials on ocular growth, emmetropization and form deprivation myopia in young chicks. Vision Res 35:1141–1152
36. McLean RC, Wallman J (2003) Severe astigmatic blur does not interfere with spectacle lens compensation. Invest Ophthalmol Vis Sci 44:449–457
37. Mon-Williams M, Tresilian JR, Strang NC, Kochhar P, Wann JP (1998) Improving vision: neural compensation for optical defocus. Proc R Soc Lond B Biol Sci 265:71–77
38. Moore SE, Irving EL, Sivak JG, Callender MG (1998) Decreased light levels affect the emmetropization process in chickens. In: Vision science and its application, vol 1, OSA Technical Digest Series, pp 202–205
39. Morgan I, Rose K (2005) How genetic is school myopia? Review article. Progr Ret Eye Res 24:1–38
40. Mulvihill A, MacCann A, Flitcroft I, O'Keefe M (2000) Outcome in refractive accommodative esotropia. Br J Ophthalmol 84:746–749
41. Mutti DO, Zadnik K (1996) Is computer use a risk factor for myopia? J Am Optom Assoc 67:521–530
42. Mutti DO, Zadnik K, Adams AJ (1996) Myopia. The nature versus nurture debate goes on. Invest Ophthalmol Vis Sci 37:952–957
43. Mutti DO, Mitchell GL, Moeschberger ML, Jones LA, Zadnik K (2002) Parental myopia, near work, school achievement, and children's refractive error. Invest Ophthalmol Vis Sci 43:3633–3640

44. Nickla DL, Wildsoet CF, Troilo D (2001) Endogenous rhythms in axial length and choroidal thickness in chicks: implications for ocular growth regulation. Invest Ophthalmol Vis Sci 42:584–588
45. Nickla DL, Wildsoet CF, Troilo D (2002) Diurnal rhythms in intraocular pressure, axial length, and choroidal thickness in a primate model of eye growth, the common marmoset. Invest Ophthalmol Vis Sci 43:2519–2528
46. Norton TT, Essinger JA, McBrien NA (1994) Lid-suture myopia in tree shrews with retinal ganglion cell blockade. Vis Neurosci 11:143–153
47. Ohngemach S, Hagel G, Schaeffel F (1997) Concentrations of biogenic amines in fundal layers in chickens with normal visual experience, deprivation, and after reserpine application. Vis Neurosci 14:493–505
48. Papastergiou GI, Schmid GF, Laties AM, Pendrak K, Lin T, Stone RA (1998) Induction of axial eye elongation and myopic refractive shift in one-year-old chickens. Vision Res 38:1883–1888
49. Parssinen O, Lyyra AL (1993) Myopia and myopic progression among schoolchildren: a three-year follow-up study. Invest Ophthalmol Vis Sci 34: 2794–2802
50. Perrigin J, Perrigin D, Quintero S, Grosvenor T (1990) Silicone-acrylate contact lenses for myopia control: 3-year results. Optom Vis Sci 67:764–769
51. Qiao-Grider Y, Hung LF, Kee CS, Ramamirtham R, Smith EL 3rd (2004) Recovery from form-deprivation myopia in rhesus monkeys. Invest Ophthalmol Vis Sci 45:3361–3372
52. Quinn GE, Shin CH, Maguire MG, Stone RA (1999) Myopia and ambient lighting at night. Nature 399:113–114
53. Rucker FJ, Kruger PB (2001) Isolated short-wavelength sensitive cones can mediate a reflex accommodation response. Vision Res 41:911–922
54. Saw SM, Chua WH, Hong CY, Wu HM, Chan WY, Chia KS, Stone RA, Tan D (2002) Nearwork in early-onset myopia. Invest Ophthalmol Vis Sci 43:332–339
55. Schaeffel F, Diether S (1999) The growing eye: an autofocus system that works on very poor images. Vision Res 39:1585–1589
56. Schaeffel F, Glasser A, Howland HC (1988) Accommodation, refractive error and eye growth in chickens. Vision Res 28:639–657
57. Schaeffel F, Howland HC (1991) Properties of the feedback loops controlling eye growth and refractive state in the chicken. Vision Res 31:717–734
58. Schaeffel F, Burkhardt E, Howland HC, Williams RW (2004) Measurement of refractive state and deprivation myopia in two strains of mice. Optom Vis Sci 81:99–110
59. Seidemann A, Schaeffel F (2002) Effects of longitudinal chromatic aberration on accommodation and emmetropization. Vision Res 42:2409–2417
60. Seidemann A, Schaeffel F (2003) An evaluation of the lag of accommodation using photorefraction. Vision Res 43:419–430
61. Seidemann A, Guirao A, Artal P, Schaeffel F. (1999) Relation of peripheral refraction to refractive development? Invest Ophthalmol Vis Sci 40 [Suppl], # 2362 (ARVO abstract)
62. Shih YF, Chen CH, Chou AC, Ho TC, Lin LL, Hung PT (1999) Effects of different concentrations of atropine on controlling myopia in myopic children. J Ocul Pharmacol Ther 15:85–90
63. Siegwart JT, Norton TT (1993) Refractive and ocular changes in tree shrews raised with plus and minus lenses. Invest Ophthalmol Vis Sci 34 [Suppl], # 2482 (ARVO abstract)
64. Schmid, KL, Wildsoet, CF (1996) Effects on the compensatory responses to positive and negative lenses of intermittent lens wear and ciliary nerve section in chicks. Vision Res 36:1023–1036
65. Simon P, Feldkaemper M, Bitzer M, Ohngemach S, Schaeffel F (2004) Early transcriptional changes of retinal and choroidal TGFbeta-2, RALDH-2, and ZENK following imposed positive and negative defocus in chickens. Mol Vis 10:588–597
66. Smith EL 3rd, Hung LF (1999) The role of optical defocus in regulating refractive development in infant monkeys. Vision Res 39:1415–1435
67. Smith EL 3rd, Hung LF (2000) Form-deprivation myopia in monkeys is a graded phenomenon. Vision Res 40:371–381
68. Smith EL 3rd, Bradley DV, Fernandes A, Boothe RG (1999) Form deprivation myopia in adolescent monkeys. Optom Vis Sci 76:428–432
69. Smith EL 3rd, Bradley DV, Fernandes A, Hung LF, Boothe RG (2001) Continuous ambient lighting and eye growth in primates. Invest Ophthalmol Vis Sci 42:1146–1152
70. Smith EL 3rd, Hung LF, Kee CS, Qiao Y (2002) Effects of brief periods of unrestricted vision on the development of form-deprivation myopia in monkeys. Invest Ophthalmol Vis Sci 43:291–299
71. Stone RA, Lin T, Laties AM, Iuvone PM (1989) Retinal dopamine and form-deprivation myopia. Proc Natl Acad Sci U S A 86:704–706
72. Stone RA, Lin T, Laties AM (1991) Muscarinic antagonist effects on experimental chick myopia. Exp Eye Res 52:755–758
73. Stone RA, Sugimoto R, Gill AS, Liu J, Capehart C, Lindstrom JM (2001) Effects of nicotinic antagonists on ocular growth and experimental myopia. Invest Ophthalmol Vis Sci 42:557–565

74. Tigges M, Iuvone PM, Fernandes A, Sugrue MF, Mallorga PJ, Laties AM, Stone RA (1999) Effects of muscarinic cholinergic receptor antagonists on postnatal eye growth of rhesus monkeys. Optom Vis Sci 76:397–407
75. Tokoro T, Kabe S (1965) Treatment of the myopia and the changes in optical components. Report II. Full-or under-correction of myopia by glasses (in Japanese). Nippon Ganka Gakkai Zasshi 69:140–144
76. Troilo D, Gottlieb MD, Wallman J (1987) Visual deprivation causes myopia in chicks with optic nerve section. Curr Eye Res 6:993–999
77. Wallman J, Turkel J, Trachtman J (1978) Extreme myopia produced by modest change in early visual experience. Science 201:1249–1251
78. Wallman J, Gottlieb MD, Rajaram V, Fugate-Wentzek LA (1987) Local retinal regions control local eye growth and myopia. Science 237:73–77
79. Wallman J, Winawer J (2004) Homeostasis of eye growth and the question of myopia. Neuron 43:447–468
80. Wallman J, Wildsoet C, Xu A, Gottlieb MD, Nickla DL, Marran L, Krebs W, Christensen AM (1995) Moving the retina: choroidal modulation of refractive state. Vision Res 35:37–50
81. Webster MA, Georgeson MA, Webster SM (2002) Neural adjustments to image blur. Nat Neurosci 5:839–840
82. Weiss S, Schaeffel F (1993) Diurnal growth rhythms in the chicken eye: relation to myopia development and retinal dopamine levels. J Comp Physiol [A] 172:263–270
83. Whatham AR, Judge SJ (2001) Compensatory changes in eye growth and refraction induced by daily wear of soft contact lenses in young marmosets. Vision Res 41:267–273
84. Wiesel TN, Raviola E (1977) Myopia and eye enlargement after neonatal lid fusion in monkeys. Nature 266:66–68
85. Wildsoet C (2003) Neural pathways subserving negative lens-induced emmetropization in chicks – insights from selective lesions of the optic nerve and ciliary nerve. Curr Eye Res 27:371–378
86. Wildsoet C, Wallman J (1995) Choroidal and scleral mechanisms of compensation for spectacle lenses in chicks. Vision Res 35:1175–1194
87. Winawer J, Wallman J (2002) Temporal constraints on lens compensation in chicks. Vision Res 42:2651–2668
88. Zadnik K, Mutti DO, Friedman NE, Adams AJ (1993) Initial cross-sectional results from the Orinda Longitudinal Study of Myopia. Optom Vis Sci 70:750–758
89. Zadnik K, Jones LA, Irvin BC, Kleinstein RN, Manny RE, Shin JA, Mutti DO (2000) Myopia and ambient night-time lighting. CLEERE Study Group. Collaborative Longitudinal Evaluation of Ethnicity and Refractive Error. Nature 404:143–144
90. Zhong X, Ge J, Smith EL 3rd, Stell WK (2004) Image defocus modulates activity of bipolar and amacrine cells in macaque retina. Invest Ophthalmol Vis Sci 45:2065–2074
91. Zhu X, Winawer JA, Wallman J (2003) Potency of myopic defocus in spectacle lens compensation. Invest Ophthalmol Vis Sci 44:2818–2827

Preschool Vision Screening: Is It Worthwhile?

Josefin Ohlsson, Johan Sjöstrand

Core Messages

- Vision screening in childhood aims to detect several disorders resulting in vision defects. Vision screening programs usually consist of examinations in the newborn period, surveillance via Child Heath Care centers, and preschool vision screening
- Preschool vision screening aims to detect amblyopia and related conditions such as strabismus, anisometropia, and refractive errors. Due to lack of predictive and easily identifiable risk factors, population-based screening is recommended
- High participation rates are of utmost importance for an effect to be garnered from a population-based point of view. By combining preschool vision screening with other well-known and well-attended systems, such as school entry or vaccination programs, high participation rates may be facilitated
- Visual acuity testing is recommended due to high sensitivity and specificity. Moreover, it is reliable, safe, and repeatable. It is easy to perform and has been shown to be cost-efficient. Charts in logMAR steps and with crowded optotypes are recommended
- Current knowledge points toward a possible age effect in amblyopia treatment, with better outcome in younger children. The dividing line seems to be at age 4–5 years
- The "best buy" for preschool vision screening seems to be vision screening at age 4–5 years when visual acuity testing can be reliably performed and successful treatment is still achievable
- Preschool vision screening and treatment for amblyopia is probably cost-effective, but depends on whether amblyopia is connected to loss in utility and whether treatment restores utility
- Further knowledge on the relationship between amblyopia and quality of life/utility is needed

2.1 Introduction

2.1.1 Definition of Screening

The United States Commission of Chronic Illness [10] defined screening in 1957 as "the presumptive identification of unrecognized disease or defect by the application of tests, examinations, or other procedures which can be applied rapidly. Screening tests sort out apparently well persons who probably have a disease from those who probably do not. A screening test is not intended to be diagnostic. Persons with positive or suspicious findings must be referred to their physician for diagnosis and necessary treatment." This description is still highly accurate.

Screening refers to the application of a test (or tests) to people who are asymptomatic, for the purpose of classifying them with respect to their likelihood of having a particular disease.

As indicated above, screening does not claim to find all affected subjects, or correctly diagnose those with disease. The aim of a screening program is to correctly identify as many individuals affected by the target condition as possible while minimizing the numbers of healthy individuals who are incorrectly suspected of having the disorder.

In 1968, Wilson and Jungner [52] added criteria about the disorder screened for and the treatment. They state that the conditions screened for needs to have a high prevalence in the population, it has to be significantly disabling, it has to have a known natural history, and it should have a presymptomatic phase. Moreover, there has to be an accessible treatment, which is effective and acceptable to the participants.

In recent years, the potential negative effects of screening programs have received attention. These include the risk of imposing anxiety upon the identified individual and his or her family. False-negative cases may be erroneously reassured that they are healthy and false-positive cases are exposed to unnecessary investigation. Some screening programs also involve potentially hazardous examinations, such as X-rays. Moreover, there may be legal risks involved, with subjects missed at screening suing health care professionals.

In a world with limited economic resources and ever-growing expenses for medical services, the demand for evaluation, evidence of benefit, and proof of cost-effectiveness for government-financed screening programs has also increased.

2.1.2 Aims of Vision Screening

Screening programs generally aim to detect a specific disease. Vision screening in childhood differs from this since it detects a range of ophthalmologic disorders related to different visual problems.

Population-based vision screening in the newborn period normally includes examination of the red reflex. It aims to detect structural abnormalities and serious conditions, which threaten vision, or even life, such as congenital cataracts and retinoblastoma.

In most screening statements on preschool vision screening, the purpose of the programs has been to identify and treat amblyopia and related conditions, holding a gain for the society in reduction of visual loss in the population.

In many industrialized countries, there is a general surveillance system for all children, with examinations throughout infancy and childhood, with the purpose of following the development of all children and detecting problems or disease. As well as noticing other problems, visual and ophthalmologic disorders with signs and symptoms, such as strabismus, are found by this surveillance system. The presence of an attentive public health system, observant parents, and the accessibility of further examinations is important for visual and ocular surveillance of infants and children.

Apart from population-based vision screening of newborn and preschool children, special risk groups may need additional examinations. These include screening for ROP (retinopathy of prematurity) in children born preterm and examinations of children with certain hereditary disorders, etc.

Summary for the Clinician

- **Screening sorts out apparently well persons who probably have a disease from those who probably do not. A screening test is not intended to be diagnostic**
- **Vision screening in childhood aims to detect vision defects. It usually consists of examination(s) in the newborn period, surveillance via child heath care centers, and preschool vision screening. Special risk groups, such as children born preterm, may need additional screening**

2.2 Preschool Vision Screening

2.2.1 Definition of Preschool Vision Screening

According to the Medical Subject Headings (MeSH) database of the United States National Library of Medicine (NLM), the term "preschool" refers to a child between the ages of 2 and 5 years. The adjacent age groups are "infant," which refers to a child between 1 and 23 months of age, and "child," which refers to a person 6–12 years of age. The MeSH thesaurus is used by NLM for indexing articles from 4,600 of the world's leading biomedical journals for the MEDLINE/PubMED database. In publications, the term "preschool" is unfortunately sometimes used with reference to the school-system in the country concerned rather than in the scientifically defined way.

In this chapter, we have used the definition of preschool age from 2 years of age to 5 years of age (i.e., before the 6th birthday).

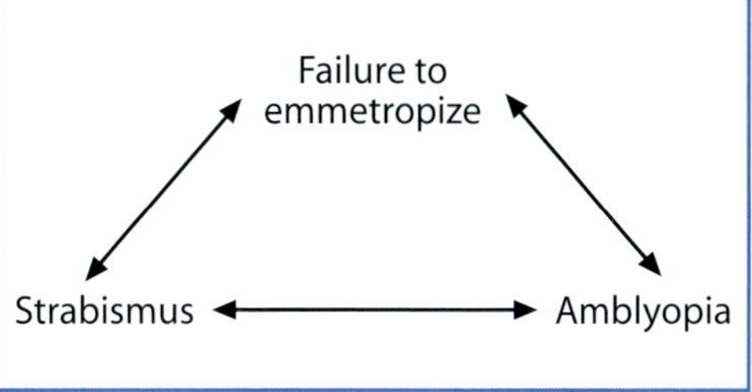

Fig. 2.1. Interrelationships and interactions between amblyopia and amblyogenic factors. No simple cause and effect connections seem to exist

2.2.2 Target Conditions for Preschool Vision Screening

Amblyopia and amblyogenic factors are the commonest target conditions for preschool vision screening. Amblyopia is normally defined as a reduction of visual acuity, despite optimal optical correction and without any signs of organic cause. The reduction in visual acuity is commonly unilateral, but it can be bilateral. Amblyopia can only develop during the sensitive period for visual development, which stretches over the first decade of life.

Amblyopia is associated with conditions depriving the visual system of normal visual experience. Campos [6] suggests three groups of amblyogenic factors: (1) strabismus, (2) anisometropia, and (3) form vision deprivation. The causes of unilateral form deprivation amblyopia include complete ptosis, media opacities, unilateral occlusion, and cycloplegia caused by pharmacological agents such as atropine. Bilateral amblyopia may in addition be associated with uncorrected high bilateral hyperopia, astigmatism (meridional amblyopia), and nystagmus.

Strabismus and anisometropia are the two dominating amblyogenic factors. The causes for strabismus and anisometropia are obscure and possibly even entangled. It is far from established what comes first in amblyopia. Does anisometropia come first and lead to the development of amblyopia, or is it amblyopia that causes the abnormal refraction? It has been shown that in unilateral amblyopia associated with hyperopia and strabismus, the fixating eye becomes more myopic with time, while the amblyopic eye remains hyperopic. Moreover, anisometropia can lead to development of strabismus and amblyopia formation. In normal visual development, the refractive status of the eye approaches emmetropia during childhood, a process known as emmetropization. Failure to emmetropize has been shown to be highly associated with development of amblyopia [1, 43] (Fig. 2.1).

Treatment of amblyopia generally consists of occlusion of the better eye with an adhesive patch, combined with optical correction when needed. Recent reports have also boosted the use of atropine drops, an old clinical method that had fallen into oblivion.

Considering the criteria suggested by Wilson and Junger for screening programs (see Sect. 2.1.1), preschool vision screening only fulfill some. Amblyopia affects 2–4% of the population, giving it a considerable prevalence. The natural history of amblyopia is insufficiently known (see Sect. 2.2.3), as well as the possible attributable disability (see Sect. 2.7.2). Amblyopia is usually asymptomatic, and there is accessible treatment, which (provided good compliance) is effective in general. The acceptability of the treatment has been debated, but recent data indicate that the psychosocial impact of treatment is less than feared.

Table 2.1. Prevalence of amblyopia in previous studies of screened and unscreened populations

Author:	Screened	Sample	Age (years)	Definition	Prevalence
Köhler and Stigmar (1978) [24]	Yes	2,178	7	?	0.8%
Jensen and Goldschmidt (1986) [21]	Yes	8,769	5 to 13	≤0.5	1.1%
Kvarnström et. al. (1998) [28]	Yes	3,126	10	≤0.5	0.9%
Ohlsson et al. (2001) [34]	Yes	1,046	12–13	≤0.5	1.1%
McNeil (1955) [30]	No	6,965	9–15	≤20/30	2.7%
Vinding et al. (1991) [49]	No	1,000	60–80	6/9	2.9%
Attebo et al. (1998) [4]	No	3,654	49	≤0.5	2.5%
Ohlsson et al. (2003) [35]	No	1,035	12 to 13	≤0.5	2.5%

2.2.3 Natural History of Untreated Amblyopia

There are no longitudinal studies that have investigated the natural history of untreated amblyopia. From an ethical point of view, it would be very difficult to withhold treatment from a child with detected amblyopia. Studies on natural history of amblyopia due to noncompliance have shown that the visual acuity of the amblyopic eye deteriorates during childhood [42] as well as during adolescence [13]. Studies on prevalence of amblyopia in countries without vision screening and studies on prevalence in nonscreened older age-cohorts in countries with vision screening have consistently shown higher prevalences than in vision-screened populations (Table 2.1). These facts strongly indicate that amblyopia does not spontaneously resolve with increasing age.

2.2.4 Whom to Screen?

Screening can be applied either to all (population-based screening) or to high risk groups (selective screening). In the presence of certain risk factors, such as increasing astigmatism or strabismus, the risk for amblyopia development is markedly increased compared to that of the general population [43]. This makes it tempting to suggest selective screening, e.g., for siblings of children with strabismus or children of parents with amblyopia. Unfortunately, less than half of children with strabismus have a family history of this disorder. Moreover, amblyopia and amblyogenic factors such as microstrabismus and anisometropia are asymptomatic, making it almost impossible for the child or parent to detect it. Inversely, far from all children with significant ametropia or anisometropia become amblyopic, and refractive development has been shown to be surprisingly dynamic [1].

In consequence, the lack of highly predictive and easily identifiable risk factors for a majority of amblyopic subjects makes population-based screening the only plausible choice for preschool vision screening [43].

Summary for the Clinician

- **Preschool refers to a child between the ages of 2 and 5 years**
- **Preschool vision screening aims to detect amblyopia and related conditions, such as strabismus and anisometropia. Population-based screening is recommended since highly predictive and easily identifiable risk factors are lacking**
- **The natural history of untreated amblyopia is insufficiently studied, but current knowledge strongly indicates that it does not spontaneously resolve**

Table 2.2. Definitions of sensitivity, specificity, positive and negative predictive value

	Truly diseased	Truly healthy	Total
Positive screening test	a	b	a + b
Negative screening test	c	d	c + d
Total	a + c	b + d	

a = the number of subjects who have the disease and for whom the screening test is positive (true positive); *b* = the number of subjects who are healthy, but for whom the screening test is positive (false positive); *c* = the number of subjects who have the disease, but for whom the screening test is negative (false negative); *d* = the number of subjects who are healthy and for whom the screening test is negative (true negative); Sensitivity: a/ a+c; specificity: d / b+d; positive predictive value: a / a+b; negative predictive value: d / c+d

2.3 Vision Screening Methodology

2.3.1 What Test to Use for Screening?

The capacity of a test to correctly identify subjects in a screening situation is described as sensitivity and specificity. The sensitivity of a test is the ability to detect subjects who truly are affected by the target condition ("truly diseased"). The specificity of a test is the ability to correctly identify subjects free of the target condition ("truly healthy") (Table 2.2). A test with low sensitivity fails to detect a substantial part of affected individuals ("under-referrals"). A test with low specificity wrongly suspects disease in a large number of healthy subjects ("over-referrals"). Sometimes the qualities of a screening test are also described in terms of positive predictive value, which is the proportion of subjects found positive upon testing who truly are affected with the target condition. A low positive predictive value means that few of those found positive at screening actually are affected by the disease. This might lower the confidence of the screening result among the public and can lead to low compliance with referral for more specialized care.

2.3.2 Visual Acuity

Visual acuity testing has been shown to be very sensitive in detecting amblyopia [23, 28]. Specificity is high and it is relatively easy to carry out, but also has the disadvantage of being time-consuming and sensitive to simple refractive errors. Visual acuity testing should preferably be performed with age-appropriate visual charts in logMAR steps. Each step/line (0.1) in the logMAR system is equally large physiologically speaking, in contrast to Snellen lines. Crowded visual charts have been shown to be more sensitive in detecting amblyopia. If single optotypes are used, products with crowding bars surrounding the optotype should be chosen.

When testing a child monocularly, the examiner must ensure that the occluded eye is totally covered in order to avoid peeking. An adhesive occluder is more reliable than a "pirate-patch."

2.3.3 Stereo Tests

Theoretically, stereo tests are attractive to use in a screening situation. They are less time-consuming than most other test methods, less sensitive to simple refractive errors, and may offer a "system" test of both optical and motor as well as neuronal components of vision. Unfortunately, several authors have found disappointing results with unacceptably high under-referral rates.

2.3.4 Orthoptic Assessment

An orthoptic examination usually includes cover-uncover testing at near and far, examination of eye motility and head posture and sometimes evaluation of fixation. In most screening settings where the examination is carried out by orthoptists, the assessment also includes stereo testing and monocular visual acuity.

2.3.5 Photorefractive Screening

Autorefraction at an early age has been suggested as a method of detecting strabismus and preventing amblyopia formation by correcting ametropia and anisometropia with glasses. Theoretically, photorefraction is an attractive method since it can detect amblyogenic factors and thus constitute a system of primary prevention. Drawbacks include difficulties in detecting microstrabismus and defining when a refractive error is highly amblyogenic for an individual child, especially during infancy or early preschool age. Furthermore, the risk of unnecessary treatment is marked in many children. Emmetropization has been shown to be a very dynamic process, and by correcting all children who on one occasion are found to have ametropia and/or anisometropia, large numbers will be subjected to unnecessary treatment. Early optical correction has moreover been accused of disturbing emmetropization. Current knowledge is contradictory.

2.3.6 Cost-Effectiveness of Different Tests

The cost-effectiveness of different methods of screening for amblyopia in preschool children has been compared in a study by König and Barry [25]. They found that visual acuity screening, with re-screening of inconclusive cases, was most favorable from a cost-benefit point of view. By adding additional testing (cover testing, motility test, and head posture), only a few additional cases were detected while the costs increased dramatically. Refractive screening was on average 60 % more expensive than other methods (average cost per detected case) due to large numbers of false-negative, false-positive, and inconclusive results.

2.3.7 Who Should Perform the Screening?

The cost and accessibility of vision screening is highly dependent on the profession of the personnel who conduct the tests. The level of training needed for the screening also depends on the test used in the program. Stereo testing, autorefractor readings, and visual acuity testing can be done by ophthalmologically unskilled personnel with only a minimum of training. Cover testing and other orthoptic assessment, on the other hand, requires highly skilled personnel. Moreover, one should not blink at the fact that strong occupational groups may have a major impact on decisions taken regarding vision screening. Government-financed examinations of an entire population naturally involves economic interests.

In Sweden, nurses in Child Health Care Centers do the screening (visual acuity testing), while in the UK, the testing is usually performed by orthoptists. In the United States, pediatricians or general practitioners often carry out vision screening. There are also programs in the US that have volunteers conducting the examination (autorefractor photographs) and the interpretation of the results is done by trained specialists.

2.3.8 At What Level Should Pass/ Fail Criteria Be Set?

Independent of the screening method chosen, the pass/fail criteria established are essential for the sensitivity and specificity of the test. A low (i.e., 0.5 instead of 0.8) pass/fail threshold will lower the number of over-referrals, but it will also increase the number of under-referrals and vice versa. Both under- and over-referrals are considered disadvantages in a screening system. Under-referrals give a false impression of visual and ocular health, while over-referrals lead to an unnecessarily large number of subjects referred for more specialized examinations.

In a recent policy statement by the American Academy of Pediatrics, visual acuity of less than 20/40 in either eye, or a two-line interocular difference irrespective of visual acuity, at age 3–5 years is suggested for referral criteria [11]. For children 6 years and older, visual acuity less than 20/30 in either eye, or a two-line interocular difference irrespective of visual acuity, is suggested. For both age groups, any abnormalities of ocular alignment or ocular media also constitute reasons for referral.

In Scandinavia, the visual acuity criteria have traditionally been stricter. In Sweden the referral criteria for 4-year-olds has been less than 0.8 (20/25) in either eye, or two lines of interocular difference. For 5.5-year-olds, the criteria has been less than 1.0 (20/20) in either eye, or two lines interocular difference [28]. Due to large numbers of over-referrals, a project was carried out in the Göteborg region with less strict referral criteria [15]. Children with visual acuity (0.65 in each eye or 0.65 in one eye and 0.8 in the other) where re-tested at age 5.5 years and then referred if visual acuity is less than 0.8 in either eye. The project showed that few children with slightly reduced visual acuity at age 4 years had conditions needing specialized ophthalmologic care. For those requiring treatment, outcome was good.

In a study on randomized treatment of unilateral visual impairment detected at preschool vision screening in 3- to 5-year-old children, Clarke et al. [9] found no difference in outcome for children with initial visual acuity 0.5–0.67, when comparing subjects who received treatment to those who did not receive any treatment. They argue that "... children with 6/9 (approximately 0.65) in one eye no longer constitute screen failures and do not justify treatment, even with glasses."

Summary for the Clinician

- **The ability of a test to correctly identify affected subjects is termed sensitivity.**
- **The ability of a test to correctly identify healthy subjects is termed specificity.**
- **The cost and accessibility of vision screening depends on the profession conducting the test. By using tests that can be administered by personnel with only a minimum of ophthalmologic training, costs for screening can be kept low.**
- **Choosing appropriate pass/fail criteria is crucial for a screening system to be efficient. Referral criteria for visual acuity at preschool screening differ between countries. Recent studies suggest that 3- to 5-year-old children with moderately reduced visual acuity (0.65) should not be considered screening failures due to lack of effect on outcome compared to controls.**

2.4 When to Screen?

2.4.1 Treatment Outcome and Age

For many years, there has been a general belief among ophthalmologists that early detection of amblyopia gives better treatment outcome. Recent studies have shown contradictory results.

Williams et al. [50] compared an extensive program with orthoptist examinations on six occasions from age 8 months to age 37 months, with one orthoptist examination at age 37 months. Results showed that children subjected to the intensive screening protocol had a lower prevalence of amblyopia at age 7.5 years. Interestingly, more than half of amblyopic subjects in the intensive groups were found at 37 months, despite five previous examinations. A major drawback of the study is the large number of dropouts at the final examination; only slightly more than half attended at age 7.5 years, which makes the representativeness of the results questionable.

In two studies by the US-based Pediatric Eye Disease Investigator Group on moderate amblyopia (VA 0.2–0.5) in children aged 3–7 years, no association was found between age and treatment effect [38, 39]. In a study on severe amblyopia (VA 0.05–0.2) by the same group [18], no significant age effect was found when comparing all age groups, but when pooling data and comparing younger children (<5 years old) to older children (5 to <7 years old), a significant age effect was found with a larger improvement in younger children.

In a study of children aged 3–5 years, Clarke et al. [9] found no negative effect when treatment was delayed until age 5 years. Surprisingly, their data even showed that deferring treatment nearly halved the proportion of children needing patching treatment at all.

Results from the Monitored Occlusion Treatment of Amblyopia Study (MOTAS) [46] found a significant difference in improvement of visual acuity following occlusion with greater improvement for age less than 4 years, compared to age 4–6 years and over 6 years.

All in all, the results indicate a possible small age effect with better outcome for children younger than 4–5 years of age.

2.4.2 Testability and Age

Visual acuity testing is feasible from around 3 years of age in most children. Visual acuity testing requires cooperation from the child in order to be practicable and reliable. Around 80% of 3-year-old children are testable with visual acuity charts. This number increases with nearly 10% for each additional year, with only a small percentage being untestable at age 5 years.

Simple stereo tests, such as the Titmus fly can sometimes be used for small children, but for tests requiring more cooperation, such as the TNO test, subjects needs to be at least 3–4 years of age for the results to be reliable.

Orthoptic examination can be done in infancy, although examination of a cooperative child is more reliable.

Hand-held photorefractive instruments or devices operating at some distance from the child can be used regardless of age.

2.4.3 Age at Vision Screening and Risk of New Cases or Rebounding Amblyopia

Basic neurophysiologic research on amblyopia performed by Hubel and Wiesel showed that there is an upper age limit for the development of amblyopia in animals. Keech and Kutschke [22] studied the upper age limit for development of amblyopia in humans and found that no subject developed amblyopia after age 6 years. By placing vision screening in the late preschool period, few cases of amblyopia will develop after screening. If vision screening is performed early, a second screening session might be necessary in order to detect cases developing after the first vision screening.

Amblyopic children who are treated and cured may need re-institution of treatment and are often supervised until early school age (generally around 8–9 years of age). Previous studies has shown that subjects who did not need re-institution of treatment therapy were older at end of treatment than those patients who did need maintenance therapy [19, 36]. It could be argued that children who are diagnosed with amblyopia at late preschool age still have a possibility for good treatment outcome and after treatment they will need supervision and possibly maintenance therapy for only a short period of time. The burden of occlusion therapy will thereby be minimized.

2.4.4 Age and Psychosocial Impact of Treatment

In a report on amblyopia and disability from 1997, Snowdon and Stewart-Brown [45] reported that subjects who had received treatment for amblyopia in many cases had experienced this as very problematic (psychologically, socially, and practically). Searle et al. [41] confirmed this in a qualitative study on the psychological effects of patching. They concluded that "eye patching has adverse psychological effects for both the child and family" and that "the restrictions imposed on a child through wearing a patch are disabling in themselves due to the impaired ability to engage in certain activities."

Two recent studies on the impact of occlusion therapy for amblyopia, Hrisos et al. [19] and Holmes et al. [17] both found that occlusion treatment and (in Holmes et al.) atropine treatment for amblyopia is associated with psychosocial distress. The effect was minor in both studies and Hrisos et al. found no effect on the child's global well-being. Interestingly, neither of the studies found any age effect in the distress of treatment. There has been a general belief that older children are more bothered by treatment and it would thereby be more beneficial to treat early. Hrisos et al. even found parents of 4-year-olds more upset than parents of older children.

Choong et al. [7] also reports on psychosocial implications of childhood amblyopia. Contrary to Hrisos et al. [19], they found no effect of occlusion on carer's stress or child's psychosocial well-being when comparing amblyopic non-occluded and occluded children. The majority of children in the study were treated with glasses prior to occlusion and no more than around 50% needed occlusion after the initial phase with optical correction only. Following onset of optical correction, carers felt significantly more negative toward their child. Surprisingly, this effect was reversed at onset of occlusion therapy.

Summary for the Clinician

- Recent studies on the relationship between treatment outcome and age for amblyopia has shown contradictory results. Put together, the results indicate a possible small age effect with better outcome for children younger than 4–5 years of age
- Visual acuity testing and stereo testing require the child to cooperate. Some children can perform the tests at around 3 years, but the number of children testable increases rapidly. At age 4–5 years, the majority of children can be tested reliably. Orthoptic examination and distant photorefraction can be performed irrespective of age
- Amblyopia can only form up to approximately age 6 years. Early vision screening may involve a risk of new cases of amblyopia developing after screening
- Studies on the psychosocial impact of amblyopia treatment have not been able to demonstrate an age effect, i.e., older children are not more bothered by amblyopia treatment than younger children

2.4.5 Current Recommendations on Suitable Age for Vision Screening

In a policy statement from pediatricians, orthoptists, and ophthalmologists in the US [11], vision screening with visual acuity testing is requested to be performed at "the earliest possible age that it is practical (usually at approximately 3 years of age)." A recent report from the UK [14] suggests vision screening to be carried out with visual acuity testing at age 5 years. In Sweden, visual acuity is tested at 4 years of age at the Child Health Care centers. The policy on timing of retesting differs between regions, and varies from retesting within 6 months to retesting at age 5.5 years.

2.5 The Effect of Preschool Vision Screening

2.5.1 The Necessity of High Participation Rates

The participation frequency of a screening program is crucial for its effectiveness. This was shown by Williams et al. [51] in a study on prevalence of amblyopia in 7.5 year old children with and without screening at 37 months. When comparing those who actually attending screened with those who were not screened, there was a small, but statistically significant difference in outcome. Comparing those offered screening (67% actually participated) with those not offered screening, this difference disappeared. This points to the need for high attendance rates in order for a screening system to be effective and worthwhile from a population point of view, which was addressed in the editorial by Moseley and Fielder in the same issue. In Sweden, where 99% of 4- to 5-year-olds participate in vision screening, deep amblyopia (visual acu-

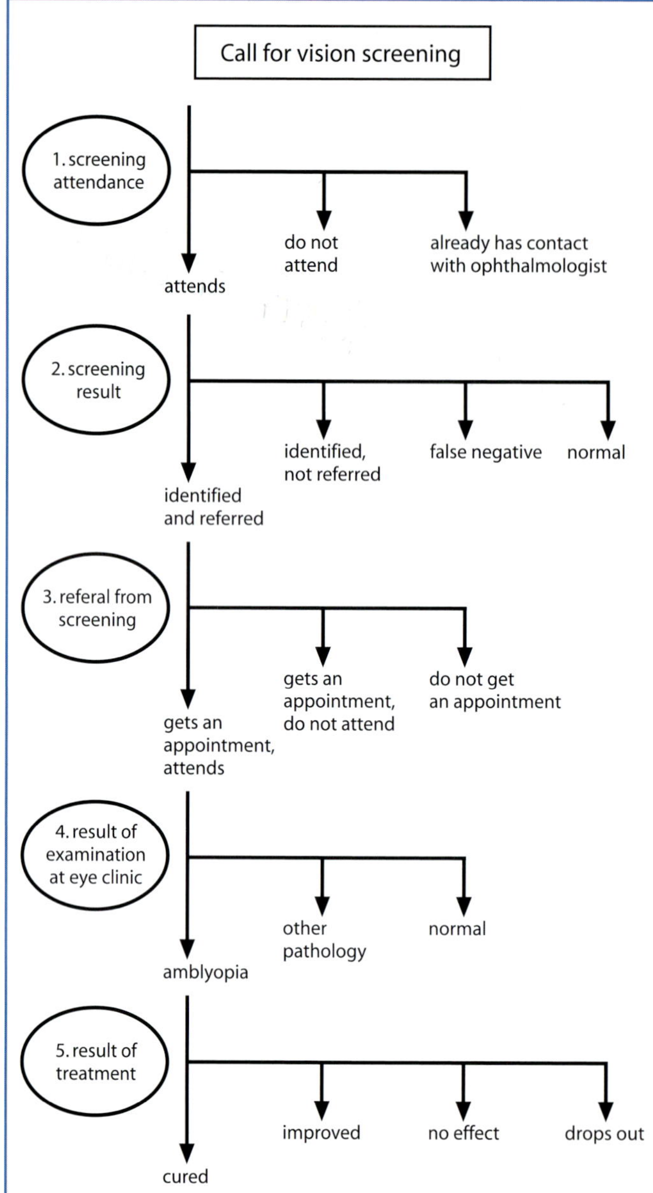

Fig. 2.2. Suggested flowchart for evaluating preschool vision screening programs

ity <0.3) has been shown to decrease to a tenth of that in unscreened age groups [28].

The best way to reach acceptable participation frequencies for vision screening programs is probably to incorporate the program into an already existing system with a high participation rate, e.g., vaccination programs or school entry. The vision screening system in Sweden is one part of the 4-year check-up at the Child Health Care centers, with retesting of inconclusive and borderline cases.

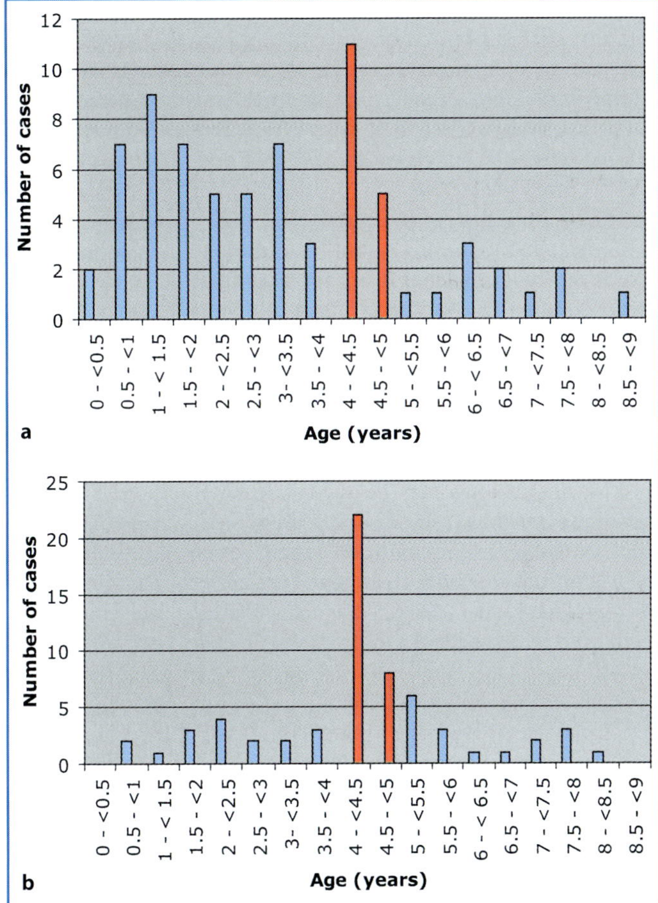

Fig. 2.3. **a** The age at which strabismus is diagnosed by an ophthalmologist at the Eye Clinic in the city of Västerås, Sweden, for all children born 1979–1980. Note that only 22% (16/72) is detected at preschool vision screening (*red bars*). (Reprinted from Sjöstrand and Abrahamsson [44] with kind permission of Georg Thieme Verlag.) **b** The age at which amblyopia (visual acuity ≤0.5) is diagnosed by an ophthalmologist at the Eye Clinic in the city of Västerås, Sweden, for all children born 1979–1980. Slightly less than half of children with amblyopia (30/64) are detected at preschool vision screening (*red bars*). (Reprinted from Sjöstrand and Abrahamsson [44] with kind permission of Georg Thieme Verlag)

2.5.2 Evaluating the Effect of Preschool Vision Screening

In evaluating a screening system, the entire process has to be mapped out and the effect on the population has to be assessed. How many cases of amblyopia are found before screening is carried out? Do a substantial number of cases present anyway? If so, are they referred by other clinics or do the parents individually contact the eye clinic? Do children found to be abnormal at screening reach ophthalmologic clinics and treatment? Is treatment successful? Figure 2.2 maps out the flow, and possible pitfalls, of a vision screening system.

Sjöstrand and Abrahamsson [44] studied the ophthalmologic hospital records of all children born between 1979 and 1980 in the community of Västerås, Sweden. They found that only 22% of strabismic children are detected at vision screening. The remaining 78% are diagnosed before, but also after, vision screening. Amblyopia found at screening was mainly associated with anisometropia and microstrabismus (Fig. 2.3 a, b). Consequently, the presence of an active child health care system (monitoring) has an effect on lowering the prevalence of amblyopia (compare Fig. 2.2, number 1).

The transfer of children from screening to ophthalmologic care can be a problem, as shown by preliminary results from the Dutch study RAMSES (Rotterdam Amblyopia Screening Effectiveness Study), where only 63% of children referred from vision screening actually visited an ophthalmologist (personal communication)! More encouraging numbers are found in a study by Newman et al. [33], where children referred from vision screening to hospital eye care were followed. In this study, out of 348 children referred, 15 failed to attend follow up, 10 defaulted follow up, 6 moved, and for 13 records where unavailable. Accordingly, at least 7% (25 children) where lost to follow-up (compare Fig. 2.2, number 3)

Vision screening seems to lower the prevalence of amblyopia ≤0.5 to between one-third and one-half the prevalence of that in an unscreened population (Table 2.1). The prevalence of residual amblyopia may be due to cases not attending screening, cases missed in the screening at 4 years of age, the condition having developed later, unsuccessful treatment (including noncompliance) or incorrect diagnosis. Out of 11 children with residual amblyopia ≤0.5 in a Swedish study [34], eight reported having had previous contact with an ophthalmologist, but only five of these before age 7 years. The six cases without contact before age 7 years consisted of three cases of anisometrope, one of microesotropia, one of esotropia, and one of high hyperopia.

Even though the primary aim for preschool vision screening is to reduce amblyopia and amblyogenic factors, it is important to recognize other beneficial effects. These include detection of visual disorders other than amblyopia, such as organic disorders, and conditions that may impede schoolwork, such as high hyperopia.

Summary for the Clinician

- **In order for preschool vision screening to have an effect on a population basis, the participation rate needs to be very high. A participation rate of 67% was not sufficient in a recent study. One method to enable a high participation rate is to combine preschool vision screening with other well-known and well-attended systems, such as school entry or vaccination programs**
- **A majority of subjects with cosmetically obvious strabismus present before age 4 years. Preschool vision screening mainly detects amblyopia associated with anisometropia and microstrabismus**
- **Vision screening seems to lower the prevalence of amblyopia (≤0.5) to between one-third and one-half of that in an unscreened population**

2.6 What is the "Best Buy" for Vision Screening?

2.6.1 Early Versus Late Vision Screening

Supporters of early visual screening argue that by finding and treating precursors for strabismus and amblyopia, visual disorders may be prevented, and early treatment of already present amblyopia leads to better outcome. Extensive studies aiming at primary prevention of amblyopia and strabismus have shown some effect on preventing visual loss in children with significant refractive errors; the effect on prevention of strabismus development has been inconsistent [2, 3]. Advocates for late preschool vision screening reason that only a minority of children with ametropia and/or anisometropia really develop amblyopia. Rather than overtreating large numbers of children, it is better to treat those who really develop amblyopia. At late preschool age, successful treatment is still achievable: the possible age effect in outcome of amblyopia treatment is minor, if any at all, up to age 5 years.

Examinations on more than one occasion usually lead to detection of more cases affected by disease. Consequently, it could be argued that vision screening at several ages during infancy and childhood would most likely lead to better outcome from a population-based point of view. Unfortunately, by adding additional testing methods and/or additional testing occasions, the cost per detected case increases substantially. Considering the stretched economy of most public health care systems, it is probably not realistic to suggest preschool vision screening on more than one occasion.

2.6.2 What Test Should Be Used?

In order for a test method to be accepted as a screening tool, many qualities have to be fulfilled. Wilson and Jungner [52] suggested the following criteria in 1968:

The screening test needs to:

- Be reliable, valid, and repeatable
- Be acceptable to the study population, safe, and easy to perform
- Have a high positive predictive value
- Be sensitive and specific
- Be cost-effective

Visual acuity testing has been shown to have very high sensitivity and specificity for amblyopia [23, 28]. It is also sensitive to refractive errors, especially myopia, but myopia is uncommon in preschool children. Visual acuity testing can be reliably performed from age 4–5 years, and it is safe and repeatable. Visual charts in logMAR steps are recommended, preferably with crowded optotypes. Visual acuity testing is relatively easy to perform. It can carried out by nonophthalmologic personnel, as shown at the Swedish Health Care centers where nurses perform the testing after minor training. Visual acuity screening, with rescreening of inconclusive cases, has also been shown to be favorable from a cost-benefit point of view.

Conditions not affecting visual acuity might naturally elude observation in a setting with visual acuity-based screening, e.g., strabismus with normal visual acuity, minor ptosis, or small partial cataracts. On the other hand, without impact on visual acuity these disorders do not require treatment in preschool children. Strabismus may represent a cosmetic problem, though, but that is beyond the aim of vision screening.

2.6.3 What Age Is the "Best Buy" for Preschool Vision Screening?

Considering the issues discussed in the sections above, it does not seem possible to find an age that is optimal in all aspects. Put together, with a major emphasis on reaching a high participation frequency, preschool vision screening at age 4–5 years seems to be the "best buy." At this age, a majority of children are reliably testable with visual acuity charts, which have shown to be sensitive and cost-effective. There is a very small risk of new cases developing after vision screening, and monitoring after treatment and possible maintenance therapy will be needed for a minimal time period. Moreover, many countries can combine vision screening with other services with high participation frequencies, such as child health care programs (including vaccination) or school entry. Recent reports (see Sect. 2.4.1) have demonstrated a possible age effect for amblyopia treatment, with better outcome for younger children. The effect shown has not been very large though, and the dividing line between "young" and "old" children seems to be around 5 years of age.

Summary for the Clinician

- **Vision screening for amblyopia at more than one occasion during the preschool years does not seem plausible due to increasing costs per detected case**
- **Visual acuity testing has a high sensitivity and specificity for amblyopia. Visual acuity testing can be reliably performed from age 4–5 years; it is safe and repeatable. Visual acuity testing is relatively easy to perform, it can carried out by nonophthalmologic personnel. Charts in logMAR steps and crowded optotypes are recommended. Visual acuity screening has also been shown to be favorable from a cost-benefit point of view**
- **At age 4–5 years, a majority of children are reliably testable with visual acuity charts. There is a very small risk of new cases developing after vision screening, and surveillance after treatment and possible mainte-**

nance therapy will be needed a minimal time period. The possible age-effect for amblyopia treatment has been small, and the dividing line seems to be around 5 years of age

2.7 Is Preschool Vision Screening Worthwhile?

The negative impact of amblyopia from a population perspective is associated with two issues. First, the risk of losing the better eye, and second, the possible disability caused by monocular amblyopic visual loss.

2.7.1 The Risk of Losing the Nonamblyopic Eye

If a person with amblyopia loses the better eye due to trauma or ocular disease the disadvantage of having an amblyopic eye is obvious. If the remaining amblyopic eye is severely amblyopic, the subject will become visually disabled. Increase in visual acuity after loss of the better eye has been shown, even in older persons, but acceptable visual acuity outcome is highly dependent on central fixation [12, 48].

A frequently cited paper by Tommila and Tarkkanen [47] showed that the risk of injuring the nonamblyopic eye in an amblyopic individual was almost three times that in the normal population. In a recent paper, Chua and Mitchell [8] found the 5-year incidence of visual impairment in the better seeing eye to be 2.7 times higher for an amblyopic subject compared to subjects without amblyopia.

Jakobsson et al. [20], analyzing all patients in four vision rehabilitation centers in southern Sweden, report that the prevalence of visual disability (VA ≤0.3) with amblyopia as the main cause was 0.023% among the general population. By comparing this rate with data from a previous Swedish study, the authors calculated that about 1.2% of subjects with amblyopia of ≤0.3 visual acuity will eventually become visually handicapped. In a subsequent study [28], the same group showed that the Swedish vision screening program lowers the prevalence of visual acuity ≤0.3 by a factor of 10. Considering that approximately 100,000 children are born in Sweden each year, this suggests that vision screening could save approximately 20 persons per year from becoming visually disabled. Jakobsson et al. do point out, however, that about 60% of the diseases affecting nonamblyopic eyes and leading to visual impairment are inherently bilateral, and will therefore subsequently affect the amblyopic eye as well. In the UK, Rahi et al. [40], analyzing loss of vision in the nonamblyopic eye, found the same prevalence as reported by Jakobsson's group; they suggest that the lifetime risk of serious vision loss in an individual with amblyopia is 1.2%. According to Rahi et al. [40], in individuals up to 64 years old, trauma is the leading cause of visual loss, whereas in individuals 65 years and older, age-related macular degeneration (AMD) ranks highest. One year after presentation, 73% were still classified as visually impaired or blind and only 35% of patients in previous paid employment were able to continue working. Only 10% improved two lines in visual acuity.

2.7.2 Is It Disabling to Be Amblyopic?

Several studies have given amblyopia as a major cause for monocular visual loss in industrialized countries. Mulvihill et al. [31] found amblyopia to be the third most frequent cause for uniocular blindness in childhood. A study by the National Eye Institute (The Visual Acuity Impairment Study) [32], found amblyopia to be the leading cause of monocular visual loss in the age group 25–64 years. But despite theoretical support for disturbance of binocularity and visual experience in amblyopia, no objective study has been able to show that it is in fact disabling to be unilaterally amblyopic. Packwood et al. [37] in a survey of 25 straight-eye amblyopes focused on quality of life issues and psychosocial difficulties. Their results show that approximately 50% of subjects felt that their amblyopia interfered with work or school and generally affected their lifestyle. Amblyopic subjects also experienced significantly more psychological distress than control subjects. In analyzing results such as these, it is important to consider the fact that strabismus and other ocular pathologies are not independent variables, but are all associated with other morbidity, especially neurological diseases, which may confound the results.

Snowdon and Stewart-Brown [45] interviewed health care professionals, adults with amblyopia, and children in amblyopia treatment to gain an understanding of how amblyopia and treatment for amblyopia affects people's lives. Their conclusion was that health care professionals consider amblyopia to be disabling, while amblyopic subjects do not.

In a study on the relationship between amblyopia and academic performance in school children, Helveston et al. [16] could not find any connection. Regarding possible professional consequences of amblyopia, Chua and Mitchell [8] found a borderline significant effect of amblyopia on higher university degrees, but no effect on lifetime occupational class.

There are, all the same, several careers which unilateral amblyopes may be debarred from. In many countries, the army, police force, transport sector, aviation, and fire brigade all have vision requirements. Whether these demands are based on real evidence of true inability, or on general assumptions, is more uncertain. There have even been lawsuits with individuals not fulfilling vision requirements demanding antidiscriminatory laws.

2.7.3 Cost-Effectiveness of Screening and Treatment for Amblyopia

In two cost-utility studies on screening and treatment for amblyopia in 3-year-old children, König and Barry [26, 27] conclude that screening and treatment for amblyopia is likely to be cost-effective. In their conclusion, they express some reservations because of the uncertainty relating to the connection between quality of life and amblyopia. The utility (quality of life) values in the reports are drawn from a study on quality of life associated with unilateral and bilateral good vision [5]. This study does not deal with amblyopic subjects, but with subjects affected with progressive ophthalmic disease, some of whom have unilateral impaired vision. These subjects differ from unilateral amblyopes in that they had previously had healthy eyes and normal vision. In many ophthalmic diseases, there are additional visual problems such as reduction of visual field and reduced contrast sensitivity, which amblyopes usually do not suffer from. König and Barry [27] conclude that the risk of losing the better eye alone would not justify vision screening from a cost-effective point of view. But if amblyopia is associated with even minor loss in utility, vision screening would be justified provided that amblyopia treatment restores utility.

There is a clear need for objective studies on the relationship of unilateral amblyopia and disability. In such a study, a comparison should if possible be made between three groups: (1) nonamblyopes, (2) amblyopes without/before treatment, and (3) amblyopes after successful treatment.

Cost-utility studies assume that successfully treated amblyopes have the same utility value as healthy subjects. If it is shown that amblyopia is related to some kind of disability or loss of utility, then it is important to establish whether successful treatment reduces this disability or utility loss.

In discussing whether vision screening is worthwhile, it is also important to recognize that in real life vision screening detects more than amblyopia and amblyogenic factors. Vision screening at or before school entry enables detection of important nonamblyopic conditions, such as high hypermetropia (which can disturb reading and other near activities) or visual and ocular disorders requiring spectacles or other visual aids.

Summary for the Clinician

- **The lifetime risk for visual disability due to loss of the better eye is 1.2% for an amblyopic subject. The leading cause of vision loss in the nonamblyopic eye is ophthalmic disease that will subsequently affect also the amblyopic eye. Few subjects spontaneously recover visual function in the amblyopic eye**

- **The risk of injuring the nonamblyopic eye for an amblyopic subject is around three times that of the general population**
- **There is little evidence that unilateral amblyopia is disabling, but knowledge is scarce**
- **Amblyopes may be debarred from certain professions, but evidence for an effect on the academic career is uncertain**
- **Preschool vision screening for amblyopia is likely to be cost-effective, but the conclusion requires that amblyopia is associated with loss of utility, and that treatment restores utility**

2.8 Future Evidence Needed

Several important and well designed studies on amblyopia and preschool vision screening have been published in recent years, and the field has advanced significantly. More evidence is needed, however, in order to demonstrate that preschool vision screening is worthwhile and establish which method and age is optimal. More data is needed on the relationship between amblyopia and real life measures such as quality of life and/or utility, and the effect treatment has on restoring the possible deficit. Current knowledge is contradictory on whether there is an age-effect in amblyopia treatment, and if so, where the break-point is. The pathophysiology of amblyopia and the connection between precursors/amblyogenic factors and development of amblyopia are still obscure in many respects. Further understanding of these relationships may enable better treatment and possible prevention of amblyopia.

In order for preschool vision screening to have an effect on a population basis, a high participation frequency has been shown to be requisite. Further studies are needed on how to enhance participation in vision screening. Studies should also be initiated locally to fully evaluate the complete preschool vision screening system (see Fig. 2.2) and search for pitfalls for successful outcome. An aim should be that all vision screening programs fulfill defined quality standards and proves to be of benefit for the population.

References

1. Abrahamsson M, Fabian G, Andersson AK, Sjöstrand J (1990) A longitudinal study of a population based sample of astigmatic children. Acta Ophthalmol (Copenh) 68:428–440
2. Anker S, Atkinson J, Braddick O, Nardini M, Ehrlich D (2004) Non-cycloplegic refrcative screening can identify infants whose visual outcome at 4 years is improved by spectacle correction. Strabismus 12:227–245
3. Atkinson J, Braddick O, Robier B et al (1996) Two infant vision screening programmes: prediction and prevention of strabismus and amblyopia from photo- and videorefractive screening. Eye 10:189–198
4. Attebo K, Mitchell P, Cumming R, Smith W, Jolly N, Sparkes R (1998) Prevalence and causes of amblyopia in an adult population. Ophthalmology 105:154–159
5. Brown MM, Brown GC, Sharma S, Busbee B, Brown H (2001) Quality of life associated with unilateral and bilateral good vision. Ophthalmology 108:643–648
6. Campos E (1995) Amblyopia. Surv Ophthalmol 40:23–39
7. Choong YF, Lukman H, Martin S, Laws DE (2004) Childhood amblyopia treatment: psychosocial implications for patients and primary carers. Eye 18:369–375
8. Chua B, Mitchell P (2004) Consequences of amblyopia on education, occupation, and long term vision loss. Br J Ophthalmol 88:1119–1121
9. Clarke MP, Wright CM, Hrisos S, Anderson JD, Henderson J, Richardson SR (2003) Randomised controlled trial of treatment of unilateral visual impairment detected at preschool vision screening. BMJ 327:1251
10. Commission on Chronic Illness (1957) Chronic illness in the United States. Vol I. Prevention of chronic illness. Harvard University Press, Cambridge
11. Committee on Practice and Ambulatory Medicine, Section on Ophthalmology. American Association of Certified Orthoptists; American Association for Pediatric Ophthalmology and Strabismus; American Academy of Ophthalmology (2003) Eye examination in infants, children, and young adults by pediatricians. Pediatrics 111: 902–907
12. El Mallah MK, Chakravarthy U, Hart PM (2000) Amblyopia: is visual loss permanent? Br J Ophthalmol 84:952–956

13. Haase W, Wenzel F (1996) The natural course of untreated functional amblyopia: does it progress between childhood and adulthood? Binoc Vis Strab Quart 12:17–24
14. Hall D, Elliman D (eds) (2003) Health for all children. Oxford University Press, Oxford
15. Hård AL, Sjödell L, Borres MP, Zetterberg I, Sjöstrand J (2002) Preschool vision screening in a Swedish city region: results after alteration of criteria for referral to eye clinics. Acta Ophthalmol Scand 80:608–611
16. Helveston EM, Weber JC, Miller K et al (1985) Visual function and academic performance. Am J Ophthalmol 99:346–355
17. Holmes JM, Beck RW, Kraker RT et al (2003) Impact of patching and atropine treatment on the child and family in the amblyopia treatment study. Arch Ophthalmol 121:1625–1632
18. Holmes JM, Kraker RT, Beck RW et al (2003) A randomized trial of prescribed patching regimens for treatment of severe amblyopia in children. Ophthalmology 110:2075–2087
19. Hrisos S, Clarke MP, Wright CM (2004) The emotional impact of amblyopia treatment in preschool children: randomized controlled trial. Ophthalmology 111:1550–1556
20. Jakobsson P, Kvarnström G, Abrahamsson M, Bjernbrink-Hörnblad E, Sunnqvist B (2002) The frequency of amblyopia among visually impaired persons. Acta Ophthalmol Scand 80:44–46
21. Jensen H, Goldschmidt E (1986) Visual acuity in Danish school children. Acta Ophthalmol (Copenh) 64:187–191
22. Keech RV, Kutschke PJ (1995) Upper age limit for the development of amblyopia. J Pediatr Ophthalmol Strabismus 32:89–93
23. Köhler L, Stigmar G (1973) Vision screening of four-year-old children. Acta Paediatr Scand 62:17–27
24. Köhler L, Stigmar G (1978) Visual disorders in 7-year-old children with and without previous vision screening. Acta Paediatr Scand 67:373–377
25. König HH, Barry JC (2002) Economic evaluation of different methods of screening for amblyopia in kindergarten. Pediatrics 109:e59.
26. König HH, Barry JC (2004) Cost effectiveness of treatment for amblyopia: an analysis based on a probabilistic Markov model. Br J Ophthalmol 88:606–612
27. König HH, Barry JC (2004) Cost-utility analysis of orthoptic screening in kindergarten: a Markov model based on data from Germany. Pediatrics 113:e95–108
28. Kvarnström G, Jakobsson P, Lennerstrand G (1998) Screening for visual and ocular disorders in children, evaluation of the system in Sweden. Acta Paediatr 87:1173–1179
29. Levartovsky S, Gottesman N, Shimshoni M, Oliver M (1992) Factors affecting long-term results of successfully treated amblyopia: age at beginning of treatment and age at cessation of monitoring. J Pediatr Ophthalmol Strabismus 29:219–223
30. McNeil NL (1955) Patterns of visual deficits in children. Br J Ophthalmol 39:688–701
31. Mulvihill A, Bowell R, Lanigan B, O'Keefe M (1997) Uniocular childhood blindness: a prospective study. J Pediatr Ophthalmol Strabismus 34:111–114
32. National Eye Institute Office of Biometry and Epidemiology. Report on the National Eye Institute's Visual Acuity Impairment Survey Pilot Study. Department of Health and Human Services,Washington, DC, pp 81–84
33. Newman DK, Hitchcock A, McCarthy H, Keast-Butler J, Moore AT (1996) Preschool vision screening: outcome of children referred to the hospital eye service. Br J Ophthalmol 80:1077–1082
34. Ohlsson J, Villarreal G, Sjöström A, Abrahamsson M, Sjöstrand J (2001) Visual acuity, residual amblyopia and ocular pathology in a screened population of 12–13-year-old children in Sweden. Acta Ophthalmol Scand 79:589–595
35. Ohlsson J, Villarreal G, Sjöström A, Cavazos H, Abrahamsson M, Sjöstrand J (2003) Visual acuity, amblyopia and ocular pathology in 12–13-year-old children in northern Mexico. J AAPOS 7:47–53
36. Oster JG, Simon JW, Jenkins P (1990) When is it safe to stop patching? Br J Ophthalmol 74:709–711
37. Packwood EA, Cruz OA, Rychwalski PJ, Keech RV (1999) The psychosocial effects of amblyopia study. J AAPOS 3:15–17
38. Pediatric Eye Disease Investigator Group (2003) The course of moderate amblyopia treated with patching in children: experience of the amblyopia treatment study. Am J Ophthalmol 136:620–629
39. Pediatric Eye Disease Investigator Group (2003) The course of moderate amblyopia treated with atropine in children: experience of the amblyopia treatment study. Am J Ophthalmol 2003; 136:630–639
40. Rahi J, Logan S, Timms C, Russell-Eggitt I, Taylor D (2002) Risk, causes, and outcomes of visual impairment after loss of vision in the non-amblyopic eye: a population-based study. Lancet 360:597–602
41. Searle A, Vedhara K, Norman P, Frost A, Harrad R (2000) Compliance with eye patching in children and its psychosocial effects: a qualitative application of protection motivation theory. Pshychol Health Med 5:43–54

42. Simons K, Preslan M (1999) Natural history of amblyopia untreated owing to lack of compliance. Br J Ophthalmol 83:582–587
43. Sjöstrand J, Abrahamsson M (1990) Risk factors in amblyopia. Eye 4:787–793
44. Sjöstrand J, Abrahamsson M (1996) Can we identify risk groups for the development of amblyopia and strabismus? (in German) Klin Monatsbl Augenheilkd 208:23–26
45. Snowdon S, Stewart-Brown S (1997) Amblyopia and disability. A qualitative study. Health Services Research Unit, University of Oxford, Oxford
46. Stewart CE, Moseley MJ, Stephens DA, Fielder AR (2004) Treatment dose-response in amblyopia therapy: the Monitored Occlusion Treatment of Amblyopia Study (MOTAS). Invest Ophthalmol Vis Sci 45:3048–3054
47. Tommila V, Tarkkanen A (1981) Incidence of loss of vision in the healthy eye in amblyopia. Br J Ophthalmol 65:575–577
48. Vereecken EP, Brabant P (1984) Prognosis for vision in amblyopia after the loss of the good eye. Arch Ophthalmol 102:220–224
49. Vinding T, Gregersen E, Jensen A, Rindziunski E (1991) Prevalence of amblyopia in old people without previous screening and treatment. Acta Ophthalmol (Copenh) 69:796–798
50. Williams C, Northstone K, Harrad RA, Sparrow JM, Harvey I (2002) Amblyopia treatment outcomes after screening before or at age 3 years: follow-up from randomised trial. BMJ 324:1549
51. Williams C, Northstone K, Harrad RA, Sparrow JM, Harvey I (2003) Amblyopia treatment outcomes after preschool screening v school entry screening: observational data from a prospective cohort study. Br J Ophthalmol 87:988–993
52. Wilson JM, Jungner G (1968) Principles and practice of screening for disease. World Health Organization, Geneva

Modern Treatment of Amblyopia

Michael Clarke

Core Messages

- Amblyopia is a form of reversible cerebral visual impairment
- Amblyopia is caused by a disturbance of vision during a sensitive period of development
- Amblyopia may be treated by modulation of visual input during this sensitive period
- Amblyopia is always associated with disease of the visual system

3.1 Introduction

Although amblyopia has been recognised since ancient times, has been treated for over 200 years, and is a fundamental part of all paediatric ophthalmology practice, we have yet to arrive at a consensus about its definition, never mind its treatment. In this chapter, I am going to explore the definition of amblyopia and discuss the rationale behind amblyopia treatment before going on to discuss how traditional treatment concepts should be modified in the light of recent work on the subject. I hope that this will encourage the reader to think for themselves about these issues and apply relevant clinical evidence to the patients they see everyday in practice.

3.2 What Is Amblyopia?

Amblyopia has traditionally been defined by what it is not, rather than what it is. This is a hangover from the original description of amblyopia as a condition in which "the patient sees little, and neither does the physician".

We know now, from animal experimentation [12] as well as functional human neuroimaging [7], that amblyopia is a condition in which there is dysfunction of the processing of visual information resulting in a range of abnormalities of visual function. Whereas ocular examination and initial retinal function are normal in amblyopia, processing abnormalities have been shown to be present in humans in the retina and primary visual cortex, and in animals in the lateral geniculate bodies. Amblyopia always results from degradation of the retinal image during a sensitive period of visual development (which may not be the same as the sensitive period during which treatment is effective). In other words, amblyopia never occurs in isolation. It is not the cause, but the effect of another pathology.

Amblyopia may be completely or partially treated by modulation of the visual input during a sensitive period of visual development. The duration of this period varies depending on the cause of the amblyopia. Causes, which severely degrade the retinal image early in infancy, require early, vigorous treatment. Causes with a later onset, particularly if image degradation is mild, may respond to treatment up to and beyond the age of 7 years.

3.3 Should Amblyopia Be Treated?

There has been a debate, in public health circles at least, about whether amblyopia should be treated at all [30]. It has been argued that individuals with amblyopia show little functional disability and that treatment with patching is psychologically distressing. In this context, it is worth considering why any medical condition or state of health merits treatment.

States of health are considered abnormal, and so worth treating, when they impact adversely, or threaten to impact in the future, on an individual's duration or quality of life. Quality of life encompasses both the individual's functioning, and the presence of distressing symptoms. Functioning includes the ability of an individual to perform activities they either enjoy, or are necessary for the economic and social well-being of themselves or their dependents. Distressing symptoms include such things as pain, breathlessness or anxiety.

It is an important principle of modern medicine that, apart from rare instances where there is a threat to public health, treatment is offered, not imposed. Furthermore, the treating physician should inform him- or herself, and the patient, of the available evidence about the risks and benefits of the possible alternative treatments before making a decision about which to use, if any, in an individual case.

An abnormal state of health may be demonstrated either because the individual presents to medical attention with symptoms, or because it is found as a result of a medical examination (e.g. screening, case finding, clinical surveillance).

When an individual presents with symptoms, it can usually be assumed that he or she wants to be relieved of them. For example, a patient with ischaemic heart disease may be offered treatment because they wish to be rid of their chest pain, which limits exercise tolerance and so function. Treatment may also be justified to prevent death of cardiac muscle and, ultimately, of the individual. The discussion which then takes place between the physician and the patient is then about whether quality of life is better with the symptoms, or with ameliorated or abolished symptoms plus treatment side effects. In these cases, the risks of possible future treatment side effects are balanced against symptoms, which are real and current.

Other conditions (such as high blood pressure or asymptomatic malignancy) are treated because they pose a future risk to duration or quality of life. In these cases, it is the risks of future adverse events which are balanced against the risks of treatment. It is important to recognise that while the risk of stroke in the population has been shown to be reduced by the treatment of hypertension, many individuals who would never have suffered the adverse event, in this case, stroke, endure side effects from medication. These considerations need to be explained to patients, although if many opt not to have treatment then this will limit the ability of the screening programmes to modify the risk of disease in the population.

In ophthalmology, conditions are usually treated because they affect sight, or threaten to do so, or because they cause pain, or both. Patients may present with symptoms, such as poor vision from cataracts or pain from a corneal abrasion; or may be referred because of a risk factor for future visual loss, such as high intraocular pressure.

Bilateral eye disorders affect quality of life more significantly than unilateral ones. For example, a patient with a cataract in one eye may be able to function well, because the vision in the other eye remains good. Such a patient may opt to have treatment either because they perceive a disability caused by the poor vision in one eye, or because they fear a future disability should a cataract or some other visually disabling condition develop in the fellow eye. Alternatively, after consideration of the risks and benefits of treatment, their current state of visual functioning, and their overall current health and socioeconomic state, the patient may reasonably decide to defer treatment.

Summary for the Clinician

	Factors favouring treatment	Factors favouring no treatment
•	Disability	Adequate function
•	High risk of future disability	Low risk of future disability
•	Symptoms, e.g. pain	Absence of distressing symptoms
•	Low risk of side effects	High risk of side effects
•	High risk of progression	Low risk of progression

3.4 What Difference Does It Make When the Patient Is a Child?

The autonomy of a child is limited, particularly with respect to decisions about medical treatment. While the condition and its treatment should be explained to the child where possible, usually the treatment decision is arrived at as a result of discussion between the child's physician and his or her carers. Further, the child is often not in a position to report side effects from treatment. This renders children vulnerable to inappropriate, excessive or inadequate treatment.

In the context of amblyopia, it has often been stated that treatment is ineffective after the age of 7 years. While this may be true for some types of amblyopia, for example complete unilateral congenital cataract, where treatment must be commenced within a few weeks of birth to be effective [34], for other causes of amblyopia there is increasing evidence that treatment may be effective beyond this age [20]. The reluctance to contemplate treatment beyond the age of 7 may have been due, in part, to the effect of blurring vision in the better eye on educational and social functioning in the older child. In other words, the side effects of treatment may have been considered too severe at this age for treatment even to be worth trying. While these effects may be more obvious in the older child, the effects on the development of the younger child have not been systematically studied, and may be significant.

Table 3.1. Causes of amblyopia

Causes of amblyopia
Sensory deprivation
Ptosis
Orbital haemangioma
Corneal opacity
Iris cysts
Cataract
Vitreous haemorrhage and other opacity
Retinoblastoma
Optic nerve hypoplasia
Strabismic
Constant esotropia
Infantile
Microtropia
Partially accommodative
Consecutive
Acute
VIth nerve palsy
Constant exotropia
Infantile
Microtropia
Consecutive
Constant cyclovertical strabismus
Decompensated IVth nerve palsy
Severe Brown's syndrome
IIIrd nerve palsy
Refractive
Bilateral hypermetropia (>+4 dioptres)
Bilateral myopia (>–3 dioptres)
Bilateral astigmatism (>1.5 dioptres)
Anisohypermetropia (>0.75 dioptres)
Anisomyopia (>2 dioptres)
Anisoastigmatic (>0.75 dioptres)

3.5 Why Treat Amblyopia?

Impaired vision in both eyes does pose a threat to life in countries without a well-developed system of health and social care [26]. While amblyopia can affect both eyes in such conditions as bilateral congenital cataracts and bilateral high refractive errors, usually amblyopia only affects the vision in one eye, usually as a result of constant strabismus or unilateral refractive errors. For other causes see Table 3.1.

There is no evidence that unilateral amblyopia affects duration of life.

The potential effects of poor vision in one eye on quality of life include reduced binocular visual acuity and reduced binocular cooperation, causing for example reduced stereoacuity. These effects will vary depending on the degree of amblyopia with, for example an acuity of 6/9 in the amblyopic eye, causing much less disability than an amblyopic eye with an acuity of 6/60. Visual acuity in the majority of amblyopic eyes is 6/12 or better. This said, it would seem that most adults with amblyopia are less affected by their long-standing impairment of acuity than adults who have recently suffered a loss of acuity.

There is little evidence that unilateral amblyopia significantly affects quality of life provided vision in the normal eye remains good. Children with amblyopia have been found to have slightly reduced intelligence in one study [33]; however this may have been confounded by the effect of strabismus as a marker for subtle neurodevelopmental defects. The same study concluded that the majority of visual defects did not affect children's learning. Chua and Mitchell, in a recent study from the Blue Mountains Eye Study [6] found that amblyopia in individuals 49 years or older did not affect lifetime occupational class, but that fewer individuals with amblyopia completed university degrees.

Assuming normal vision in the fellow eye, reduced binocular visual acuity may result either from the loss of an additive effect of two normally seeing eyes or from temporary or permanent loss of acuity in the normal eye. Temporary loss of acuity in the normal eye may occur as a result of pathology, such as a corneal abrasion, or trauma. This may be the reason why reduction in unilateral visual acuity precludes individuals from such professions as the fire service and armed forces [1]. The reasoning behind this may be in that such occupations there is a risk of trauma to one eye during the course of dangerous duties which would put the life of the individual at risk because they would then be relying on the vision in the amblyopic eye. It is difficult to comment on whether these risks are theoretical rather than actual as there is little information on the subject.

Permanent loss of acuity in the normal eye will result in reduced quality of life. It is important to remember, however, that many of the diseases which affect vision in the normal eye, such as age-related macular degeneration, would also tend to affect vision in the amblyopic eye. In a widely quoted Finnish study, Tommila and Tarkkanen found in 20-year period between 1958 and 1978, a rate of loss of vision in the healthy eye of 1.75 per 1,000. In more than 50%, the cause was traumatic. During the same period, the overall blindness rate was 0.11 per thousand in children and 0.66 per thousand in adults. They concluded that subjects with amblyopia are at higher risk of blindness [37]. Rahi et al., in a UK national survey of the incidence of visual loss in the normal eye in the UK estimated a 1.2% risk of loss of vision in the normal eye to 6/12 or below (below the UK driving standard) during the working lifetime of an individual with amblyopia [27]. The increase in the risk of loss of vision in the better eye in individuals with amblyopia compared to the risk of bilateral blindness in normal individuals is a consistent finding [6, 27, 37]. The explanation may be simply that damage to one eye renders a subject with amblyopia visually impaired; however the reasons for this finding have yet to be fully explored. Clearly, prevention of such future disability is an important argument for the treatment of amblyopia in childhood.

The effect of amblyopia on binocular cooperation is difficult to disentangle from the effect of the strabismus which often accompanies it. Strabismus may cause amblyopia, or be caused by it, as for example in the case of a unilateral congenital cataract. Imposed refractive blur is known to reduce stereoacuity, and to do so to a greater extent than equivalent degrees of amblyopia [22]. Nevertheless, amblyopia does appear to reduce binocular cooperation to a degree dependent on the depth of the amblyopia [36].

3.6 What Are Patient Perceptions of the Disability Due to Amblyopia?

Membreno et al. calculated the effect of unilateral amblyopia on quality of life by estimating utility values for the effect of poor vision in one eye [19]. In this approach, a panel of patients or other lay individuals are asked to quantify the effect of the condition. This can be done either by a "standard gamble" or "time trade-off". In the standard gamble approach, the panel member asks what level of risk the individual would be prepared to run in order to be cured of the condition. So, for example, the question would be posed as "would you be prepared to have a treatment which carried a mortality of, for example, 10 % in order to be cured of the condition?" In the time trade-off approach, the question would be "how much duration of life would you be prepared to give up in order to live the rest of your life without the condition?" Membreno et al. used the time trade-off approach and used values derived from previous work to make their calculations. Perhaps because of confusion on the part of panel members about the true disability associated with unilateral visual loss, the values associated with an acuity of 6/12 in the source paper indicated that this was a worse disability than a unilateral visual loss of 6/18. Unpublished values were therefore used by the authors (G. Brown, personal communication) to calculate the difference in trade-off from a mean pre- to a mean post-treatment visual acuity. Although this difference was small, the presence of the condition from childhood resulted in a significant lifetime gain in quality of life years from treatment. This work needs to be corroborated by further studies which should try to educate panel members about the real implications of unilateral loss of acuity, perhaps by a period of imposed refractive blur. Even so, this is likely to overestimate the disability seen in adults with, by definition, long-standing amblyopia.

Summary for the Clinician

- **Monocular amblyopia does not significantly affect quality of life provided vision in the fellow eye is normal**
- **Monocular amblyopia is a bar to entry into certain occupations**
- **The projected lifetime risk of vision loss in the fellow eye is at least 1.2 %**

3.7 Identification of Amblyopia

The diagnosis of amblyopia is not straightforward because of the difficulties in testing vision in small children and uncertainties about the contribution made to any visual abnormality by refractive error and ocular pathology.

Visual acuity measurements in infants and children are confounded by the normal process of visual development, including emmetropisation of physiological refractive errors, the inability of the child to report accurately what he or she sees, and inattention.

The normal adult human visual system is capable of resolving targets of one minute of arc. This is the basis of Snellen, and to an extent, LogMAR, visual acuity tests. Other visual function tests such as contrast sensitivity and vernier acuity are not currently used for the clinical diagnosis of amblyopia.

Like all biological parameters, there is a range of normal functioning in the population [16, 18, 31], which is affected by the frequency of minor refractive errors. This range has been difficult to determine, partly because of the imperviousness of the commonly used Snellen-based tests to statistical analysis. Nevertheless, the range of normal acuity seems to be tight in visually normal adults.

The resolving power of the infant visual system is not known precisely. It seems likely from studies of retinal anatomy in infants, and also from consideration of the developing infant brain, that resolving power in infancy is less than in adulthood. Behavioural studies in infants using visual evoked potential measurements and preferential looking show a normal range which is wider and lower in younger children. These tests are limited by the problems of reporting and attention, and may underestimate true acuity.

From around a developmental age of 3 years, children are able to match letter optotypes. Using Snellen based tests, it has been widely assumed that if acuity is not 6/6 using these measures then the resolving power of the system is abnormal. However, the use of LogMAR tests has enabled normal ranges to be calculated. The mean visual acuity using these tests in 4-year-olds is around 0.1 LogMAR, with a normal range, as measured by 2 standard deviations from the mean, extending from 0.0 to 0.2 [31]. In other words, the visual system is not fully developed at age 3 years. Further evidence for lack of maturation is the crowding phenomenon. Crowding was first described in relation to amblyopia and is defined as the inability to resolve an optotype which is surrounded by other optotypes or bars, when that optotype is capable of being resolved when presented in isolation. In 3- to 5-year-olds, ranges of normal visual acuity are lower on crowded than on uncrowded tests [31].

Crowding is also seen in cases of cerebral visual impairment, whether due to neonatal encephalopathy, meningitis or other causes. Here it is described as the inability to pick single objects out of complex scenes, when the single object can be recognised in isolation. So crowding seems to be a normal feature of the developing visual system, which persists in amblyopia and cerebral visual impairment.

It is clear, then, that amblyopia should only be diagnosed when there is evidence that visual acuity measurements fall outside the normal range for age, as defined as 2 standard deviations below the mean. This implies that vision tests used for the diagnosis of amblyopia should be capable of statistical analysis, and that normal ranges should be known. Although some progress has been made towards this ideal, many children are still being inappropriately treated for amblyopia on the basis that their Snellen-based acuity measurement is not 6/6.

The normal infant eye is commonly from +2 to +4 dioptres hypermetropic, as a result of an imbalance between the refractive power of the cornea and lens, and the axial length of the eye. As ocular growth proceeds, this imbalance is normally corrected, with this physiological refractive error approaching zero by age 8 years [17]. This process is known as emmetropisation.

Symmetrical, spherical hypermetropic refractive errors of this magnitude should not represent a barrier to clear vision in childhood, as they can easily be overcome by a child's powerful accommodation, but it remains unclear if and when such errors should be corrected. Early correction has been reported to encourage the development of normal acuity [8], prevent strabismus [2, 3] and reduce learning difficulties [29]. There are, however, concerns that early refractive correction may impede the process of emmetropisation [13].

Summary for the Clinician

- **The normal range of visual acuity in a 4-year-old is from 0.0 to 0.2 LogMAR**
- **Amblyopia should only be diagnosed when corrected visual acuity is below the normal range for age**

3.8 Treatment of Amblyopia

Amblyopia is treated by modulating the visual input into the amblyopic eye. In the case of stimulus deprivation amblyopia, the cause of the visual deprivation, for example ptosis or cataract, needs to be dealt with. In refractive and strabismic amblyopia, significant refractive errors need to be corrected and abnormal fixation patterns overcome. Persistent visual deficit may be treated by depriving the normal eye of visual input by means of a patch or optical/pharmaceutical penalisation.

3.8.1 Evidence for Effectiveness of Amblyopia Treatment

That visual acuity improved following amblyopia treatment was demonstrated in a number of case series, such as that of Lithander [17]. However, Woodruff and colleagues in a retrospective study of treatment outcomes in the UK found only 48% of 894 patients to achieve 6/9 with the amblyopic eye at the end of treatment [38]. Neither of these studies was controlled for the effects of spontaneous improvement. The evidence base for amblyopia treatment was questioned in a government-sponsored UK report in 1997 [30]. The report pointed out that there had been no randomised controlled trials of treatment and that views of treatment efficacy based on clinical experience and teaching might be biased.

That amblyopia treatment does work, for most patients, has been demonstrated by a series of papers produced, in part, as a response to this report. These papers have considerably advanced our knowledge of the clinical response of patients with amblyopia to treatment and consideration of them forms the core of this chapter.

Clarke et al. showed that, in a population of children who had failed preschool screening (at a mean age of 4 years) on account of poor vision in one eye, treatment resulted in a significant improvement in acuity [5]. Subgroup analysis showed this benefit to be confined to children with acuity of 6/18 or worse at presentation. Other studies, particularly those by the US Pediatric Eye Disease Investigator Group (PEDIG) and the Monitored Occlusion Treatment for Amblyopia Study (MOTAS) cooperative have advanced our knowledge of how much treatment is required for amblyopia and are considered below.

3.8.2 Correction of Refractive Error

The degrees of refractive error which are thought capable of inducing amblyopia are summarised in Table 3.1. Lower degrees of myopic refractive error need to be corrected before an accurate measure of distance visual acuity can be obtained.

It might be assumed that once refractive error has been corrected, any residual visual deficit is due to amblyopia, needing treatment with other measures; however the reality is more complex. Residual apparent visual discrepancy between the two eyes following refractive correction may be due to imperfect correction of the refractive error, or due to "noise" (test-test variation, expanded normal ranges), inherent in visual acuity testing in young children.

Moseley et al. have shown a progressive improvement in acuity for up to 22 weeks in some patients after refractive correction, prior to implementation of other measures [21]. This period of "refractive adaptation" is almost certainly a form of amblyopia treatment.

Clarke et al. showed that refractive correction alone resulted in a significant improvement in acuity in a group of children failing preschool vision screening, compared to no treatment, but that further significant gains in acuity were obtained in a group receiving additional treatment with patching [5].

3.8.3 Patching

Although there are some with a prior claim, the person usually credited with proposing patching as a treatment for amblyopia is George-Louis LeClerc, Compte de Buffon, an eighteenth century polymath also credited with inventing the binomial theorem. It appears, however, that patching was not widely used until the time of Claude Worth, and then mainly in strabismic individuals where it was intended mainly to alter abnormal binocular correspondence. As a treatment for amblyopia, patching became widespread following the work of Hubel and Wiesel [12].

Patches with an adhesive rim, stuck directly onto the periorbital skin, are the most commonly used. There are two significant problems with such patches – first, they may cause allergy, and second, they are easy for a child to remove. Allergy to the constituents of the patch or the adhesive is uncommon and may be dealt with by sticking the patch on the glasses, trying a different type of patch, for example a hypoallergenic brand or by using atropine instead. The second problem is commoner and more difficult to deal with. As it is the parents or carers who will have to deal with the distressed, uncomfortable, visually impaired child who is wearing the patch, it is clearly important that they are both convinced of the need for treatment and appropriately motivated to carry it out. Giving older children a stake in their own treatment, for example with the use of patching diaries with stickers, helps. It is the active, unreasonable toddler who poses the biggest challenge.

Patches can also be stuck onto glasses, but this gives the child the opportunity to look round them. Extension patches slide over the glasses lens and have a side piece which helps prevent the child looking around the patch, but is cosmetically obtrusive. Translucent material such as Blenderm is more cosmetically acceptable, but will not completely obscure vision in the covered eye, limiting its efficacy in the treatment of severe amblyopia.

For some types of early onset amblyopia, where there is a continuing amblyogenic stimulus, such as a unilateral congenital cataract (where despite removal of the cataract the lack of accommodation puts the eye at a disadvantage compared to its fellow), reasonable levels of visual acuity can only be achieved by intensive, long-term patching [34]. Regimes for unilateral congenital cataract initially consisted of full-time patching from removal of the cataract up until the age of 7, with short breaks to try to prevent induced amblyopia in the normal eye. While these regimes were shown to result in good acuity in some cases, this was at the expense of severely disrupting binocularity and most patients had large angle divergent and vertical strabismus. Wright showed that it was possible, with lesser amounts of occlusion, especially in the 1st year of life, to achieve binocularity in some patients [39]. Subsequent regimes of occlusion for unilateral congenital cataract have made use of improved visual acuity tests for infants [35], but if reasonable levels of visual acuity are to be obtained in these cases, the burden of long-term occlusion remains substantial.

For children with amblyopia detected later, usually due to strabismus or refractive error, the amount of patching prescribed has been, until recently, a matter of individual practice. Some have argued for full-time (in practice 75% or greater of waking hours) occlusion, with commonly used regimes recommending 1 week of full time occlusion per year of age. Three such cycles have been recommended before treatment is abandoned because of a lack of effect [14]. What is less clear is how much treatment should be given in a case where vision initially improves and then appears to plateau. This raises the question of whether amblyopia should be treated indefinitely until visual acuity reaches the normal range or whether there should be a predetermined end point of treatment below this acuity.

Others have preferred to patch less intensively, recognising that treatment will take longer, but arguing that it will be less disruptive.

The US Pediatric Eye Disease Investigator Group (PEDIG) have tested two patching regimens for the treatment of moderate amblyopia [25]. One hundred and eighty-nine children under 7 years (all but two over 3 years) with unilateral amblyopia, from strabismus or refractive error or both, of between 20/40 and 20/80 were randomised to either 2 h or 6 h of patching with both groups also spending 1 h per day doing near visual activities. At the 4-month outcome examination, improvement averaged 2.4 lines in each group: mean acuity was 20/32 or improved from baseline by 3 lines in 62% in each group. The investigators pointed out that their study was not designed to test the maximum possible treatment benefit, and speculated that a further line of improvement might be possible with further treatment.

In a subsequent study of severe amblyopia, 175 children between 3 and 7 years with acuities of between 20/100 and 20/400 in the amblyopic eye were randomised to either 6 h a day or all but 1 waking hour per day patching plus 1 h spent per day on a near vision task [10]. Mean acuity at enrolment was 20/160. At the 4-month outcome visit, mean difference in acuity in the amblyopic eye between groups was only 0.03 LogMAR. Improvement from baseline averaged 4.8 lines in the 6-h group and 4.7 lines in the full-time group; 85% in the 6-h group and 84% in the full-time group had improved by 3 or more lines.

Patching treatment is by nature difficult to implement as the majority of children object to occlusion of their better-seeing eye. This has led to concerns about the emotional impact of amblyopia treatment [30], but these were not borne out by a recent study [11].

The uncertainty in practice regarding the optimal amount of patching to prescribe and the difficulties in monitoring what is achieved in practice may result in over-treatment and the development of iatrogenic amblyopia in the originally better-seeing eye. This appears more likely in younger children undergoing intense occlusion and should be preventable by careful instruction and regular review.

3.8.4 Atropine

Atropine derives from the highly toxic alkaloid substance found in *Atropa belladonna*. It works by blocking the action of acetylcholine, relaxing cholinergically innervated muscles. In the eye it blocks parasympathetic innervation of the pupil and ciliary muscle, causing pupillary dilatation and loss of accommodation.

The use of atropine in the treatment of amblyopia was first described in the French literature in 1963 [4]. It is inserted into the normal eye to blur the vision and so encourage the use of the amblyopic eye. The blurring which occurs is much greater in eyes with hypermetropic refractive errors, as these can no longer be physiologically corrected for by accommodation.

The choice between patching and atropine as an amblyopia treatment has been at the discretion of the treating physician, with most opting for patching. This has partly been based on a belief that patching is the more effective treatment, and atropine has often been reserved for cases where the child is intolerant of patching, thus selecting cases where the outcome is predestined to be less successful.

Patching is also a more flexible method of treatment. Should iatrogenic amblyopia, for example, develop in the patched eye, the patch can be removed immediately, whereas the effects of atropine will last for up to 2 weeks.

The required dose of atropine to treat amblyopia is not known. A common regime is to instil one drop of 1% atropine daily into the normal eye for a period of 1 week per year of age of the child. Given that the effects of atropine last for up to 2 weeks, it may be that less frequent instillation would suffice. This was borne out by a recent study which showed twice weekly instillation of atropine to be as effective as daily instillation [28].

Reducing the hypermetropic correction in the atropinised eye will augment the effect of atropine on visual acuity in the normal eye. The vision in the atropinised eye needs to be checked regularly to ensure it has not suffered iatrogenic amblyopia. This poses a difficulty, as aberrations caused by pupillary dilatation will result in a slight reduction in acuity even if accommodative factors are corrected for by full hypermetropic correction. A further reason for the relative underuse of atropine has been a perception that the treatment would not be effective unless, in cases of strabismus, fixation switched to the amblyopic eye. Consequently it was felt that atropine was unlikely to be effective in cases of severe amblyopia. Studies by the PEDIG group and others have shown these concepts to be flawed, and that atropine is as effective as occlusion for most cases of amblyopia and that fixation swap is not necessary for atropine to be effective. This may be due to blurring of higher spatial frequencies in the atropinised eye.

In the PEDIG trial of atropine vs patching [24], 419 children under 7 years of age with acuities of 20/40 to 20/100 were enrolled and randomised to either atropine or patching. Mean improvement was 3.16 lines in the patching group and 2.84 lines in atropine group. The study concluded that atropine was as effective as patching but took longer to work.

Pros and cons of patching vs. atropine are shown in Table 3.2.

Atropine drops or ointment have potentially serious side effects, which are said to be more

Table 3.2. Comparison of atropine and patching

	Patching	Atropine
Cosmesis	Obtrusive	Unobtrusive
Reversibility	Often poor	Effects last for up to 2 weeks
Systemic side effects	None	Rare but potentially dangerous
Compliance	Easy to remove	Once instilled, compliance is assured
Binocularity	Impaired during treatment	Allowed

frequent in children with Down's syndrome. Side effects are rare and relate to systemic parasympathetic blockade. They include flushing, dry mouth, hyperactivity, tachycardia and rarely seizures. Side effects appear to be dose-related and so are more common in infants and smaller children. Atropine ointment has been used instead of drops, and pressure on the lacrimal sac after instillation has been recommended, in an attempt to reduce systemic absorption in the nose, but will not prevent systemic absorption through conjunctival vessels.

3.8.5 Why Does Amblyopia Treatment Not Always Work?

Amblyopia treatment sometimes has no effect and frequently does not improve visual acuity to normal levels. This is often assumed to be because treatment has been started too late to be effective or is unable to be implemented at the prescribed level. While this may often be the case, it is important to realise that subtle ocular and cerebral pathology may also underlie failure to respond to treatment. Optic nerve hypoplasia is easily missed on indirect ophthalmoscopy and should be specifically excluded. Inaccurate refractive correction, which inevitably occurs during periods of emmetropisation, should also be checked for.

Lack of compliance has been shown, using electronic monitors of patching compliance, to be a frequent occurrence in children undergoing patching treatment. In one study, concordance with patching was 48% (2.8 h vs 6 h prescribed) and acuity gain was linearly correlated with occlusion dose [32]. All improvement occurred within 12 weeks of patching.

Summary for the Clinician

- **Randomised controlled trials have demonstrated amblyopia treatment to be effective**
- **Refractive correction alone may improve visual acuity in amblyopic eyes for up to 22 weeks**
- **2 h of effective patching per day is adequate for most cases of amblyopia**
- **Atropine is an effective alternative to patching**

3.9 New Developments

3.9.1 L-DOPA

Oral levodopa has been used experimentally in the treatment of amblyopia and has been shown to have some clinical effect mirrored by changes seen on functional magnetic resonance imaging (fMRI) [40]. The effect on amblyopia does not persist after treatment is discontinued [23]. The neuropsychiatric side effects of levodopa mean that this drug is unlikely to ever be used in routine clinical practice for amblyopia treatment, but the studies do demonstrate the potential for such an approach to treatment.

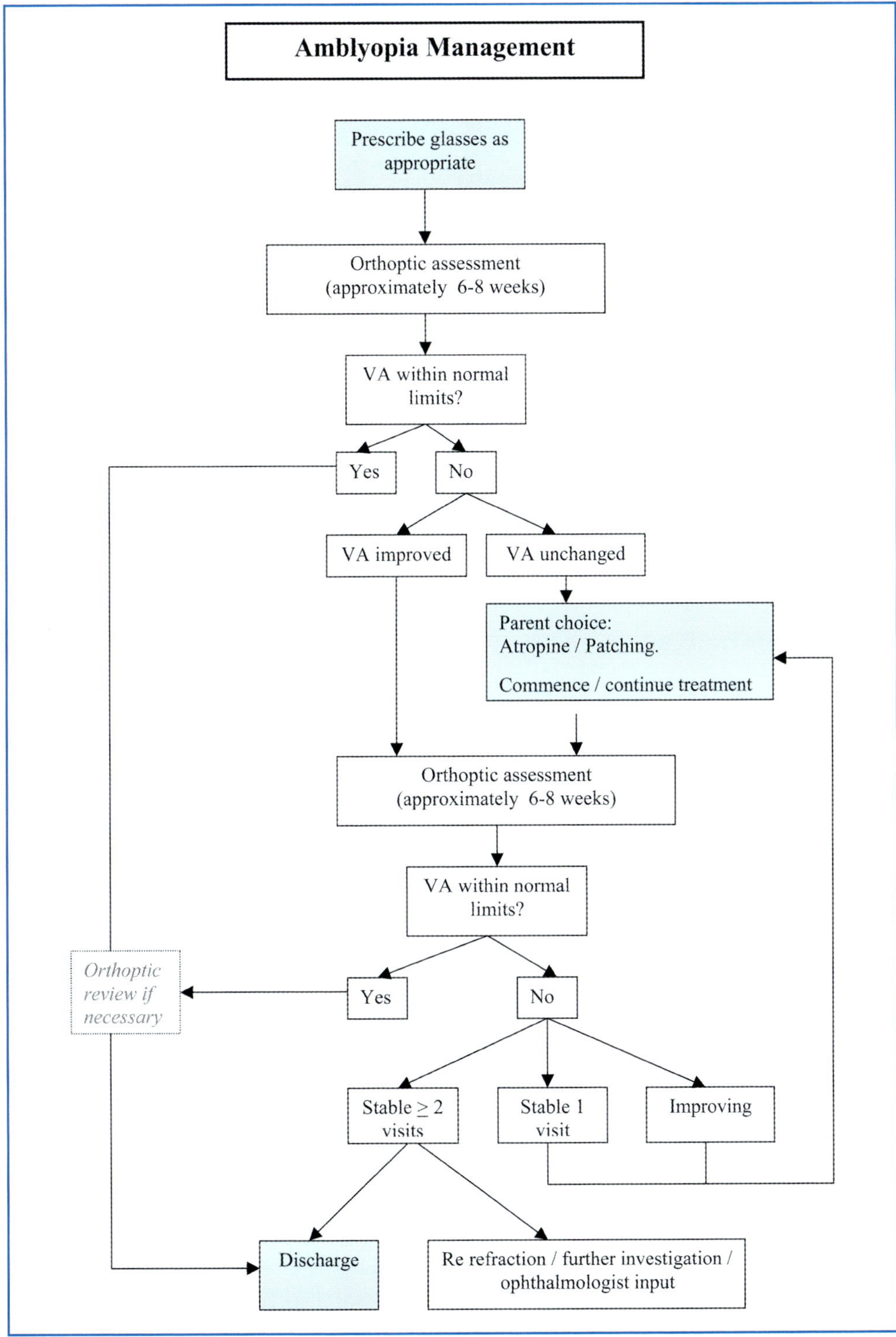

Fig. 3.1. Amblyopia management

3.9.2 Visual Stimulation

There has been interest in the use of positive visual stimulation, as opposed to occlusion or penalisation, since the days of the CAM stimulator, and near visual tasks have been a feature of some recent treatment studies. While, unfortunately, the CAM stimulator did not prove a useful treatment for amblyopia [15], there is currently interest in a computer-based Interactive Binocular Treatment (IBIT) system developed at Nottingham University, UK (R. Gregson, personal communication). This apparatus seems to produce significant effects on acuity in children who are beyond the normal age for occlusion treatment and in a shorter time period than occlusion. This system is currently undergoing trials and may transform amblyopia treatment in the future.

3.10 Translation into Practice

How can this new information be translated into practice? First, clinicians treating children with visual defects should use LogMAR acuity tests, as these enable more accurate interpretation of results by establishing and applying known normal ranges for different ages of children. Treatment should only be considered for those children who clearly fall outside the normal range for their age group.

If there is any significant refractive error, this should be corrected and the child left in the refractive correction for a period of 16–20 weeks before further treatment is considered. Parents and carers should then be offered an informed choice between occlusion and atropine drops or ointment. Occlusion regimes for strabismic and anisometropic types of amblyopia of more than 2 h patching a day, and lasting for more than 6 months, need to be carefully justified. A suggested scheme is shown in the flow diagram (Fig. 3.1).

Acknowledgements. The author would like to thank Sarah Richardson, Jugnoo Rahi and Philip Griffiths for reading drafts of this chapter and for their constructive comments.

References

1. Adams G, Karas M (1999) Effect of amblyopia on employment prospects. Br J Ophthalmol 83:380
2. Atkinson J (1993) Infant vision screening: prediction and prevention of strabismus and amblyopia from refractive screening in the Cambridge photorefraction programme. Oxford University Press, New York
3. Atkinson J, Braddick O, Bobier B (1996) Two infant vision screening programmes: predication and prevention of strabismus and amblyopia from photo and video refractive screening. Eye 10:189–198
4. Baldone J (1963) Combined atropine-fluoropyl treatment for selected children with suppression amblyopia. J La State Med Soc 115:420–422
5. Clarke M, Wright C, Hrisos S, Anderson J, Henderson J, Richardson S (2003) Randomised controlled trial of treatment of unilateral visual impairment detected at preschool vision screening. BMJ 327:1251–1256
6. Chua B, Mitchell P (2004) Consequences of amblyopia on education, occupation and long term vision loss. Br J Ophthalmol 88:1119–1121
7. Goodyear B, Nicolle D, Humphrey G, Menon R (2000) BOLD fMRI response of early visual areas to perceived contrast in human amblyopia. J Neurophysiol 84:1907–13
8. Friedberg D, Kloppel KP (1996) Early correction of hyperopia and astigmatism in children leads to better development of visual acuity. Klin Monatsbl Augenheilkd 209:21–24
9. Gwiazda J, Thorn F, Bauer J, Held R (1993) Emmetropization and the progression of manifest refraction in children followed from infancy to puberty. Clin Vision Sci 8:337–344
10. Holmes J, Kraker R, Beck R et al (2003) A randomized trial of patching regimens for the treatment of severe amblyopia in children. Ophthalmology 110:2075–2087
11. Hrisos S, Clarke MP, Wright C (2004) The emotional impact of amblyopia treatment in preschool children. Ophthalmology 111:1550–1556
12. Hubel DH, Wiesel TN (1970) The period of susceptibility to the physiological effects of unilateral eye closure in kittens. J Physiol 206:419–436
13. Ingram R, Gill L, Lambert T (2000) Effect of spectacles on changes of spherical hypermetropia in infants who did, and did not, have strabismus. Br J Ophthalmol 84:324–326
14. Keech R, Ottar W, Zhang L (2002) The minimal occlusion trial for the treatment of amblyopia. Ophthalmology 109:2261–2264

15. Keith C, Howell E, Mitchell D, Smith S (1980) Clinical trial of the use of rotating grating patterns in the treatment of amblyopia. Br J Ophthalmol 64:597–606
16. Kheterpal S, Jones H, Moseley M (1996) Reliability of visual acuity in children with reduced vision. Ophthal Physiol Opt 16:447–449
17. Lithander J, Sjøstrand J (1991) Anisometropic and strabismic amblyopia in the age group 2 years and above: a prospective study of the results of treatment. Br J Ophthalmol 75:111–116
18. McGraw P, Winn B, Gray LS, Elliot DB (2000) Improving the reliability of visual acuity measures in young children. Ophthal Physiol Opt 3:173–184
19. Membreno J, Brown M, Brown G, Sharma S, Beauchamp G (2002) A cost-utility analysis of therapy for amblyopia. Ophthalmology 109:2265–2271
20. Mohan K, Saroha V, Sharma A (2004) Successful occlusion therapy for amblyopia in 11- to 15-year-old children. J Ped Ophth Strabismus 41:89–95
21. Moseley MJ, Neufeld M, McCarry B et al (2002) Remediation of refractive amblyopia by optical correction. Ophthal Physiol Opt 22:296–299
22. Noorden GV (1996) Binocular vision and ocular motility: theory and management of strabismus, 5th edn. CV Mosby, St Louis
23. Pandey P, Chaudhuri Z, Kumar M, Satyabala K, Sharma P (2002) Effect of levodopa and carbidopa in human amblyopia. J Ped Ophth Strabismus 39:81–89
24. PEDIG (2002) A randomized controlled trial of atropine vs patching for treatment of moderate amblyopia in children. Arch Ophthalmol 120: 268–278
25. PEDIG (2003) A randomized trial of patching regimens for treatment of moderate amblyopia in children. Arch Ophthalmol 121:603–611
26. Pion SD, Kamgno J, Demanga-Ngangue MB (2002) Excess mortality associated with blindness in the onchocerciasis focus of the Mbam Valley, Cameroon. Ann Trop Med Parasitol 96: 181–189
27. Rahi J, Logan S, Timms C, Eggitt IR, Taylor DSI (2002) Risk, causes, and outcomes of visual impairment after loss of vision in the non-amblyopic eye: a population based study. Lancet 360: 597–602
28. Repka M, Cotter S, Beck R et al (2004) A randomized trial of atropine regimens for treatment of moderate amblyopia in children. Ophthalmology 111:2076–285
29. Rosner J, Rosner J (1986) Some observations of the relationship between visual perceptual skills development of young hyperopes and the age of first lens correction. Clin Exp Optom 69:166–168
30. Snowdon SK, Stewart-Brown SL (1997) Preschool vision screening. York: NHS Centre for Reviews and Dissemination, University of York, pp 1–83
31. Stewart C (2000) Comparison of Snellen and log based acuity scores for school aged children. Br Orthopt J 57:32–38
32. Stewart C, Moseley M, Stephens D, Fielder A (2004) Treatment dose-response in amblyopia therapy: The Monitored Occlusion Treatment of Amblyopia Study (MOTAS). Invest Ophthalmol Vis Sci 45:3048–3054
33. Stewart-Brown SL, Haslum MN, Butler N (1985) Educational attainment of 10-year-old children with treated and untreated visual defects. Dev Med Child Neurol 27:504–513
34. Taylor D (1998) The Doyne Lecture. Congenital cataract: the history, the nature and the practice. Eye 12:9–36
35. Taylor D, Wright K, Amaya L et al (2001) Should we aggressively treat unilateral congenital cataracts? Br J Ophthalmol 85:1120–1126
36. Tomac S, Birdal E (2001) Effects of anisometropia on binocularity. J Pediatr Ophthalmol Strabismus 38:27–33
37. Tommila V, Tarkkanen A (1981) Incidence of loss of vision in healthy eye in amblyopia. Br J Ophthalmol 65:575–577
38. Woodruff G, Hiscox F, Thompson JR, Smith LK (1994) Factors affecting the outcome of children treated for amblyopia. Eye 8:627–631
39. Wright K, Matsumoto E, Edelman P (1992) Binocular fusion and stereopsis associated with early surgery for monocular congenital cataracts. Arch Ophthalmol 110:1607–1609
40. Yang C, Yang M, Huang J et al (2003) Functional MRI of amblyopia before and after levodopa. Neurosci Lett 339:49–52

Retinopathy of Prematurity: Molecular Mechanism of Disease

4

Lois E.H. Smith

Core Messages

- ROP continues to be a blinding disease despite current treatment, so understanding the molecular basis of the disease is important to the development of medical treatment
- ROP is a two-phase disease, beginning with delayed retinal vascular growth after premature birth (phase I)
- Phase II follows when phase I-induced hypoxia releases factors to stimulate new blood vessel growth
- Both oxygen-regulated and non-oxygen-regulated factors contribute to normal vascular development and retinal neovascularization
- Vascular endothelial growth factor (VEGF) is an important oxygen-regulated factor
- A critical non-oxygen-regulated growth factor is insulin-like growth factor-I (IGF-I)
- Lack of IGF-I prevents normal retinal vascular growth, despite the presence of VEGF, important to vessel development
- Premature infants who develop ROP have low levels of serum IGF-I compared to age-matched infants without disease
- Low IGF-I predicts ROP in premature infants
- Restoration of IGF-I to normal levels might prevent ROP

4.1 Introduction

Retinopathy of prematurity (ROP) was first described in the late 1940s as retrolental fibroplasia. The disease was soon associated with excessive oxygen use [12, 14, 50]. As a result, supplemental oxygen is now delivered to premature infants to maintain adequate blood levels, but it is monitored carefully [36]. Nonetheless, even with controlled oxygen use, the number of infants with ROP has increased further [54], due most likely to the increased survival rate of very low birth weight infants [22].

ROP is still a major cause of blindness in children in the developed and developing world [66], despite current treatment of late-stage ROP. Although laser photocoagulation or cryotherapy of the retina reduces the incidence of blindness by approximately 25%, the visual outcomes after treatment are often poor. Preventive therapy for ROP is sorely needed. To develop such treatments, we need to understand the pathogenesis of the disease and develop medical interventions based on this understanding to prevent or treat ROP.

4.2 Pathogenesis: Two Phases of ROP

ROP is a biphasic disease consisting of an initial phase of vessel loss followed by vessel proliferation. To understand this puzzle, it is important to understand retinal vascular development. In the human fetus, retinal blood vessel development begins during the 4th month of gestation [26, 62] and reaches the ora serrata, the most anterior aspect of the retina just before term. Therefore, the retinas of infants born prematurely are incompletely vascularized, with a peripheral avascular zone, the area of which depends on the gestational age at birth.

4.2.1 Phase I of ROP

In the first phase of ROP, the normal retinal vascular growth that would occur in utero slows or ceases, and there is loss of some of the developed vessels. This is thought to be due in part to the influence of oxygen given to premature infants to overcome poor oxygenation secondary to lung immaturity but in part because of the relative hyperoxia of the extrauterine environment. With maturation of the premature infant, the resulting nonvascularized retina becomes increasingly metabolically active and without a blood supply, increasingly hypoxic. This phase occurs from birth to postmenstrual age (PMA): approximately 30–32 weeks.

4.2.2 Phase II of ROP

Retinal neovascularization, the second phase of ROP, is hypoxia-induced [11, 45] and occurs between roughly 32 and 34 weeks PMA. The neovascularization phase of ROP is similar to other proliferative retinopathies such as diabetic retinopathy. The new blood vessel formation occurs at the junction between the nonvascularized retina and the vascularized retina. These new vessels are leaky and can cause tractional retinal detachments leading to blindness. If we could allow the normal growth of blood vessels after preterm birth, the second destructive phase would not occur. Alternatively, if we could attenuate the rapid proliferation of abnormal blood vessels in the second phase and allow controlled vascularization of the retina, retinal detachments could be prevented.

To accomplish these goals, it is necessary to understand the growth factors involved in all aspects of ROP, both in normal retinal vascular development and in the development of neovascularization. The two phases of ROP are mirror images. The first involves growth inhibition of neural retina and the retinal vasculature, and the second involves uncontrolled proliferative growth of retinal blood vessels. The controlling growth factors are likely to be deficient in phase I and in excess in phase II. Therefore control of the disease is likely to be complex and will likely require careful timing of any intervention.

4.3 Mouse Model of ROP

To study the molecular pathways in retinal vascular development and in the development of ROP, we developed a mouse model of the disease to take advantage of the genetic manipulations possible in the murine system [67]. The eyes of animals such as mice, rats and cats – though born full term – are incompletely vascularized at birth and are similar to the retinal vascular development of premature infants. When these neonatal animals are exposed to hyperoxia there is induced loss of some vessels and cessation of normal retinal blood vessel development, which mimics phase I of ROP [10, 11, 44, 52, 67].

When mice return to room air, the nonperfused portions of the retina become hypoxic, similar to phase II of ROP and of other retinopathies. The ischemic portions of the retina produce angiogenic factors that result in neovascularization [11, 45]. Hypoxia-inducible factors appear to be common to the proliferative phase of many eye diseases [25, 37] such as retinopathy of prematurity and diabetic retinopathy, as well as in tumor growth and wound healing. This model has been useful to delineate the growth factor changes in both phases of neovascular eye diseases.

4.4 Vascular Endothelial Growth Factor and Oxygen in ROP

The risk factors of ROP are oxygen and prematurity itself. We first studied oxygen-regulated factors. In the 1940s and 1950s, Michaelson and Ashton [11, 45] postulated that retinal neovascularization was caused by release of a "vasoformative factor" from the retina in response to hypoxia. Since these initial hypotheses, it has become widely accepted that retinal hypoxia results in the release of factors that influence new blood vessel growth [51]. Not only is hypoxia a driving force for proliferative retinopathy, or phase II of ROP, but excess oxygen is also associated with phase I with loss of vessels and cessation of normal retinal vascular development. Therefore it is likely that a growth factor or factors regulated by hypoxia and hyperoxia is important in the development of ROP.

Vascular endothelial growth factor (VEGF) is a such a hypoxia/oxygen-inducible cytokine [35, 57, 65]. It was first described as a vascular permeability factor (VPF) and later described as a vascular proliferative factor [21, 63]. VEGF is a vascular endothelial cell mitogen, which is required for tumor-associated angiogenesis [35]. Several different types of cultured retinal cells have been found to secrete VEGF under hypoxic conditions [1, 4, 5]. These characteristics make VEGF an ideal candidate for Michaelson's retinal vasoformative factor.

4.4.1 VEGF and Phase II of ROP

The first demonstration that VEGF was required for retinal neovascularization (phase II of ROP) came from studies of the mouse model of proliferative retinopathy [67]. The location and time course of VEGF expression in association with retinal neovascularization was found to correlate with disease in the mouse ROP model. After oxygen-induction of vessel loss and subsequent hypoxia, there is an increase in the expression of VEGF mRNA in the retina within 12 h. The increased expression is sustained until the development of neovascularization [55, 67]. This occurs in the ganglion cell layer and in the inner nuclear layer consistent with expression in astrocytes and Muller cells.

To establish that a growth factor is critical for neovascularization, inhibition of the factor must inhibit the proliferation of blood vessels. Inhibition of VEGF with intravitreal injections of either an anti-VEGF antisense oligonucleotide or with a molecule to adsorb VEGF (VEGF receptor/IgG chimera) significantly decreased the neovascular response in the mouse model of ROP [6, 61], indicating that VEGF is a critical factor in retinal neovascularization. VEGF also has been associated with ocular neovascularization by other investigators in other animal models, confirming the central role of VEGF in neovascular eye disease [3, 18, 47, 72, 76]. These results correspond to what is seen clinically. VEGF is elevated in the vitreous of patients with retinal neovascularization [2, 4]. VEGF was found in the retina of a patient with ROP in a pattern consistent with mouse results [76]. Based on these and other studies an anti-VEGF aptamer is now available to treat neovascularization associated with age-related macular degeneration and is in phase III clinical trials for diabetic retinopathy. Clinical trials are planned for evaluation of treatment of the proliferative phase of ROP with anti-VEGF injections.

Summary for the Clinician

- **VEGF is an important factor for the development of retinal vascular proliferation in ROP. Inhibition of VEGF with anti VEGF treatment (Anti-VEGF aptamer or anti-VEGF antibody) has been successfully used clinically in other proliferative retinal vascular diseases such as age-related macular degeneration and diabetic retinopathy. Clinical trials are in the planning stage for anti-VEGF therapy for ROP (injection into the vitreous in phase II) to prevent retinal detachment and blindness**

4.4.2 VEGF and Phase I of ROP

In the first phase of ROP, it has been suggested that the relative hyperoxia of the extrauterine environment causes the suppression of normal vessel development and vaso-obliteration [In animal models of oxygen-induced retinopathy, a clear association between exposure to hyperoxia and vaso-obliteration has been observed (11, 13, 53, 67]. Further study of this association is important because the extent of nonperfusion in the initial phase of retinopathy of prematurity appears to determine the subsequent degree of neovascularization.

Premature infants normally experiencing low levels of oxygen in the intrauterine environment suffer cessation of normal retinal vessel growth and vaso-obliteration of some immature retinal vasculature when exposed to the relatively high levels of oxygen of the extrauterine environment. It followed logically that if hypoxia up-regulated VEGF in the retina causing vaso-proliferation then hyperoxia might down-regulate VEGF and cause vessel loss. Therefore we examined the possibility that VEGF was necessary for vessel maintenance and normal retinal vessel growth and that exposure to extrauterine oxygen causes cessation of vessel growth and vaso-obliteration.

4.4.2.1 VEGF Phase I: Vessel Loss

Indeed, in the mouse model of ROP, just as hypoxia dramatically up-regulates VEGF m RNA, hyperoxia almost totally suppresses VEGF m RNA expression. The down-regulation of VEGF m RNA with hyperoxia causes loss or vaso-obliteration of immature retinal vessels. This loss can be prevented with intravitreal injections of exogenous VEGF [7, 56]. Furthermore, hyperoxia can reverse hypoxia-induced increases in VEGF, rationalizing the therapeutic use of oxygen in premature neonates with proliferative retinopathy (as used in the multicenter clinical STOP-ROP study) [23].

4.4.2.2 VEGF Phase I: Cessation of Normal Vascular Development

VEGF is also required for normal blood vessel growth in animal models of ROP. As the retina develops anterior to the vasculature, there is increased oxygen demand, which creates localized hypoxia. Induced by a wave of "physiologic hypoxia" that precedes vessel growth [56, 71], VEGF is expressed in response to the hypoxia, and blood vessels grow toward the VEGF stimulus. As the hypoxia is relieved by oxygen from the newly formed vessels, VEGF mRNA expression is suppressed, moving the wave forward.

Supplemental oxygen interferes with that normal development in the mouse and rat models of ROP. Hyperoxia causes cessation of normal vessel growth through suppression of VEGF mRNA, causing loss of the physiological wave of VEGF anterior to the growing vascular front [7, 56]. This indicates that VEGF is required for maintenance of the immature retinal vasculature and explains, at least in part, the effect of hyperoxia on normal vessel development in ROP.

4.5 Other Growth Factors Are Involved in ROP

Although VEGF and oxygen play an important role in the development of retinal blood vessels, it is clear that other biochemical mediators also are involved in the pathogenesis. Inhibition of VEGF does not completely inhibit hypoxia-induced retinal neovascularization in the second phase of ROP. In the first phase of ROP, although hyperoxia is clearly the cause of both cessation of vascular growth and vaso-obliteration in animal models, it is clear that clinical ROP is multifactorial. Despite controlled use of supplemental oxygen, the disease persists as ever-lower gestational aged infants are saved, suggesting that other factors related to prematurity itself also are at work.

4.5.1 IGF-1 Deficiency in the Preterm Infant

The insulin-like growth factors I and II (IGFs) are important in fetal growth and development during all stages of pregnancy [41]. They are found in embryological fluids in the first trimester [46] and there is a strong association between IGF concentrations and growth in human pregnancy [8, 9, 15, 16, 20, 24, 28–30, 39, 40, 42, 48, 60, 70, 73, 74]. Fetal cordocentesis serum samples show that IGF-I concentrations, but generally not IGF-II concentrations, increase with gestational age and correlate with fetal size [8, 42, 49, 60].

IGF-1 levels rise significantly in the third trimester of pregnancy [41]. Preterm birth in the earlier stages of the third trimester is associated with a loss of maternal sources of IGF-I and lower levels of serum IGF-1 compared to in utero counterparts as preterm infants grow outside the womb [43]. IGF-I levels rise slowly after preterm birth as babies who are born very prematurely appear unable to produce adequate IGF-1 compared to term infants [28]. In premature infants, IGF-I may be reduced further by conditions such as poor nutrition [78], acidosis, hypothyroxinemia, and sepsis.

Because the third trimester is associated with the rapid development of fetal tissue, loss of IGF-1 could be critical [28] since IGF-I is important for physical growth. Although serum GH levels in extremely preterm infants are significantly higher than term infants, serum IGF-I levels in extremely preterm infants are low. IGF-I concentrations are positively related to physical growth for several months after birth, whereas no relationship is observed between GH and physical growth. [34]. In particular, IGF-1 appears important for retinal and brain growth [33]. Thus IGF-1 appears to be a pivotal growth factor in early development.

4.5.2 GH and IGF-1 in Phase II of ROP

Prematurity is the most significant risk factor for ROP, which suggests that growth factors such as GH and IGF-1 relating to development are critical to the disease process. The first study to show that IGF-1 is important in retinopathy came from work in the proliferative phase of the disease (phase II). Because GH has been implicated in proliferative diabetic retinopathy [59, 64, 75], we considered GH and IGF-I, which mediates many of the mitogenic aspects of GH, as potential candidates for one of these growth factors.

In the mouse model of ROP, proliferative retinopathy, the second phase of ROP [68], is substantially reduced in transgenic mice expressing a GH-receptor antagonist or in wild type mice treated with a somatostatin analog that decreases GH release [68]. GH inhibition of neovascularization is mediated through an inhibition of IGF-I, because systemic administration of IGF-I in transgenic mice with decreased GH action completely restores the neovascularization seen in control mice. Direct proof of the role of IGF-I in the proliferative phase of ROP in mice was established with an IGF-I receptor antagonist, which suppresses retinal neovascularization without altering the vigorous VEGF response induced in the mouse ROP model [69].

Other studies have examined the role of both IGF-1 and insulin in the vascular endothelium in the ROP mouse model using mice with a vascular endothelial cell-specific knockout of the insulin receptor (VENIRKO) or IGF-1 receptor (VENIFARKO). VENIRKO mice show a 57% decrease in retinal neovascularization as compared with controls, associated with a reduced rise in VEGF, eNOS, and endothelin-1, VENIFARKO mice showed a 34% reduction in neovascularization, suggesting that both insulin and IGF-1 signaling in endothelium play a role in retinal neovascularization [38]. Therefore, IGF-I is likely to be one of the nonhypoxia-regulated factors critical to the development of ROP.

4.5.3 IGF-1 and VEGF Interaction

During GH and IGF-I inhibition, hypoxia-induced VEGF production is unchanged, indicating that IGF-I does not directly act through VEGF under these physiological conditions. These findings suggest a more complex role for IGF-I in retinal neovascularization [68]. IGF-I regulates retinal neovascularization at least in part through control of VEGF activation of p44/42 MAPK, establishing a hierarchical relationship between IGF-I and VEGF receptors [31, 69]. IGF-I acts to allow maximum VEGF stimulation of new vessel growth. Low levels of IGF-I inhibit vessel growth despite the presence of VEGF. This work suggests that IGF-I serves a permissive function, and VEGF alone may not be sufficient for promoting vigorous retinal angiogenesis.

4.5.4 Low Levels of IGF-I and Phase I of ROP

Since suppression of IGF-1 can suppress neovascularization, in phase II of ROP we hypothesized that IGF-I is critical to normal retinal vascular development and that a lack of IGF-I in the early neonatal period is associated with poor vascular growth and with subsequent proliferative ROP. After birth, IGF-I levels decrease from in utero levels due to the loss of IGF-I provided by the placenta and the amniotic fluid.

We examined normal retinal vascular development in IGF-I knockout mice and found that IGF-I is critical in the normal development of the retinal vessels. [31]. Retinal blood vessels grow more slowly in IGF-1 knockout mice than in normal mice, a pattern very similar to that seen in premature babies with ROP. It was determined that a minimum level of IGF-I is required for maximum VEGF activation of the Akt endothelial cell survival pathway. This finding explains how loss of IGF-I could cause the disease by preventing the normal survival of vascular endothelial cells.

4.5.5 Clinical Studies: Low IGF-1 Is Associated with Degree of ROP

The degree of Phase I determines the degree of Phase II, the later destructive phase of ROP. Normal vessel development in the retina precludes the development of proliferative ROP. Because ROP is initiated by abnormal postnatal retinal development, we hypothesized that prolonged low IGF-I in premature infants might be a risk factor for ROP. We conducted a prospective, longitudinal study measuring serum IGF-I concentrations weekly in 84 premature infants from birth (postmenstrual ages: 24–32 weeks) until discharge from the hospital. Infants were evaluated for ROP and other morbidity of prematurity: bronchopulmonary dysplasia (BPD), intraventricular hemorrhage (IVH), and necrotizing enterocolitis (NEC). Low serum IGF-I values correlated with later development of ROP. The mean IGF-I level during postmenstrual ages 30–33 weeks was lowest with severe ROP, intermediate with moderate ROP, and highest with no ROP. The duration of low IGF-I also correlated strongly with the severity of ROP. Each adjusted stepwise increase of 5 μg/l in mean IGF-I during postmenstrual ages 30–33 weeks was associated with a 45% decreased risk of proliferative ROP. Other complications (NEC, BPD, IVH) were correlated with ROP and with low IGF-I levels. The relative risk for any morbidity (ROP, BPD, IVH, or NEC) was increased 2.2-fold if IGF-I was 33 μg/l at 33 weeks postmenstrual age. These results indicate that persistent low serum concentrations of IGF-I after premature birth are associated with later development of ROP and other complications of prematurity. In this study, IGF-I was at least as strong a determinant of risk for ROP as postmenstrual age at birth and birth weight. [31, 33]. These findings suggest the possibility that increasing IGF-1 to uterine levels might prevent the disease by allowing normal retinal vascular development. If phase I is aborted the destructive second phase of vasoproliferation will not occur.

4.5.6 Low IGF-1 Is Associated with Decreased Vascular Density

More recent evidence suggests that very low IGF-1 directly causes decreased vascular density [32]. Retinal vessel morphology in patients with genetic defects of the GH/IGF-I axis and low levels of IGF-I during and after normal retinal vessel growth had significantly less retinal vascularization as evidenced by fewer vascular branching points compared with the reference group of normal controls, providing genetic evidence for a role of the GH and IGF-I system in retinal vascularization in humans. This accumulated evidence suggests that low IGF-1 is associated with vessel loss and may be detrimental by contributing to early vessel degeneration in phase I that sets the stage for hypoxia leading later to proliferative retinopathy.

Summary for the Clinician

- Postnatally low levels of IGF-1 in premature infants correlate with the severity of ROP. Clinical trials are in the planning phase to supplement IGF-1and IGFBP-3 to in utero levels in premature infants to evaluate if restoration of IGF-1 to normal levels can prevent or reduce the severity of ROP

4.5.7 IGF-1 and Brain Development

Low IGF-I may also contribute to poor neural retinal development and might contribute to poor neurological development in the preterm infant. There is considerable evidence that IGF-1 is important for neural development in brain and retina is part of the central nervous system. Poor retinal function is associated with ROP [27]. During development, IGF-I and IGF-binding proteins that modify IGF-I actions, as well as the IGF-1 receptor are found throughout the brain. IGF-I is a neural mitogen in cell culture, suggesting an important role for IGF-1 in the growth and development of the central nervous system. In vivo studies of brain development in transgenic mice with over- or under-expression of IGF-I provide more evidence for the role of IGF-1 in central nervous system development. Transgenic mice with postnatal overexpression of IGF-1 have brains with increased numbers of neurons and increased myelination. Mutant mice with low IGF-1 effect (reduced IGF-I and IGF1R expression or overexpression of IGFBPs capable of inhibiting IGF actions) have inhibited brain growth. Evidence from experiments in these mouse models also indicates that IGF-I has a role in recovery from neural injury [17]. IGF-I can both promote proliferation of neural cells in the embryonic central nervous system in vivo and inhibit their apoptosis during postnatal life [58].

Reduction of IGF-1 levels through overexpression of IGFBP-1 in the liver, which reduces IGF-1 availability, in transgenic mice affect brain development [19]. With the lowest level of IGF-1 effect (homozygous for IGFBP-1 overexpression), the cerebral cortex is reduced in size with disorganized neuronal layers. Similar anomalies have been reported in mice with disruption of the IGF-I gene and in a model of transgenic mice overexpressing IGFBP-1 in all tissues, including the brain [19].

Summary for the Clinician

- Animal studies suggest that low levels of IGF-1 postnatally in preterm infants could have an effect of neural retinal development as well as on brain development and might account for abnormal neural retinal function in ROP. Increasing postnatal IGF-1 through improved nutrition or other means might improve brain and retinal development

4.6 Conclusion: A Rationale for the Evolution of ROP

A rationale for the evolution of ROP has emerged based on this new understanding of the roles of VEGF and IGF-I in both phases of ROP. Blood vessel growth is dependent on both IGF-I and VEGF. In premature infants, the absence of IGF-I (normally provided by the placenta and the amniotic fluid) inhibits blood vessel growth. As the eye matures, it becomes oxygen-starved, sending signals to increase VEGF. As the infant's organs and systems then continue to mature, IGF-I levels rise again, suddenly allowing the VEGF signal to produce blood vessels (Fig. 4.1). This neovascular proliferation of phase II of ROP can cause blindness.

Summary for the Clinician

- The discovery of the importance of VEGF and IGF-I in the development of ROP is a step forward in our understanding of the pathogenesis of the disease. These studies suggest a number of ways to intervene medically in the disease process, but also make clear that timing is critical to any intervention. Inhibition of either VEGF or IGF-I early after birth can prevent normal blood vessel growth and precipitate the disease, whereas inhibition at the second neovascular phase might prevent destruc-

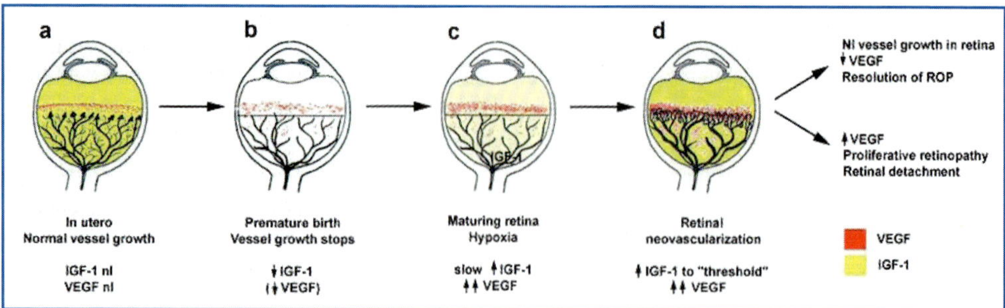

Fig. 4.1a–d. Schematic representation of IGF-I and VEGF control of blood vessel development in ROP (from [31]). **a** In utero, VEGF is found at the growing front of vessels. IGF-I is sufficient to allow vessel growth. **b** With premature birth, IGF-I is not maintained at in utero levels and vascular growth ceases, despite the presence of VEGF at the growing front of vessels. Both endothelial cell survival (Akt) and proliferation (mitogen-activated protein kinase) pathways are compromised. With low IGF-I and cessation of vessel growth, a demarcation line forms at the vascular front. High oxygen exposure (as occurs in animal models and in some premature infants) may also suppress VEGF, further contributing to inhibition of vessel growth. **c** As the premature infant matures, the developing but nonvascularized retina becomes hypoxic. VEGF increases in retina and vitreous. With maturation, the IGF-I level slowly increases. **d** When the IGF-I level reaches a threshold at 34 weeks of gestation, with high VEGF levels in the vitreous, endothelial cell survival, and proliferation driven by VEGF may proceed. Neovascularization ensues at the demarcation line, growing into the vitreous. If VEGF vitreal levels fall, normal retinal vessel growth can proceed. With normal vascular growth and blood flow, oxygen suppresses VEGF expression, so it will no longer be overproduced. If hypoxia (and elevated levels of VEGF) persists, further neovascularization and fibrosis leading to retinal detachment can occur

tive neovascularization. Similarly, replacement of IGF-I early on might promote normal blood vessel growth, whereas late supplementation with IGF-I in the neovascular phase of ROP could exacerbate the disease. In the fragile neonate, the choice of any intervention must be made very carefully to promote normal physiological development of both blood vessels and other tissue. In particular, the finding that later development of ROP is associated with low levels of IGF-I after premature birth suggests that increasing IGF-1 to physiologic levels found in utero through better nutrition or other means might prevent the disease by allowing normal vascular development

References

1. Adamis AP, Shima DT, Yeo KT, Yeo TK, Brown LF, Berse B et al (1993) Synthesis and secretion of vascular permeability factor/vascular endothelial growth factor by human retinal pigment epithelial cells. Biochem Biophys Res Comm 193:631–638
2. Adamis AP, Miller JW, Bernal MT, D'Amico DJ, Folkman J, Yeo TK et al (1994) Increased vascular endothelial growth factor levels in the vitreous of eyes with proliferative diabetic retinopathy. Am J Ophthalmol 118:445–450
3. Adamis AP, Shima DT, Tolentino MJ, Gragoudas ES, Ferrara N, Folkman J et al (1996) Inhibition of vascular endothelial growth factor prevents retinal ischemia-associated iris neovascularization in a nonhuman primate. Arch Ophthalmol 114: 66–71
4. Aiello LP, Avery RL, Arrigg PG, Keyt BA, Jampel HD, Shah ST et al (1994) Vascular endothelial growth factor in ocular fluid of patients with diabetic retinopathy and other retinal disorders [see comments]. N Engl J Med 331:1480–1487
5. Aiello LP, Northrup JM, Keyt BA, Takagi H, Iwamoto MA (1995) Hypoxic regulation of vascular endothelial growth factor in retinal cells. Arch Ophthalmol 1113:1538–1544

6. Aiello LP, Pierce EA, Foley ED, Takagi H, Chen H, Riddle L et al (1995) Suppression of retinal neovascularization in vivo by inhibition of vascular endothelial growth factor (VEGF) using soluble VEGF-receptor chimeric proteins. Proc Natl Acad Sci U S A 92:10457–10461
7. Alon T, Hemo I, Itin A, Pe'er J, Stone J, Keshet E (1995) Vascular endothelial growth factor acts as a survival factor for newly formed retinal vessels and has implications for retinopathy of prematurity. Nat Med 1:1024–1028
8. Arosio M, Cortelazzi D, Persani L, Palmieri E, Casati G, Baggiani AM et al (1995) Circulating levels of growth hormone, insulin-like growth factor-I and prolactin in normal, growth retarded and anencephalic human fetuses. J Endocrinol Invest 18:346–353
9. Ashton IK, Zapf J, Einschenk I, MacKenzie IZ (1985) Insulin-like growth factors (IGF) 1 and 2 in human foetal plasma and relationship to gestational age and foetal size during midpregnancy. Acta Endocrinol (Copenh) 110:558–563
10. Ashton N (1966) Oxygen and the growth and development of retinal vessels. In vivo and in vitro studies. The XX Francis I. Proctor Lecture. Am J Ophthalmol 62:412–435
11. Ashton N, Ward B, Serpell G (1954) Effect of oxygen on developing retinal vessels with particular reference to the problem of retrolental fibroplasia. Br J Ophthalmol 38:397–432
12. Campbell K (1951) Intensive oxygen therapy as a possible cause of retrolental fibroplasia: a clinical approach. Med J Aust 2:48–50
13. Chan-Ling T, Tout S, Hollander H, Stone J (1992) Vascular changes and their mechanisms in the feline model of retinopathy of prematurity. Invest Ophthalmol Vis Sci 33:2128–2147
14. Crosse VM, Evans PJ (1952) Prevention of retrolental fibroplasia. Arch Ophthalmol 48:83–87
15. D'Ercole AJ, Underwood LE (1985) Somatomedin in fetal growth. Pediatr Pulmonol 1 [3 Suppl]: S99–S106
16. D'Ercole AJ, Hill DJ, Strain AJ, Underwood LE (1986) Tissue and plasma somatomedin-C/insulin-like growth factor I concentrations in the human fetus during the first half of gestation. Pediatr Res 20:253–255
17. D'Ercole AJ, Ye P, O'Kusky JR (2002) Mutant mouse models of insulin-like growth factor actions in the central nervous system. Neuropeptides 36:209–220
18. Donahue ML, Phelps DL, Watkins RH, LoMonaco MB, Horowitz S (1996) Retinal vascular endothelial growth factor (VEGF) mRNA expression is altered in relation to neovascularization in oxygen induced retinopathy. Curr Eye Res 15:175–184
19. Doublier S, Duyckaerts C, Seurin D, Binoux M (2000) Impaired brain development and hydrocephalus in a line of transgenic mice with liver-specific expression of human insulin-like growth factor binding protein-1. Growth Horm IGF Res 10:267–274
20. Fant M, Salafia C, Baxter RC, Schwander J, Vogel C, Pezzullo J et al (1993) Circulating levels of IGFs and IGF binding proteins in human cord serum: relationships to intrauterine growth. Regul Pept 48:29–39
21. Ferrara N, Henzel W (1989) Pituitary follicular cells secrete a novel heparin-binding growth factor specific for vascular endothelial cells. Biochem Biophys Res Commun 161:851–858
22. Flynn JT (1983) Acute proliferative retrolental fibroplasia: multivariate risk analysis. Trans Am Ophthalmol Soc 81:549–591
23. Flynn JT, Bancalari E (2000) On "supplemental therapeutic oxygen for prethreshold retinopathy of prematurity (STOP-ROP), a randomized, controlled trial. I: Primary outcomes" [editorial]. J AAPOS 4:65–66
24. Foley TP Jr, DePhilip R, Perricelli A, Miller A (1980) Low somatomedin activity in cord serum from infants with intrauterine growth retardation. J Pediatr 96:605–610
25. Folkman J, Klagsbrun M (1987) Angiogenic factors. Science 235:442–446
26. Foos R, Kopelow S (1973) Development of retinal vasculature in perinatal infants. Surv Ophthalmol 18:117–127
27. Fulton AB, Hansen RM, Petersen RA, Vanderveen DK (2001) The rod photoreceptors in retinopathy of prematurity: an electroretinographic study. Arch Ophthalmol 119:499–505
28. Giudice LC, de Zegher F, Gargosky SE, Dsupin BA, de las Fuentes L, Crystal RA et al (1995) Insulin-like growth factors and their binding proteins in the term and preterm human fetus and neonate with normal and extremes of intrauterine growth. J Clin Endocrinol Metabol 80:1548–1555
29. Gluckman PD, Butler JH (1983) Parturition-related changes in insulin-like growth factors-I and -II in the perinatal lamb. J Endocrinol 99:223–232
30. Gluckman PD, Johnson-Barrett JJ, Butler JH, Edgar BW, Gunn TR (1983) Studies of insulin-like growth factor -I and -II by specific radioligand assays in umbilical cord blood. Clin Endocrinol (Oxf) 19:405–413
31. Hellstrom A, Perruzzi C, Ju M, Engstrom E, Hard AL, Liu JL et al (2001) Low IGF-I suppresses VEGF-survival signaling in retinal endothelial cells: direct correlation with clinical retinopathy of prematurity. Proc Natl Acad Sci U S A 98: 5804–5808

32. Hellstrom A, Carlsson B, Niklasson A, Segnestam K, Boguszewski M, de Lacerda L et al (2002) IGF-I is critical for normal vascularization of the human retina. J Clin Endocrinol Metab 87:3413–3416
33. Hellstrom A, Engstrom E, Hard AL, Albertsson-Wikland K, Carlsson B, Niklasson A et al (2003) Postnatal serum insulin-like growth factor I deficiency is associated with retinopathy of prematurity and other complications of premature birth. Pediatrics 112:1016–1020
34. Hikino S, Ihara K, Yamamoto J, Takahata Y, Nakayama H, Kinukawa N et al (2001) Physical growth and retinopathy in preterm infants: involvement of IGF-I and GH. Pediatr Res 50: 732–736
35. Kim KJ, Li B, Winer J, Armanini M, Gillett N, Phillips HS et al (1993) Inhibition of vascular endothelial growth factor-induced angiogenesis suppresses tumour growth in vivo. Nature 362: 841–844
36. Kinsey VE, Arnold HJ, Kalina RE, Stern L, Stahlman M, Odell G et al (1977) PaO2 levels and retrolental fibroplasia: a report of the cooperative study. Pediatrics 60:655–668
37. Knighton D, Hunt T, Scheuenstuhl H (1993) Oxygen tension regulates the expression of angiogenesis by macrophages. Science 221:1283–1285
38. Kondo T, Vicent D, Suzuma K, Yanagisawa M, King GL, Holzenberger M et al (2003) Knockout of insulin and IGF-1 receptors on vascular endothelial cells protects against retinal neovascularization. J Clin Invest 111:1835–1842
39. Kubota T, Kamada S, Taguchi M, Aso T (1992) Determination of insulin-like growth factor-2 in feto-maternal circulation during human pregnancy. Acta Endocrinol (Copenh) 127:359–365
40. Langford K, Blum W, Nicolaides K, Jones J, McGregor A, Miell J (1994) The pathophysiology of the insulin-like growth factor axis in fetal growth failure: a basis for programming by undernutrition? Eur J Clin Invest 24:851–856
41. Langford K, Nicolaides K, Miell JP (1998) Maternal and fetal insulin-like growth factors and their binding proteins in the second and third trimesters of human pregnancy. Hum Reprod 13:1389–1393
42. Lassarre C, Hardouin S, Daffos F, Forestier F, Frankenne F, Binoux M (1991) Serum insulin-like growth factors and insulin-like growth factor binding proteins in the human fetus. Relationships with growth in normal subjects and in subjects with intrauterine growth retardation. Pediatr Res 29:219–225
43. Lineham JD, Smith RM, Dahlenburg GW, King RA, Haslam RR, Stuart MC et al (1986) Circulating insulin-like growth factor I levels in newborn premature and full-term infants followed longitudinally. Early Hum Dev 13:37–46
44. McLeod D, Crone S, Lutty G (1996) Vasoproliferation in the neonatal dog model of oxygen-induced retinopathy. Invest Ophthalmol Vis Sci 37:1322–1333
45. Michaelson I (1948) The mode of development of the vascular system of the retina, with some observations in its significance for certain retinal diseases. Trans Ophthalmol Soc UK 68:137–180
46. Miell JP, Jauniaux E, Langford KS, Westwood M, White A, Jones JS (1997) Insulin-like growth factor binding protein concentration and post-translational modification in embryological fluid. Mol Hum Reprod 3:343–349
47. Miller JW, Adamis AP, Shima DT, D'Amore PA, Moulton RS, O'Reilly MS et al (1994) Vascular endothelial growth factor/vascular permeability factor is temporally and spatially correlated with ocular angiogenesis in a primate model. Am J Pathol 145:574–584
48. Nieto-Diaz A, Villar J, Matorras-Weinig R, Valenzuela-Ruiz P (1996) Intrauterine growth retardation at term: association between anthropometric and endocrine parameters. Acta Obstet Gynecol Scand 75:127–131
49. Ostlund E, Bang P, Hagenas L, Fried G (1997) Insulin-like growth factor I in fetal serum obtained by cordocentesis is correlated with intrauterine growth retardation. Hum Reprod 12:840–844
50. Patz A, Hoeck LE, DeLaCruz E (1952) Studies on the effect of high oxygen administration in retrolental fibroplasia: I. Nursery observations. Am J Ophthalmol 35:1248–1252
51. Patz A (1982) Clinical and experimental studies on retinal neovascularization. Am J Ophthalmol 94:715–743
52. Penn JS, Tolman BL, Henry MM (1994) Oxygen-induced retinopathy in the rat: relationship of retinal nonperfusion to subsequent neovascularization. Invest Ophthalmol Vis Sci 35:3429–3435
53. Penn JS, Tolman BL, Lowery LA (1993) Variable oxygen exposure causes preretinal neovascularization in the newborn rat. Invest Ophthalmol Vis Sci 34:576–585
54. Phelps DL (1981) Retinopathy of prematurity: an estimate of visual loss in the United States: 1979. Pediatrics 67:924–926
55. Pierce EA, Avery RL, Foley ED, Aiello LP, Smith LE (1995) Vascular endothelial growth factor/vascular permeability factor expression in a mouse model of retinal neovascularization. Proc Natl Acad Sci U S A 92:905–909
56. Pierce EA, Foley ED, Smith LE (1996) Regulation of vascular endothelial growth factor by oxygen in a model of retinopathy of prematurity [see comments] [published erratum appears in Arch Ophthalmol 1997 115:427]. Arch Ophthalmol 114:1219–1228

57. Plate KH, Breier G, Weich HA, Risau W (1992) Vascular endothelial growth factor is a potential tumour angiogenesis factor in human gliomas in vivo. Nature 359:845–848
58. Popken GJ, Hodge RD, Ye P, Zhang J, Ng W, O'Kusky JR et al (2004) In vivo effects of insulin-like growth factor-I (IGF-I) on prenatal and early postnatal development of the central nervous system. Eur J Neurosci 19:2056–2068
59. Poulsen JE (1953) Recovery from retinopathy in a case of diabetes with Simmonds' disease. Diabetes 2:7–12
60. Reece EA, Wiznitzer A, Le E, Homko CJ, Behrman H, Spencer EM (1994) The relation between human fetal growth and fetal blood levels of insulin-like growth factors I and II, their binding proteins, and receptors. Obstet Gynecol 84:88–95
61. Robinson GS, Pierce EA, Rook SL, Foley E, Webb R, Smith LE (1996) Oligodeoxynucleotides inhibit retinal neovascularization in a murine model of proliferative retinopathy. Proc Natl Acad Sci U S A 93:4851–4856
62. Roth AM (1977) Retinal vascular development in premature infants. Am J Ophthalmol 84:636–640
63. Senger DR, Galli SJ, Dvorak AM, Perruzzi CA, Harvey VS, Dvorak HF (1983) Tumor cells secrete a vascular permeability factor that promotes accumulation of ascites fluid. Science 219:983–985
64. Sharp PS, Fallon TJ, Brazier OJ, Sandler L, Joplin GF, Kohner EM (1987) Long-term follow-up of patients who underwent yttrium-90 pituitary implantation for treatment of proliferative diabetic retinopathy. Diabetologia 30:199–207
65. Shweiki D, Itin A, Soffer D, Keshet E (1992) Vascular endothelial growth factor induced by hypoxia may mediate hypoxia-initiated angiogenesis. Nature 359:843–845
66. Silverman WA (1980) Retrolental fibroplasia: a modern parable. Grune & Stratton, New York
67. Smith LE, Wesolowski E, McLellan A, Kostyk SK, D'Amato R, Sullivan R et al (1994) Oxygen-induced retinopathy in the mouse. Invest Ophthalmol Vis Sci 35:101–111
68. Smith LE, Kopchick JJ, Chen W, Knapp J, Kinose F, Daley D et al (1997) Essential role of growth hormone in ischemia-induced retinal neovascularization. Science 276:1706–1709
69. Smith LE, Shen W, Perruzzi C, Soker S, Kinose F, Xu X et al (1999) Regulation of vascular endothelial growth factor-dependent retinal neovascularization by insulin-like growth factor-1 receptor. Nat Med 5:1390–1395
70. Smith WJ, Underwood LE, Keyes L, Clemmons DR (1997) Use of insulin-like growth factor I (IGF-I) and IGF-binding protein measurements to monitor feeding of premature infants. J Clin Endocrinol Metab 82:3982–3988
71. Stone J, Itin A, Alon T, Pe'er J, Gnessin H, Chan-Ling T et al (1995) Development of retinal vasculature is mediated by hypoxia-induced vascular endothelial growth factor (VEGF) expression by neuroglia. J Neurosci 15:4738–4747
72. Stone J, Chan-Ling T, Pe'er J, Itin A, Gnessin H, Keshet E (1996) Roles of vascular endothelial growth factor and astrocyte degeneration in the genesis of retinopathy of prematurity. Invest Ophthalmol Vis Sci 37:290–299
73. Verhaeghe J, Van Bree R, Van Herck E, Laureys J, Bouillon R, Van Assche FA (1993) C-peptide, insulin-like growth factors I and II, and insulin-like growth factor binding protein-1 in umbilical cord serum: correlations with birth weight. Am J Obstet Gynecol 169:89–97
74. Wang HS, Lim J, English J, Irvine L, Chard T (1991) The concentration of insulin-like growth factor-I and insulin-like growth factor-binding protein-1 in human umbilical cord serum at delivery: relation to fetal weight. J Endocrinol 129:459–464
75. Wright AD, Kohner EM, Oakley NW, Hartog M, Joplin GF, Fraser TR (1969) Serum growth hormone levels and the response of diabetic retinopathy to pituitary ablation. BMJ 2:346–348
76. Young TL, Anthony DC, Pierce E, Foley E, Smith LE (1997) Histopathology and vascular endothelial growth factor in untreated and diode laser-treated retinopathy of prematurity. J Aapos 1:105–110

Screening for Retinopathy of Prematurity

5

Birgit Lorenz

Core Messages

- Retinopathy of prematurity (ROP) is still a vision-threatening condition in premature infants despite significant advances in neonatal medicine
- The proportion of childhood blindness caused by ROP goes from 8 % in high-income countries to 40 % in middle-income countries
- The incidence of severe ROP has decreased in more mature premature infants in countries with advanced neonatal care. However, the overall incidence of ROP has not changed over the years because of increasing survival rates in extreme premature infants
- The original classification and definition of treatment-requiring ROP (threshold ROP) has been refined and earlier treatment is now recommended for the most aggressive forms of ROP, namely zone I and posterior zone II disease
- The ETROP study group advocated treatment at prethreshold; this resulted in treatment as early as 30.6 weeks postmenstrual age. This suggests that national guidelines will need to be revised
- It is still unclear whether treatment at prethreshold in type 1 ROP will result in better clinical outcomes
- National guidelines for screening for ROP have to take into account potential country-specific risks related to local socioeconomic and health care conditions
- Screening for ROP needs a high degree of expertise in order to recognize ROP requiring treatment. Due to the relative rarity of ROP requiring treatment, digital photography and evaluation of the images in an expert reading center via telemedicine appear to have the potential of optimizing screening efficiency

5.1 Introduction

Retinopathy of prematurity (ROP) is a disease that occurs in premature infants and affects the postnatal maturation of the retinal blood vessels. Ultimately, it may result in the formation of vascular shunts, retinal neovascularization, and eventually tractional retinal detachment associated with severe visual handicap including blindness. The smallest infants are at highest risk for such an unfavorable anatomical and functional outcome, whereas in more mature infants ROP is usually milder and regresses spontaneously. The disease and its causative association with prematurity was first described by Terry in 1942 and 1943 [50]. Terry's initial interpretation of the disease was based on his observation of a retrolental proliferation of the embryonic hyaloid system. Therefore, he coined the term "retrolental fibroplasia." As the pathophysiology became better appreciated and improved classification systems were developed, the term "retinopathy of prematurity" (ROP) was introduced. During the 10 years following

Terry's first report, ROP was seen in epidemic proportions and became the largest cause of blindness throughout the developed world. Approximately 7,000 children in the United States alone were blinded by ROP [47]. Subsequently, oxygen therapy was identified as a major cause of ROP and its use restricted. This did in fact lead to a significant decrease in the incidence of ROP; however, this was associated with an adverse effect on the morbidity and mortality rates of the premature infants [3, 36]. In the 1970s, the development of arterial blood gas monitoring enabled more precise documentation of the premature infant's oxygen needs. Despite these improvements, a second epidemic of ROP resulted from increased survival rates of smaller and younger preterm infants. Low birth weight and low gestational age became recognized as strong risk factors for the development group. In the 1980s and 1990s, significant progress was made in reducing the complications from ROP, and numerous clinical trials were conducted evaluating the effect of various treatment modalities such as vitamin E supplementation, cryotherapy, laser photocoagulation, nursery light levels, and oxygen supplementation. This chapter will summarize current views on screening for ROP as indications for treatment evolve.

5.2 The Disease

During embryonic life, retinal vascular development begins at 16 weeks gestational age (GA) with mesenchyme as the blood vessel precursor growing from the optic disc to reach the ora nasally at 8 months GA and the ora temporally shortly after birth [2, 20, 22]. According to Ashton's theory [2], a primitive immature network of capillaries develops on the posterior edge of the advancing mesenchyme. This delicate meshwork undergoes involution and remodeling to form mature retinal arteries and veins surrounded by the capillary meshwork [2, 20, 21]. The immature incompletely vascularized retina is susceptible to oxygen toxicity. Whereas the fetus is in a hypoxic state with PaO_2 of 2–24 mmHg, full-term babies and a normal adult have a PaO_2 of 70–90 mmHg. One factor identified in recent years that stimulates the growth of immature retinal vessels to the periphery is vascular endothelial growth factor (VEGF). The amount of oxygen influences the amount of VEGF. Low oxygen levels stimulate VEGF production, high oxygen levels down-regulate VEGF production. A detailed description of the pathophysiology is given by L. Smith in Chap. 4 of this volume. Prolonged hyperoxia

Table 5.1. International Classification of ROP ICROP[a]

Stage number	Characteristics		
1	Demarcation line[b]		
2	Ridge[c]		
3	Ridge with extraretinal fibrovascular proliferation[d]		
4	Subtotal retinal detachment		
	A. Extrafoveal		
	B. Retinal detachment including fovea		
5	Total retinal detachment		
	Funnel	Anterior	Posterior
		Open	Open
		Narrow	Narrow
		Open	Narrow
		Narrow	Open

[a] Zones: I to III (see Fig. 5.1). Stages: 1–5. Plus disease: ROP in the presence of progressive dilatation and tortuosity of the retinal vessels in at least 2 quadrants of the posterior pole [9, 28]

[b] A thin, relatively flat, white demarcation line separates the avascular retina anteriorly from the vascularized retina posteriorly. Vessels that lead to the demarcation line are abnormally branched and/or arcaded

[c] The demarcation line has visible volume and extends off the retinal surface as a ridge, which may be white or pink. Retinal vessels may appear stretched locally, and vault off the surface of the retina to reach the peak of the ridge. Tufts of neovascular tissue may be present posterior to, but not attached to, the ridge

[d] Extraretinal fibrovascular (neovascular) proliferative tissue emanating from the surface of the ridge extending posteriorly along the retinal surface, or anteriorly toward the vitreous cavity. This gives the ridge a ragged appearance

will lead to vasoconstriction and vaso-obliteration. Subsequent tissue hypoxia will induce VEGF production. Normal VEGF levels will lead to normal vessel outgrowth, increased VEGF levels to arteriovenous shunting, and neovascularization. The different stages of ROP that result can be classified according to the International Classifications [9].

5.2.1 Classification

The classification of acute ROP according to the International Classification Scheme [9, 28] is given in Table 5.1 and in Figs. 5.1 and 5.2. The classification comprises three parameters: (1) the location, i.e., zone of the disease in the retina, (2) the extent by clock hours of the developing vasculature involved, and (3) the severity, i.e., stage of abnormal vascular response observed. Zone I is a posterior circle centered on the optic disc, and the radius is twice the distance from the disc to the center of the macula. The zone is defined by the most posterior location of disease. If, therefore, any ROP is found in zone I the eye is a zone I eye. A circle centered on the disc with a radius equal to the distance to the nasal ora serrata defines the boundary between zones II and III. Zone III comprises the remaining temporal crescent. As a general rule, the more posterior the disease, the more aggressive. An example is given in Fig. 5.3. Recently, it has been shown that the border of vascularization may not lie within a circle centered around the optic disc. In fact, data analysis from wide-angle images indicate that the distance to the nasal periphery may be shorter than that to the temporal periphery [23]. This may have implications for future classification schemes.

5.2.2 Treatment Requiring ROP

In the multicenter cryotherapy study for treatment of acute ROP (ICROP), threshold, i.e., treatment requiring ROP, was defined as stage 3 plus disease in zone II or zone I with at least 5 continuous clock hours or at least 8 cumulative clock hours of stage 3 disease, i.e., extraretinal proliferations (Table 5.2, Fig. 5.1b) [9]. Using this criterion, a favorable functional outcome at 1 year was achieved in 73% of zone II disease eyes, and in 12% of zone I disease eyes, compared to 46% of zone II disease eyes that were not treated, and 6% zone I disease eyes that were not treated [12]. Despite this considerable success compared to the natural history, the number of unfavorable outcomes was still high.

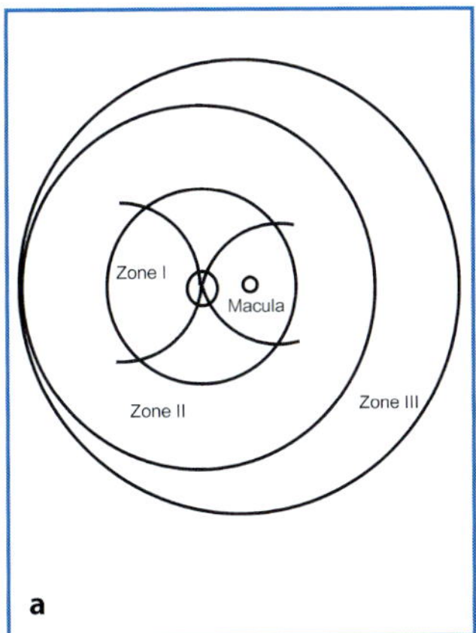

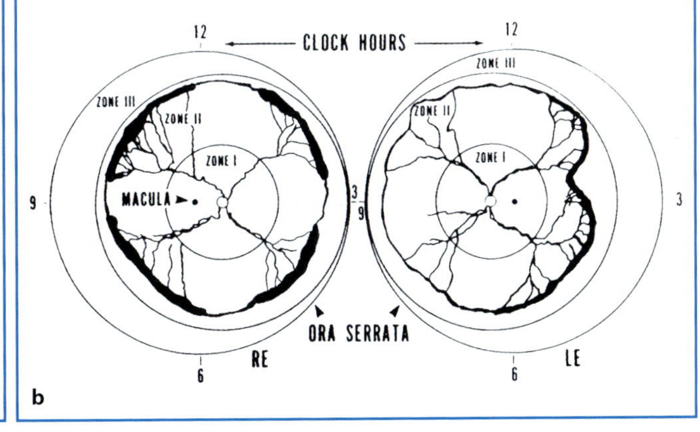

Fig. 5.1. a Classification of acute ROP according to the International Committee for the Classification of Retinopathy of Prematurity [9, 28]. Zones I–III. **b** Definition of threshold disease, with permission from *Archives of Ophthalmology* [11]

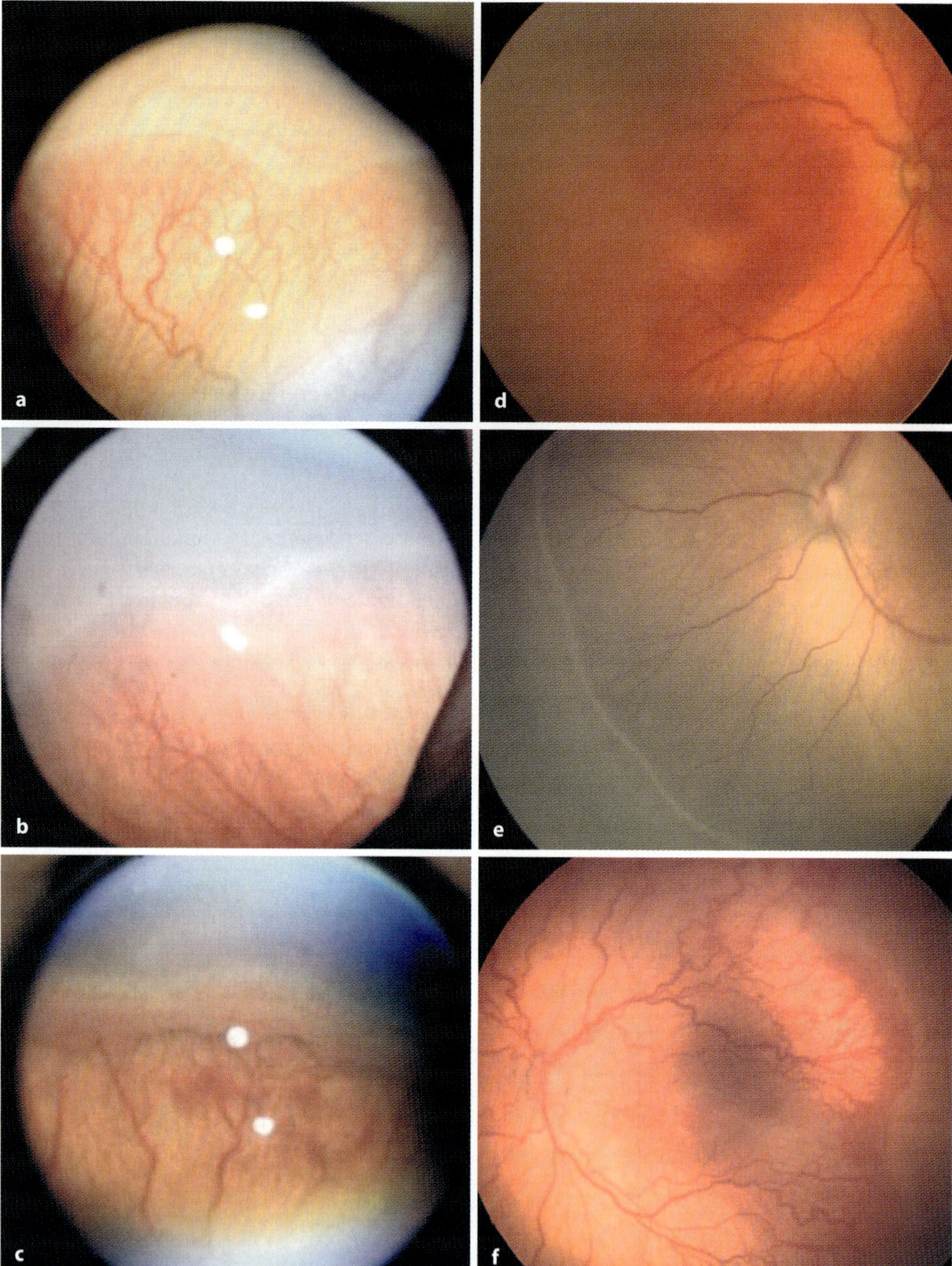

Fig. 5.2 a–f. Stages 1–3 of acute ROP as seen by indirect ophthalmoscopy (**a–c**) and with digital wide field imaging (**d–f**)

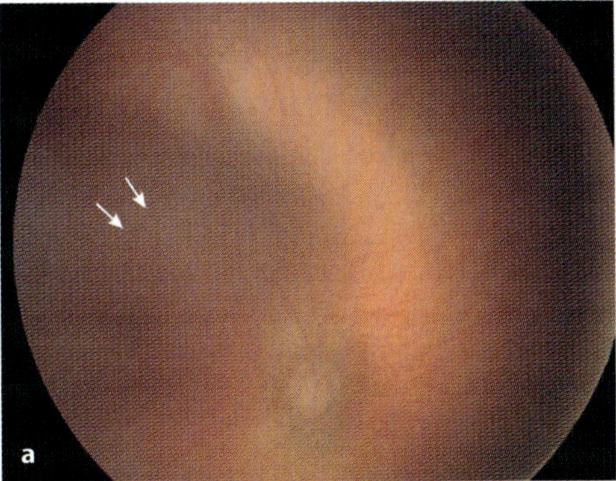

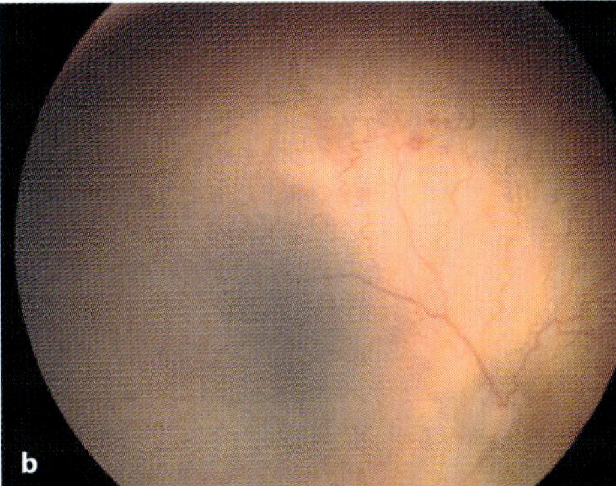

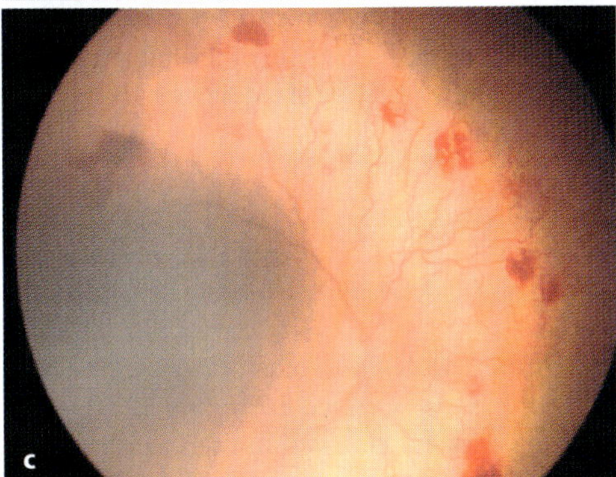

Fig. 5.3 a–c. Zone I disease in a ELBW premature (GA 25 weeks, BW 710 g). **a** First examination at postmenstrual age PMA 31 weeks/postnatal age 6 weeks. Extremely thin retinal vessels ending in zone I. Arrows highlight the extremely thin arteries visible only in zone I. **b** Two weeks later (PMA 33 weeks), compared to 1st exam now dilated retinal vessels with intraretinal proliferations in zone I. Treatment (at prethreshold) scheduled within 72 h. **c** At the time of treatment further rapid progression with widespread intraretinal hemorrhages. This is an example of a very aggressive form of zone I disease

Table 5.2. Definition of threshold disease and of prethreshold disease [9]

Threshold disease
Stage 3+ in zone I and II[a]
5 or more contiguous clock hours
8 or more cumulative clock hours
Plus disease: dilation and tortuosity of posterior pole retinal vessels in at least two quadrants meeting or exceeding that of a standard photograph.
Prethreshold disease
Zone I
Any disease below threshold
Zone II
Stage 2 with plus disease
Stage 3 without plus disease
Stage 3 with plus disease but below threshold
Plus disease: dilation and tortuosity of posterior pole retinal vessels in at least two quadrants meeting or exceeding that of a standard photograph

[a] In zone I and posterior zone II disease, vascular proliferation may be intraretinal only or very flat on the retinal surface (Fig. 5.3). There is a high risk of progression to retinal detachment without appearance of extraretinal proliferation. This fact has been accounted for in more recent national guidelines [8]

Table 5.3. RM-ROP2

$p = \{1 + exp[-(\alpha + \beta_1 x_1 + \beta_2 x_2 + \beta_k x_k)]\}^{-1}$
Each x_i is an infant that increased (or decreased) the risk p to have an unfavorable outcome. The β_i and α are coefficients in the risk model that are estimated from these data.
The β_i is the coefficient associated with x_i and α is a constant term. The function *exp* raises the expression in brackets to the base e = 2.71828...

From [25]

Table 5.4. Early treatment for retinopathy of prematurity ETROP. Classification of treatment-requiring ROP

	Type 1 ROP	Type 2 ROP
Zone I	Any stage of ROP with plus disease	Stage 1 or 2 without plus disease
Zone II	Stage 2 and 3 with plus disease	Stage 3 without plus disease
Recommendation	Laser photocoagulation (or cryo)	Follow-up examinations until type 1 ROP or threshold ROP is reached
In this classification, zone III disease is not contained as treatment is not estimated necessary		

From [16]

This led, in the following years, to a redefinition of treatment-requiring disease. The risk model RM-ROP published by Hardy in 1997 [26] consists of five mathematical equations that provide a relationship between risk factors observed concerning the infant and the infant's retina as they correlate with structural outcome. The program is based on data from 4,099 infants who weighed less than 1,251 g at birth who composed the natural history cohort of the Multicenter Trial for Cryotherapy for Retinopathy of Prematurity [40, 44]. This risk model has recently been further developed and replaced by the risk model RM-ROP2 [25], which evaluates the risk of prethreshold ROP to progress to threshold ROP and to an unfavorable outcome (Table 5.3). For eyes with a risk of 0.15–1.0, 36% had an unfavorable structural outcome at 3 months compared to 5% for eyes with a risk of less than 0.15. There is now an internet address that makes it possible to directly calculate the risk (http://www.sph.uth.tmc.edu/rmrop/riskcalc/disclaimer.aspx). The same calculation was used in the Early Treatment of ROP Study Group ETROP used this calculation. ETROP defines treatment-requiring ROP as type 1 ROP, whereas they recommend a watch and wait policy in type 2 ROP. The definition of the two types is given in Table 5.4. For eyes designated high risk, 63% progressed to the conventional threshold ROP requiring treatment, and for eyes designated low risk, 14% progressed to threshold. ETROP claims that the new definition of treatment-requiring ROP has the potential to salvage more eyes from an unfavorable outcome, and to generally improve the functional outcome. With the conventional threshold, 44.4% of eyes had a visual acuity of 20/200 or less at 10-year follow-up, and of the 55.6% with a visual acuity of better than 20/200, only 45.4% had a visual acuity of 20/40 or better, i.e., only about 25% of all infants that were treated reached a visual acuity of at least 20/40 [15]. Whether with the new definition of treatment-requiring ROP the functional outcome will be indeed improved remains to be demonstrated. This is important as on the other hand a significant number, i.e., 37% of infants will be treated unnecessarily.

Summary for the Clinician

- **Classification of the acute stages of retinopathy of prematurity ROP has been refined during the past years, in particular for zone 1 disease. Definition of treatment-requiring ROP has also evolved during the most recent years due to a still limited anatomical and functional outcome when treatment was undertaken at threshold. The new definition of treatment-requiring ROP by the ETROP study group published in 2003 is type 1 ROP, and better anatomical and functional outcomes are hoped for in the future. This, however, still remains to be demonstrated. To detect type 1 ROP at an appropriate time revision of screening guidelines is mandatory**

5.2.3 Treatment of Acute ROP

Once treatment-requiring ROP is detected, photocoagulation therapy or (mainly in earlier years or where lasers are not available) cryotherapy is recommended. Although in the American Guidelines the time to treatment is defined as within 72 h [1], it may be necessary to treat without any further delay, in particular in zone I disease with very rapid progression, or when at examination already a more advanced stage is seen than considered optimal for photocoagulation.

5.2.3.1 Treatment Options

In earlier years, cryotherapy was the standard treatment for threshold ROP once its beneficial effect had been shown in a multicenter study [10, 12–14]. Since the early 1990s, laser photocoagulation has been used [27, 29, 33, 37] and is now the preferred treatment modality, as the results are considered to be at least as good and even superior to cryotherapy [38, 41, 51]. The 810 diode laser is more widely used than the argon laser due to its portability and more favorable absorption characteristics. More advanced stages may benefit from encircling bands and/or vitrectomy. Lens-sparing vitrectomy appears to be the most promising therapy for stage 4 ROP [42]. A discussion of the various treatment options is beyond the scope of this chapter.

5.2.3.2 Treatment Results

Fallaha et al. [19] report on an overall progression rate to ROP 4 and 5 of 18.1% after diode laser photocoagulation for threshold ROP. The progression rate depended dramatically on the location of the disease: in zone I and posterior zone II disease, 44.8% progressed to ROP 4 and 5 compared to only 3.9% in anterior zone II disease. The range of progression reported by other authors goes from 0% to 29% [4–6, 10, 12, 40]. Banach [10] compared confluent vs scatter laser treatment. The retreatment rate was similar with both treatment regimes, i.e., 35% vs 37%, but near confluent laser progression to retinal detachment was observed only in 3.6% compared to 29.4% in the scatter group. In their series, Fallaha et al. had applied confluent laser spots in all patients, although some variability was in fact present, as photocoagulation was performed by six different ophthalmologists, with some using rather near confluent laser than confluent laser spots. Interestingly, a similar rate of adverse outcomes was observed in both treatment groups, i.e., approximately 30% in zone I and posterior zone II disease, and roughly 16% in anterior zone II disease. The same group had reported earlier that with confluent laser ablation there may be a higher risk for phthisis bulbi [13, 30].

Summary for the Clinician

- **Posterior forms of acute treatment-requiring ROP still have a higher risk of adverse outcome. Treatment at prethreshold in zone I disease appears to lower the risk for adverse outcome significantly. Some authors claim that confluent laser treatment may lower the risk for adverse outcome. However, confluent laser treatment may be associated with a higher risk for phthisis bulbi**

5.3 Epidemiology of ROP

About 1% of the neonates are born prematurely, with a birth weight below 1,500 g, roughly 0.5% with a birth weight below 1,000 g (extremely low birth weight, ELBW). The overall birth rate is about 1 per 100 inhabitants per year. This means that for example in Germany with over 80 million inhabitants, about 800,000 children are born per year, of whom 8,000 have a birth weight below 1,500 g, and 4,000 below 1,000 g. The relative numbers are similar in Western countries. This means that in the US with about 240 million inhabitants, about 24,000 infants per year are born with a birth weight below 1,500 g, and about 12,000 infants with a birth weight below 1,000 g.

5.3.1 Risk Factors

The main risk factors for ROP are low gestational age and low birth weight. Oxygen has been recognized as a risk factor for ROP since the 1950s, but a direct correlation of duration and concentration of oxygen with severity of ROP is not possible. ROP has been reported in the absence of supplemental oxygen. Many additional factors may contribute to the severity of the disease including degree of illness, sepsis, blood transfusions, and as observed in the CRYO-ROP study, white race, multiple births, and being born outside a study center nursery. For a more complete discussion of possible risk factors see Ober et al. [39].

5.3.2 Incidence of ROP

The incidence of ROP is dependent on birth weight and gestational age, as observed in several independent studies, and is summarized in Tables 5.5–5.8. There are many more studies reporting on a wide range on the overall incidence of ROP, and of the incidence of various stages. Variation is highest for mild disease, particularly due to its more peripheral location and hence more difficult visualization. Incidence of threshold ROP in various studies is in the order of up to 6%–8% in infants with a birth weight of 1,250 g or less [16]. Using the ETROP2003 classification of type 1 and type 2 ROP (Table 5.4), 9% of infants with a birth

Table 5.5. Percentage of patients with various categories of ROP in the Cryotherapy for Retinopathy of Prematurity Group. Incidence of retinopathy of prematurity ROP is dependent on birth weight and gestational age in different study groups

BW (g)	Any ROP	Stage 3	Prethreshold	Threshold
<750	90	37.4	39.4	15.5
750–999	78.2	21.9	21.4	6.8
1000–1250	46.9	8.5	7.3	2.0
Total group	65.8	18.3	17.8	6.0

From [40]

Table 5.6. Relation of ROP to birth weight in two consecutive groups (1998–1990 and 1998–2000) in Sweden

	Birth weight (g)					
	<750	751–1,000	>1,000			
	1990	2000	1990	2000	1990	2000
No ROP (%)	3 (23.1)	2 (8.7)	29 (47.5)	23 (34.4)	123 (66.1)	136 (83.4)
Mild ROP (%)	3 (23.1)	4 (17.4)	14 (23.0)	22 (32.8)	36 (19.4)	20 (12.3)
Severe ROP (%)	7 (53.8)	17 (73.9)	18 (29.5)	22 (32.8)	27 (14.5)	7 (4.3)
Total ROP (%)	10 (76.9)	21 (91.3)	32 (52.5)	44 (65.6)	63 (33.9)	27 (16.6)
Totals	13	23	61	67	186	163

From [32], mild ROP is defined as stages 1 and 2, severe ROP is defined as stages 3 (even in the absence of "plus disease") to 5

Table 5.7. Relation of ROP to gestational age at birth in two consecutive groups (1988–1990 and 1998–2000) in Sweden

	Gestational age at birth (weeks)							
	≤ 26		27–29		30–32		>33	
	1990	2000	1990	2000	1990	2000	1990	2000
No ROP (%)	10 (28.6)	6 (10.5)	72 (57.6)	73 (69.5)	53 (67.9)	73 (89.0)	20 (90.9)	9 (100)
Mild ROP (%)	9 (25.7)	16 (28.1)	30 (24.0)	23 (21.9)	12 (15.4)	7 (8.6)	2 (9.1)	0 (0)
Severe ROP (%)	16 (45.7)	35 (61.4)	23 (18.4)	9 (8.6)	13 (16.7)	2 (2.4)	0 (0)	0 (0)
Total ROP (%)	25 (71.4)	51 (89.5)	53 (42.4)	32 (30.5)	25 (32.1)	9 (11.0)	2 (9.1)	0 (0)
Totals	35	57	125	105	78	82	22	9

From [32], mild ROP is defined as stages 1 and 2, severe ROP is defined as stages 3 (even in the absence of plus disease) to 5

Table 5.8. Comparison of overall incidence of ROP in various studies

Study	Infants	Mean GA (weeks)	Mean BW (g)	ROP (all stages)	Method
Mathew et al. 2002 [35]	205	28	1,205	31.2%	BIO
Larsson et al. 2002 [31][a]	253	28.5	1,118	36.4%	BIO
Larsson et al. 2002 [32][b]	392	29.4	1,381	25.5%	BIO
Elflein and Lorenz unpublished	249	29.8	1,297	20.9%	RetCam

[a] Born between 1998–2000, BW <1,500 g,
[b] Born between 1998–2000, GA <32 weeks
BIO binocular indirect ophthalmoscopy, *RetCam* digital wide-angle photography, *GA* gestational age, *BW* birth weight

Table 5.9. Infants at risk according to various national guidelines published by 31/02/2004

	GA (weeks)		BW (g)	Additional infants
US 2001 [58]	≤28	or	<1500	1,500 g–2,000 g with unstable course if considered high risk
UK 1996 [55]	<32	and/or	<1501	
Sweden 1993 [56]	≤ 32			
Sweden 2002 [31]	Suggestion ≤31			
Canada 2000 [57]	≤30	and	≤ 1500	Also above these limits if the neonatologist considers the premature baby at risk for ROP
Germany 1999 [18]	<32	and/or	<1500	Any preterm baby <36 completed gestational weeks who had received artificial ventilation for at least 3 days

If screening of infants with a GA of 32 weeks and above and a BW of more than 1,500 g would be omitted, about 1.5 million exams per year could be saved in the US without missing any clinically important ROP [52]

weight of 1,250 g or less will have ROP type 1 requiring treatment. In countries with different socioeconomic conditions and different standards of neonatal care, the incidence may differ considerably. This has to be taken into account when new screening programs are started in countries where screening for ROP has not yet been done routinely [24].

5.4 Screening Guidelines

Following the reports of the Multicenter Cryo Study Group showing a significant reduction in the adverse outcome of acute ROP by cryotherapy at threshold [10, 12–14], screening guide-

Table 5.10. Timing of first examination, follow-up examinations and treatment of prematures at risk as given in various national guidelines by 31/02/2004

	First exam	Follow-up	Treatment
US 2001 [58]	4–6 weeks PNA or 31–33 weeks PMA, whichever is sooner	ROP zone I or zone II: at least weekly if treatment is not yet considered ROP zone III: bimonthly If no ROP but immature retina: every 2–3 weeks until vascularization complete	Within 72 h if indicated
US 2001 [49]	ELBW 5–6 weeks (42 days)		
US 2002 [59]	4 weeks PNA or 31 weeks PMA, whichever is later![a]	Until ≥ 45 weeks PMA if not ≥ prethreshold, zone III vascularization if no previous zone II disease, full vascularization*	
UK 1996 [55]	6–7 weeks PNA	According to pathology seen	
Sweden 2002 [31]	5–6 weeks PNA	According to pathology seen	
Canada 2000 [57]	4–6 weeks PNA	Weekly if ROP Bi-monthly if no ROP until vascularization complete	
Germany 1999 [18]	4–6 weeks PNA but not before 31 weeks PMA[a, b]	Weekly if ROP in zone I or II Bi-weekly if ROP zone III or no ROP until vascularization complete or ROP resolved	

[a] In the 2003 paper of the ETROP group [16], the mean ± SD at high risk prethreshold treatment were postmenstrual age 35.2 ± 2.3 weeks, the range 30.6–42.1 weeks, and chronological age 10.0 ± 2.0 weeks. This would mean that with the US guidelines from 2002 and the German guidelines from 1999 not all infants would have been identified at high-risk prethreshold. Following the suggestion by Subhani et al. [49] to screen ELBW infants already at day 42 would most likely detect these infants, although these data are not evident from [16]

[b] The German National Guidelines are currently being revised and there is agreement among the ophthalmologists of the Committee that the first examination will be scheduled to 4 –6 weeks PNA but not before 30 weeks PMA. Thus all infants at risk should be identified at prethreshold stages according to the data of [16]

ELBW extremely low birth weight = <1,000 g (GA usually 23–25 weeks)

lines have been developed in many high income countries. Screening for ROP should be performed by an ophthalmologist with sufficient knowledge of the disease location and the sequential retinal changes, and experienced with the examination of premature infants with binocular indirect ophthalmoscopy, i.e., preferably by a pediatric ophthalmologist or a retina specialist. Data from a number of epidemiological studies have led to a continuous up-date of the guidelines. Tables 5.9 and 5.10 give an overview of the most recent guidelines from the US, the UK, Sweden, Canada, and Germany, specifying those infants at risk for acute ROP, the timing of screening for ROP, and its endpoint. Although the numbers do not appear to differ significantly, they have significant implications as to the total number of examinations required and the probability of identifying stages that are considered to profit from treatment in a timely manner. Very recently, earlier treatment has been advocated by the Early Treatment of ROP Study Group ETROP, to further improve the anatomical and functional outcomes [16]. These data will have implications as to updating national guidelines. Physicians involved in screening and treating infants at risk for ROP should therefore keep themselves constantly updated with the current literature.

Summary for the Clinician

- **Evolving knowledge on the anatomical and functional outcome of treated ROP has recently led to new definitions of treatment-requiring ROP. Currently, national guidelines need to be modified to take account of the ETROP study. Specific socioeconomic and health care conditions may require adaptation of national guidelines, e.g., including infants with a higher gestational age and/or birth weight**

5.5 Screening Methods

Treatment-requiring ROP is a relatively rare yet potentially blinding disease. Therefore, screening should be undertaken by ophthalmologists who are experienced in examining premature infants and who can recognize the different stages of ROP.

5.5.1 Conventional Screening

It is crucial to achieve good pupillary dilation in order to allow examination of the retinal periphery in addition to the posterior pole. Recommended eye drops are tropicamide 0.5% together with phenylephrine 2.5% applied two to three times every 5–10 min. As an alternative, custom-made atropine 0.1% eye drops applied also two to three times every 5–10 min may be used, as they provide good mydriasis for about 3 h, thus requiring a less stringent planning of the exact consultation time by the ophthalmologist in charge of the screening. In order to avoid potentially harmful light exposure, the incubator should in this case be covered by a cloth. The nurses are asked to check pupil size, and to repeat the application of cycloplegic agents whenever needed. Immediately prior to the ophthalmic examination, local anesthetic eye drops are instilled (e.g., oxybuprocaine), and a sterile lid speculum for premature infants is gently inserted. The examination is best performed in a darkened room using a binocular indirect ophthalmoscope (BIO) together with a 28-diopter (D) lens (for a good peripheral view and to classify the disease by zones) and a 20-D lens (for more detailed evaluation). To visualize the peripheral retina out to the ora serrata, rotation of the globe together with gentle indentation is needed, e.g., with a squint hook or a lens wire loop. It is advisable to have a nursing staff member present during the examination to assist in physically restraining the infant, and to monitor the infant's vital signs and airway. Bradycardia due to the oculocardiac reflex is a recognized complication of the examination [7]. The examination should be thorough yet rapid. It is not sufficient to only examine the temporal periphery, as in particular in zone I and posterior zone II disease, acute ROP may be more advanced in the nasal periphery, and also in the upper and lower periphery [16]. An important sign is the presence of plus disease. Prior to the formation

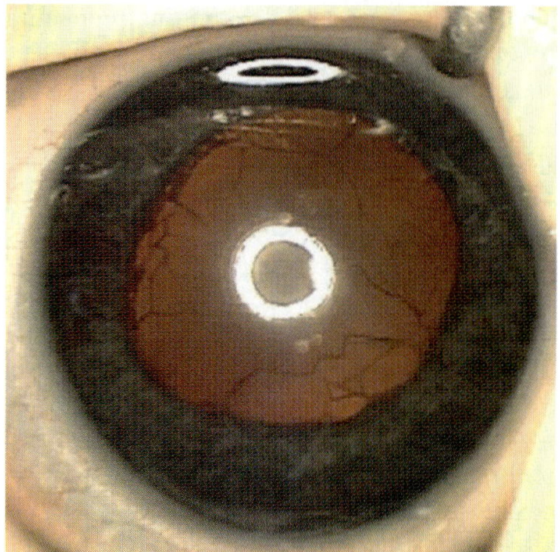

Fig. 5.4. Hyperemia of the iris and dilated persistent Tunica vasculosa lentis associated with ROP stage 3+, posterior zone II

of plus disease, significant vasoconstriction may be present. If the vasculature is very immature, i.e., limited to zone I or posterior zone II disease, the presence of vasoconstriction should prompt weekly follow-up examinations. Anterior segment changes should also be carefully evaluated as the presence of a persistent and dilated tunica vasculosa lentis and overt hyperemia of the iris vessels are a clear indicator of severe retinal disease that may require treatment (Fig. 5.4). The findings must be documented in a written report specifying the location, extent, and severity of the disease, and also recommendations as to follow-up or therapy. A scheme for follow-up examinations in the presence of ROP is given in Tables 5.9 and 5.10. Care must be taken that recommended follow-up examinations also take place once the infant is discharged from the NICU.

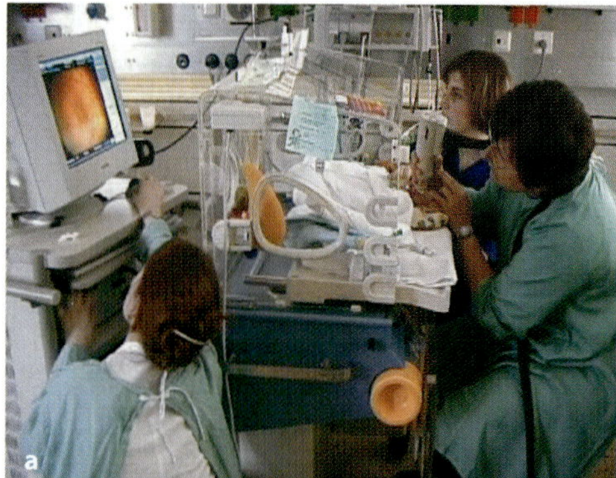

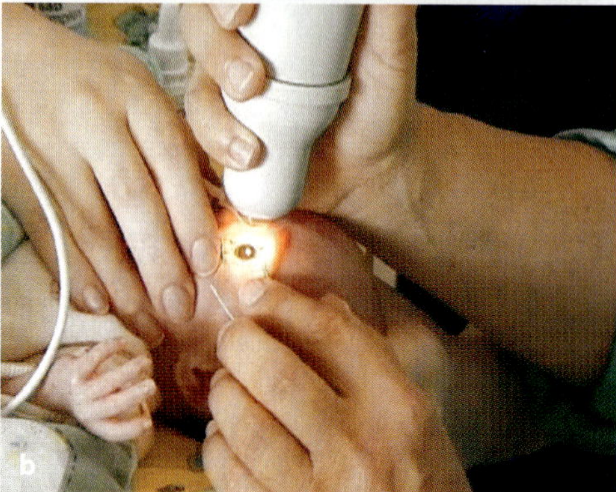

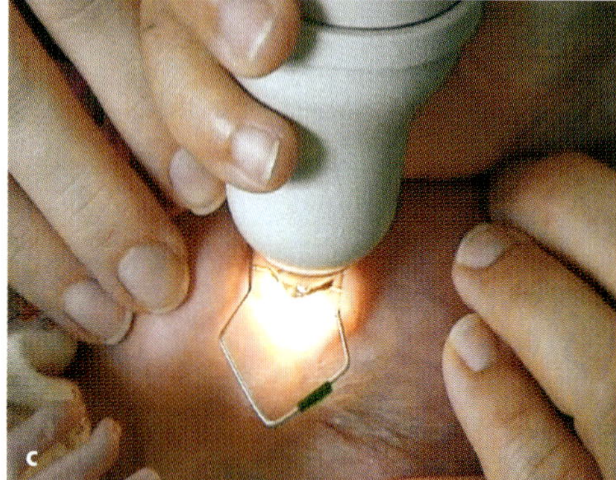

Fig. 5.5 a–c. Digital wide-field imaging. **a** Examination of infant in incubator. **b** Non-contact imaging of the anterior segment. **c** Imaging of the retina in contact mode. Pressure-free contact of the nose piece of the camera to the eye is established by a cushion of transparent highly viscose gel on the corneal surface

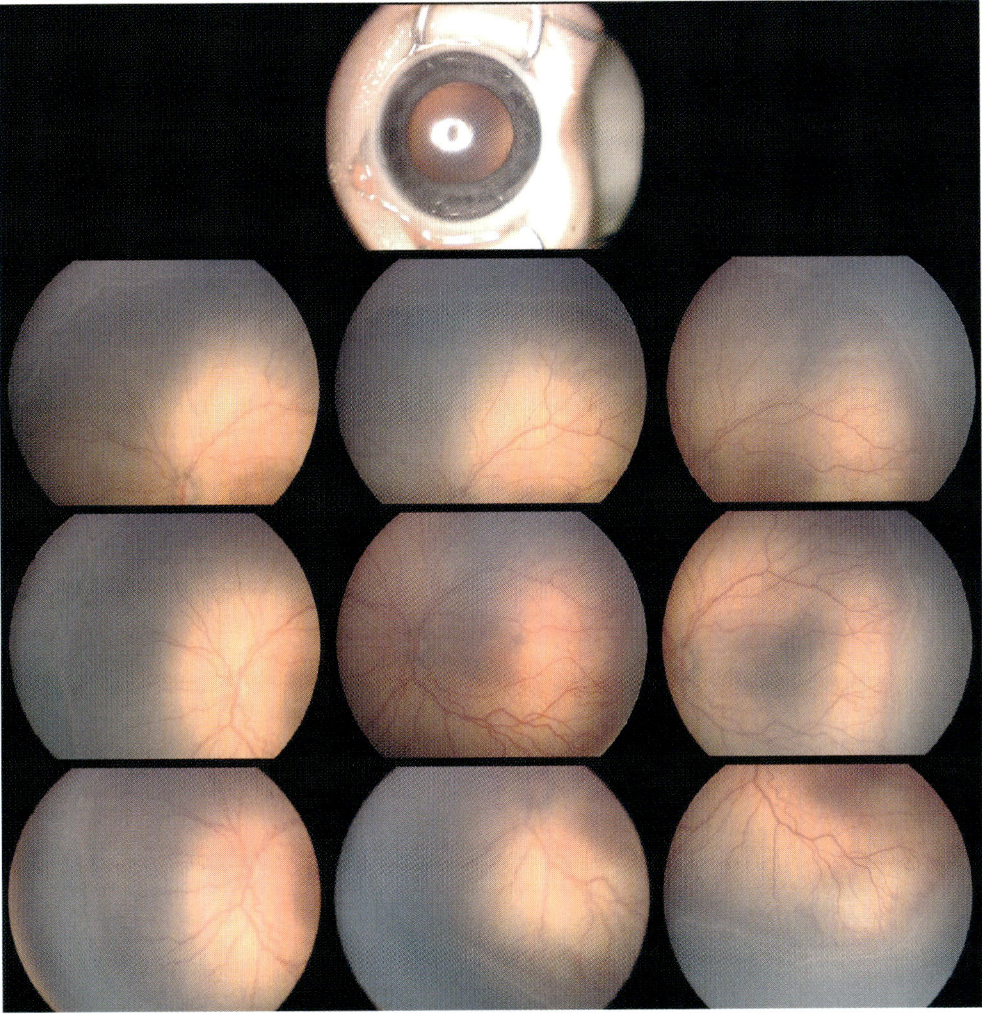

Fig. 5.6. Standard image set for imaging premature infants at risk for ROP

5.5.2 Digital Photography

The RetCam120, a digital retinal wide-field imaging system, has been used for several years to image the retina of premature infants and detect ROP (Fig. 5.5) [43, 45, 46, 53]. It can document large parts of the retina within minutes. Just as with conventional screening, it is advisable to have a nursing staff member present during the examination to assist in physically restraining the infant, and to monitor the infant's vital signs and airway. Good mydriasis is crucial, just as with BIO. With one central and eight peripheral images and an additional image of the anterior segment, all structures are visualized that are essential to detect serious, i.e., eventually treatment-requiring disease (Fig. 5.6). Indentation usually does not improve visibility of the peripheral retina, and is therefore not advised. Evaluation of the shape, degree of arborization, and diameter of retinal vessels at the border of vascularization or at the peripheral border of the images estimate the severity of the disease even in the absence of complete imaging, in particular of zone III, which technically often is not feasible. There is also skill involved with reading the images. Compared with BIO, one does not get a three-dimensional view. Being familiar with both the funduscopic aspect and the RetCam image is important for correct interpretation of the images. Digital imaging also offers the opportunity of improved education for students, doctors, and parents.

Several studies have investigated different issues surrounding the use of the RetCam 120 in the management of ROP. In the Yen et al. study, ROP screening with the RetCam in preterm babies at risk was performed by neonatal nurses [53, 54]. Different from the recommended screening schedule, and in an attempt to reduce the number of examinations needed to reliably identify infants at risk for treatment-requiring ROP, in this study pictures of the retina were taken only at two points of time in the neonatal phase: examination 1 at a PMA of 32–34 weeks, examination 2 at 38–40 weeks PMA. Masked readers evaluated the images as to ROP and determined whether each eye would progress to threshold disease or not. The sensitivity of this approach was not high enough to be recommended as a substitute for conventional screening. Two recent papers have evaluated the value of the RetCam120 in screening for ROP using serial examinations, just as with conventional screening with binocular ophthalmoscopy. In a French study, in one NICU, RetCam images of 145 premature infants at risk were assessed by neonatologists and by ophthalmologists [48]. They reported no false-positive results, and an exact correlation between observers in all cases of acute ROP. In a Canadian study, comparing the RetCam to binocular indirect ophthalmoscopy in 44 premature infants at risk, the sensitivity to detect severe ROP was shown to be 100% for the RetCam [18]. Very recently, the data of the ongoing Photo-ROP study were presented at the Annual Meeting of the Association for Research in Vision and Ophthalmology ARVO 2005. Again, very high sensitivity and specificity were reported for the RetCam 120 images.

5.5.3 Telemedicine

The advent of telemedicine offers the opportunity for improved ROP screening in remote areas and thus has the potential to reduce the risk of avoidable severe visual impairment [34, 45]. In our prospective study, the RetCam120 has been used for ROP screening in five Bavarian NICUs since 2001. To date, in 2005, more than 600 infants at risk have been examined. Four of these NICUs are peripheral sites, with ROP screening performed by general ophthalmologists. All images are transferred to the Reading Center at the University of Regensburg for evaluation. The objective of this screening program is targeted at detection of the need for a specialist consult to make the final treatment decision in the presence of referral-warranted ROP and thereby ideally eliminate late referrals. Thus, the sensitivity to detection of inconsequential disease is not at issue. In this program, digital imaging using the RetCam 120 was successful in detecting all referral-warranted ROP stages, with no incidents where treatment-requiring disease was missed of referred late, and with no false-negative or false-positive results in a subset of patients where digital imaging and BIO were directly compared, i.e., the sensitivity and the specificity to detect referral-warranted ROP were both 100% [17].

Summary for the Clinician

- **Effective screening for ROP requires skill with BIO and experience with the extent and sequential retinal changes of ROP. Digital imaging allows objective documentation of large parts of the retina and of the anterior segment. Expert reading is essential for correct interpretation of the images. Digital imaging allows improved education of students, junior doctors, pediatricians, and parents. Digital imaging-based telemedicine offers the opportunity for standardized evaluation of ROP irrespective of local circumstances**

5.6 Conclusions

Prerequisites for effective prevention of severe visual handicap in premature children are adequate screening and correct interpretation of the findings. National evidence-based guidelines have been developed from multicenter studies. Because of increasing knowledge with the natural course of the disease and the anatomical and functional outcome with actual treatment regimes, new treatment recommendations have recently evolved that eventually may modify actual guidelines. Because of late sequelae such as ametropia, amblyopia, strabismus, secondary glaucoma, and secondary retinal detachment, life-long ophthalmological examinations are mandatory.

References

1. Anonymous (1997) Screening examination of premature infants for retinopathy of prematurity. A joint statement of the American Academy of Pediatric, the American Association for Pediatric Ophthalmology and Strabismus, and the American Academy of Ophthalmology. Ophthalmology 104:888–889
2. Ashton N (1966) Oxygen and the growth and development of retinal vessels. In vivo and in vitro studies. The XX Francis I. Proctor Lecture. Am J Ophthalmol 62:412–435
3. Avery ME, Oppenheimer EH (1960) Recent advances in mortality from hyaline membrane disease. J Pediatr 57:553–559
4. Brown GC, Tasman WS, Naidoff M, Schaffer DB, Quinn G, Bhutani VK (1990) Systemic complications associated with retinal cryoablation for retinopathy of prematurity. Ophthalmology 97: 855–858
5. Campbell PB, Bull MJ, Ellis FD, Bryson CQ, Lemons JA, Schreiner RL (1983) Incidence of retinopathy of prematurity in a tertiary newborn intensive care unit. Arch Ophthalmol 101: 1686–1688
6. Capone A Jr, Diaz-Rohena R, Sternberg P Jr, Mandell B, Lambert HM, Lopez PF (1993) Diode-laser photocoagulation for zone 1 threshold retinopathy of prematurity. Am J Ophthalmol 116:444–450
7. Clarke WN, Hodges E, Noel LP, Roberts D, Coneys M (1985) The oculocardiac reflex during ophthalmoscopy in premature infants. Am J Ophthalmol 99:649–651
8. Clemens S, Eckardt C, Gerding H, Grote A, Jandeck C, Kellner U et al (1999) Augenärztliche Screening-Untersuchung von Frühgeborenen. Ophthalmologe 96:257–263
9. The Committee for the Classification of Retinopathy of Prematurity (1984) An international classification of retinopathy of prematurity. Arch Ophthalmol 102:1130–1134
10. Cryotherapy for Retinopathy of Prematurity Cooperative Group (1988) Multicenter trial of cryotherapy for retinopathy of prematurity. Preliminary results. Arch Ophthalmol 106:471–479
11. Cryotherapy for Retinopathy of Prematurity Cooperative Group (1988) Multicenter trial of cryotherapy for retinopathy of prematurity: preliminary results. Pediatrics 81:697–706
12. Cryotherapy for Retinopathy of Prematurity Cooperative Group (1990) Multicenter trial of cryotherapy for retinopathy of prematurity. One-year outcome – structure and function. Arch Ophthalmol 108:1408–1416
13. Cryotherapy for Retinopathy of Prematurity Cooperative Group (1990) Multicenter trial of cryotherapy for retinopathy of prematurity. Three-month outcome. Arch Ophthalmol 108: 195–204
14. Cryotherapy for Retinopathy of Prematurity Cooperative Group (1993) Multicenter trial of cryotherapy for retinopathy of prematurity. 3 1/2-year outcome – structure and function. Arch Ophthalmol 111:339–344
15. Cryotherapy for Retinopathy of Prematurity Cooperative Group (2001) Multicenter Trial of Cryotherapy for Retinopathy of Prematurity: ophthalmological outcomes at 10 years. Cryotherapy for Retinopathy of Prematurity Cooperative Group. Arch Ophthalmol 119:1110–1118
16. Early Treatment for Retinopathy of Prematurity Cooperative Group (2003) Revised indications for the treatment of retinopathy of prematurity: results of the early treatment for retinopathy of prematurity randomized trial. Arch Ophthalmol 121:1684–1694
17. Elflein H, Lorenz B (2005) Improved screening for retinopathy of prematurity – demonstration of telemedical solution. In: Yogi S, Len J (eds) Teleophthalmology. Springer, New York, Berlin, Heidelberg
18. Ells AL, Holmes JM, Astle WF, Williams G, Leske DA, Fielden M et al (2003) Telemedicine approach to screening for severe retinopathy of prematurity: a pilot study. Ophthalmology 110:2113–2117

19. Fallaha N, Lynn MJ, Aaberg TM Jr, Lambert SR (2002) Clinical outcome of confluent laser photoablation for retinopathy of prematurity. J AAPOS 6:81–85
20. Flynn JT (1987) Retinopathy of prematurity. Pediatr Clin North Am 34:1487–1516
21. Flynn JT, O'Grady GE, Herrera J, Kushner BJ, Cantolino S, Milam W (1977) Retrolental fibroplasia: I. Clinical observations. Arch Ophthalmol 95:217–223
22. Foos RY, Kopelow SM (1973) Development of retinal vasculature in paranatal infants. Surv Ophthalmol 18:117–127
23. Gallagher K, Moseley MJ, Tandon A, Watson MP, Cocker KD, Fielder AR (2003) Nasotemporal asymmetry of retinopathy of prematurity. Arch Ophthalmol 121:1563–1568
24. Gilbert C, Fielder A, Gordillo L, Quinn G, Semiglia R, Visintin P et al (2005) Characteristics of infants with severe retinopathy of prematurity in countries with low, moderate, and high levels of development: implications for screening programs. Pediatrics 115:e518–e525
25. Hardy RJ, Palmer EA, Dobson V, Summers CG, Phelps DL, Quinn GE et al (2003) Risk analysis of prethreshold retinopathy of prematurity. Arch Ophthalmol 121:1697–1701
26. Hardy RJ, Palmer EA, Schaffer DB, Phelps DL, Davis BR, Cooper CJ (1997) Outcome-based management of retinopathy of prematurity. Multicenter Trial of Cryotherapy for Retinopathy of prematurity Cooperative Group. J AAPOS 1:46–54
27. Hunter DG, Repka MX (1993) Diode laser photocoagulation for threshold retinopathy of prematurity. A randomized study. Ophthalmology 100: 238–244
28. The International Committee for the Classification of the Late Stages of Retinopathy of Prematurity (1987) An international classification of retinopathy of prematurity. II. The classification of retinal detachment. Arch Ophthalmol 105:906–912
29. Iverson DA, Trese MT, Orgel IK, Williams GA (1991) Laser photocoagulation for threshold retinopathy of prematurity. Arch Ophthalmol 109:1342–1343
30. Lambert SR, Capone A Jr, Cingle KA, Drack AV (2000) Cataract and phthisis bulbi after laser photoablation for threshold retinopathy of prematurity. Am J Ophthalmol 129:585–591
31. Larsson E, Holmstrom G (2002) Screening for retinopathy of prematurity: evaluation and modification of guidelines. Br J Ophthalmol 86:1399–1402
32. Larsson E, Carle-Petrelius B, Cernerud G, Ots L, Wallin A, Holmstrom G (2002) Incidence of ROP in two consecutive Swedish population based studies. Br J Ophthalmol 86:1122–1126
33. Laser ROP Study Group (1994) Laser therapy for retinopathy of prematurity. Arch Ophthalmol 112:154–156
34. Lorenz B, Bock M, Müller HM, Massie NA (1999) Telemedicine based screening of infants at risk for retinopathy of prematurity. Stud Health Technol Inform 64:155–163
35. Mathew MR, Fern AI, Hill R (2002) Retinopathy of prematurity: are we screening too many babies? Eye 16:538–542
36. McDonald AD (1963) Cerebral palsy in children of very low birth weight. Arch Dis Child 38:579–588
37. McNamara JA, Tasman W, Brown GC, Federman JL (1991) Laser photocoagulation for stage 3+ retinopathy of prematurity. Ophthalmology 98: 576–580
38. O'Keefe M, O'Reilly J, Lanigan B (1998) Longer-term visual outcome of eyes with retinopathy of prematurity treated with cryotherapy or diode laser. Br J Ophthalmol 82:1246–1248
39. Ober RR, Palmer EA, Drack AV, Wright KW (2003) Retinopathy of prematurity. In: Wright KW, Spiegel PH (eds) Pediatric Ophthalmology and strabismus. Springer, Berlin Heidelberg New York, pp 600–628
40. Palmer EA, Flynn JT, Hardy RJ, Phelps DL, Phillips CL, Schaffer DB et al (1991) Incidence and early course of retinopathy of prematurity. The Cryotherapy for Retinopathy of Prematurity Cooperative Group. Ophthalmology 98:1628–1640
41. Pearce IA, Pennie FC, Gannon LM, Weindling AM, Clark DI (1998) Three year visual outcome for treated stage 3 retinopathy of prematurity: cryotherapy versus laser. Br J Ophthalmol 82:1254–1259
42. Prenner JL, Capone A Jr, Trese MT (2004) Visual outcomes after lens-sparing vitrectomy for stage 4A retinopathy of prematurity. Ophthalmology 111:2271–2273
43. Roth DB, Morales D, Feuer WJ, Hess D, Johnson RA, Flynn JT (2001) Screening for retinopathy of prematurity employing the RetCam 120: sensitivity and specificity. Arch Ophthalmol 119:268–272
44. Schaffer DB, Palmer EA, Plotsky DF, Metz HS, Flynn JT, Tung B et al (1993) Prognostic factors in the natural course of retinopathy of prematurity. The Cryotherapy for Retinopathy of Prematurity Cooperative Group. Ophthalmology 100:230–237

45. Schwartz SD, Harrison SA, Ferrone PJ, Trese MT (2000) Telemedical evaluation and management of retinopathy of prematurity using a fiberoptic digital fundus camera. Ophthalmology 107:25–28
46. Seiberth V, Woldt C (2001) Weitwinkelfundusdokumentation bei Retinopathia praematurorum. Ophthalmologe 98:960–963
47. Silverman W (1980) Retrolental fibroplasia: a modern parable. Grune & Stratton, New York
48. Sommer C, Gouillard C, Brugniart C, Talmud M, Bednarek N, Morville P (2003) Dépistage et suivi de la rétinopathie du prématuré par camera de rétine (Retcam 120) : expérience d'une équipe de néonatalogistes à propos de 145 cas. Arch Pediatr 10:694–699
49. Subhani M, Combs A, Weber P, Gerontis C, DeCristofaro JD (2001) Screening guidelines for retinopathy of prematurity: the need for revision in extremely low birth weight infants. Pediatrics 107:656–659
50. Terry TL (1943) Extreme prematurity and fibroblastic overgrowth of persistent vascular sheath behind each crystalline lens. II. Report of cases. Am J Ophthalmol 29:36–53
51. White JE, Repka MX (1997) Randomized comparison of diode laser photocoagulation versus cryotherapy for threshold retinopathy of prematurity: 3-year outcome. J Pediatr Ophthalmol Strabismus 34:83–87
52. Wright K, Anderson ME, Walker E, Lorch V (1998) Should fewer premature infants be screened for retinopathy of prematurity in the managed care era? Pediatrics 102:31–34
53. Yen KG, Hess D, Burke B, Johnson RA, Feuer WJ, Flynn JT (2000) The optimum time to employ telephotoscreening to detect retinopathy of prematurity. Trans Am Ophthalmol Soc 98:145–151
54. Yen KG, Hess D, Burke B, Johnson RA, Feuer WJ, Flynn JT (2002) Telephotoscreening to detect retinopathy of prematurity: preliminary study of the optimum time to employ digital fundus camera imaging to detect ROP. J AAPOS 6:64–70
55. Anonymous (1996) Report of a Joint Working Party of the Royal College of Ophthalmologists and British Association of Perinatal Medicine. Retinopathy of prematurity: guidelines for screening and treatment. Early Hum Dev 46:239–258
56. Holmström G, el Azazi M, Jacobson L et al. (1993) A population-based, prospective study of the development of ROP in prematurely born children in the Stockholm area of Sweden. Br J Ophthalmol 77:417–23.
57. Anonymous (2000) Canadian Association of Pediatric Ophthalmologists Ad Hoc Committee on Standards of Screening Examination for Retinopathy of Prematurity. Guidelines for screening examination for retinopathy of prematurity. Can J Ophthalmol 35:251–252.
58. Anonymous (2001) Screening Examination of Premature Infants for Retinopathy of Prematurity. Pediatrics, 108:809–811
59. Reynolds JD, Dobson V, Quinn GE, Fielder AR, Palmer EA, Saunders RA, Hardy RJ, Phelps EL, Baker JD, Trese MT, Schaffer D, Tung B (2002) Evidence-based Screening Criteria for retinopathy of Prematurity – Natural History Data from the CRO-ROP and LIGHT-ROP studies. Arch. Ophthalmol. 120:1470–1476

Controversies in the Management of Infantile Cataract

6

Scott R. Lambert

Core Messages

- Eyes with congenital cataracts are being more successfully rehabilitated than they were in the past
- The best visual results are achieved in children with unilateral congenital cataracts if treatment is initiated during the first 6 weeks of life
- Cataract surgery during the first 4 weeks of life may increase the risk of an eye developing aphakic glaucoma
- Intraocular lens implantation during infancy appears to increase the risk of reoperations
- The Infant Aphakia Treatment Study is a multicenter clinical trial comparing IOLs and contact lenses for the treatment of infants with unilateral congenital cataracts

6.1 Introduction

The management of infantile cataracts is one of the most controversial topics in the field of pediatric ophthalmology. Three issues in particular divide the pediatric ophthalmology community. The first issue is the optimal age to perform cataract surgery in a neonate with a cataract. While some authors have recommended performing cataract surgery as soon as possible, others have recommended waiting until a child is at least 4 weeks of age. The second issue is whether it is better to implant an intraocular lens (IOL) as a primary procedure during infancy or wait to implant an IOL as a secondary procedure later in childhood. The final issue is whether it is better to perform bilateral simultaneous cataract surgery or two separate surgeries in infants with bilateral cataracts.

6.1.1 Epidemiology

Data on the birth prevalence of infantile cataracts come from a variety of surveillance systems in the US and Europe (Table 6.1). Data from the US comes primarily from birth certificates, passive surveillance systems, such as the Birth Defects Monitoring Program (BDMP), active surveillance systems such as the Metropolitan Atlanta Congenital Defects Program (MACDP), and clinical examination of populations. Based on these studies, and the data from the British Congenital Cataract Interest Group in particular [37], the true prevalence of congenital cataracts is probably 2.5 per 10,000 live births, but it may be as high as 3.0 per 10,000. These studies suggest that 40–45% of all infantile cataracts are unilateral (Fig. 6.1). Therefore, we would expect approximately 1,000 children to be born each year in the U.S. with visually significant cataracts, of which approximately 400 would be unilateral.

Table 6.1. Prevalence of congenital cataracts reported in the literature

Study	Population	Method	Prevalence Per 10,000	% Monocular	Comments
BDMP [19]	USA	Passive	1.2	N/A	Obtained from neonatal discharge summaries. Likely to underestimate the true prevalence since only identifies those cases diagnosed at birth.
MACDP [19]	USA Metro. Atlanta	Active	1.9	56%	Cases must be diagnosed by 12 months of age. Identified by reviewing records of hospitals, therefore would miss cases not receiving surgery or in whom the surgery was done as an outpatient.
United Kingdom Birth Cohort Study [41]	United Kingdom	Clinical exam	5.6	41%	Examined all 12,853 children born in Britain between April 5 and 11, 1970. Imprecise estimate because of the small sample size.
Oxfordshire Birth Cohort Study [40]	United Kingdom	Active	3.0	N/A	The ocular records of all preschool children born in 1984 in Oxfordshire were examined. The cataracts in one patient were visually insignificant.
British Congenital Cataract Interest Group [37]	United Kingdom	Active	2.5	35%	Most comprehensive study. Ascertained an estimated 92% of all newly diagnosed cases of congenital cataract in the UK between 10/95 and 10/96.

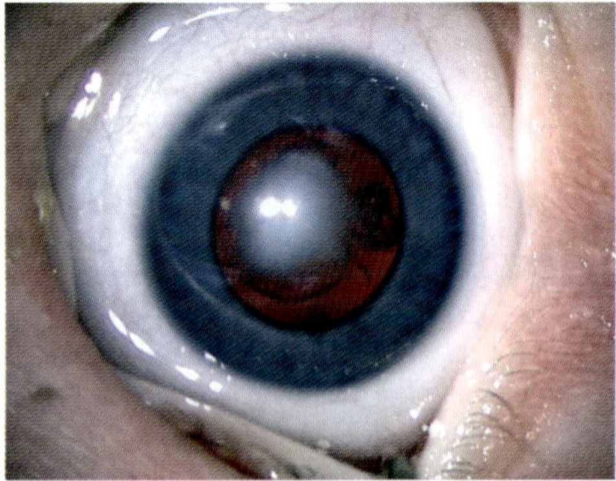

Fig. 6.1. Nuclear cataract in the right eye of a 4-week-old child. The left eye was normal

6.2 Optimal Age for Infantile Cataract Surgery

The optimal age to perform cataract surgery in an infant with an infantile cataract remains controversial. As recently as the 1970s, it was recommended that surgery be deferred until an infant was 3–6 months of age [39]. However, following the pioneering work of Wiesel and Hubel [45] on the plasticity of the visual system during infancy, the trend shifted toward performing cataract surgery at younger and younger ages. The trend climaxed in a case report of a newborn undergoing cataract surgery on the 2nd day of life [14]. Other series have also noted excellent visual outcomes in neonates undergoing cataract surgery during the 1st week of life [11]; however, an analysis of 45 children with dense unilateral cataracts who underwent cataract surgery found that the visual outcome was the same regardless of when the surgery was performed during the first 6 weeks of life [6]. It is generally accepted that a latent period exists for 6 weeks in newborns with unilateral cataracts prior to them entering a sensitive period during which time they are susceptible to visual deprivation. While in the past is was presumed that the latent period for infants with bilateral cataracts extended to 8 weeks of age [1, 30], a recent analysis found that it may even extend to 10 weeks of age [26]. While it is now generally accepted that the best visual outcomes are obtained if cataract surgery is performed during the first 6 weeks of life for an infant with a unilateral cataract and 8–10 weeks of life for an infant with bilateral cataracts, it is unclear if the visual outcome is better if surgery is performed as early as possible within this latent period. In a recent study of infants with unilateral cataracts who underwent cataract surgery during the first 6 weeks of life, the visual outcome correlated more closely with factors such as patching and contact lens compliance than the age of the child within this 6-week window [25]. In fact, very early cataract surgery may increase the risk of certain postoperative complications such as glaucoma and pupillary membranes. In addition, general anesthesia may be associated with more risks in a newborn than a 4-week-old infant.

6.2.1 Aphakic Glaucoma

One of the most serious complications that can occur following pediatric cataract surgery is glaucoma. It is usually open angle and has been reported to develop in up to one-third of children after a lensectomy and vitrectomy. Known risk factors for aphakic glaucoma include microcornea, persistent fetal vasculature, and cataract surgery during infancy. Parks and coworkers [35] reported that 54% of the children in their series who developed aphakic glaucoma underwent cataract surgery when they were younger than 2 months of age. Rabiah [36] reported that 37% of children undergoing cataract surgery when 9 months of age or younger developed glaucoma compared to only 6% of children undergoing surgery thereafter. Vishwanath and colleagues [43] noted that 50% of children undergoing bilateral lensectomies during the 1st month of life developed glaucoma in one or both eyes after a 5-year follow-up compared to only 15% of children undergoing cataract surgery when 1 month of age or older. Lundvall and Kugelberg [30] also reported that 80% of the children in their series who developed glaucoma underwent cataract surgery during the first 4 weeks of life. Finally, Watts and co-workers [44] reported that aphakic glaucoma was more prevalent in children undergoing surgery when 14–34 days of age. While it is possible that eyes with congenital cataracts requiring very early surgery are more prone to developing glaucoma than eyes that acquire cataracts later in infancy, it is more likely that very early surgery increases the risk of these eyes developing glaucoma. For this reason, Vishwanath and coworkers [43] have proposed that cataract surgery should be deferred until after the first 4 weeks of life.

6.2.2 Pupillary Membranes

Pupillary membranes are a common complication following infantile cataract surgery. When these membranes are relatively thin, they may be opened with a YAG laser. When thicker, intraocular surgery may be necessary to adequately excise them. They are particularly common in microphthalmic eyes that undergo cataract surgery coupled with IOL implantation during the neonatal period [23, 42]. The increased incidence of pupillary membranes in infants is likely related to the more exuberant inflammatory reaction occurring in infantile eyes following cataract surgery. The increased incidence in pseudophakic eyes is likely related to a tendency for fibrin to become organized on the surface of IOLs.

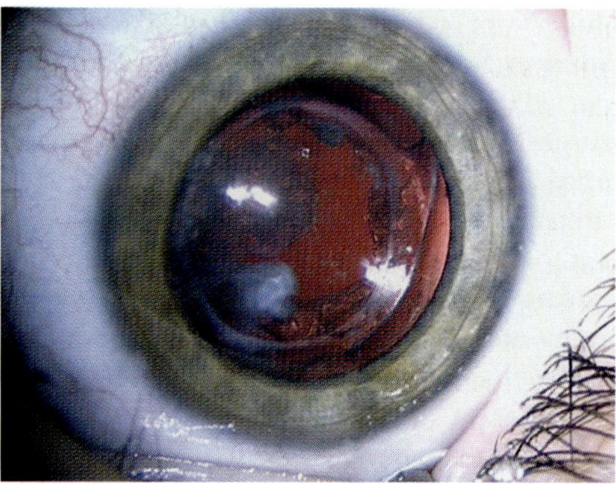

Fig. 6.2. Lens reproliferation anterior and posterior to an IOL 7 months following cataract surgery. The lens material was aspirated using a limbal approach

6.2.3
Lens Reproliferation

Lens reproliferation occurs universally in infantile eyes after cataract surgery. It usually occurs in the retroiridian space and becomes encapsulated within the remnants of the anterior and posterior lens capsules. When encapsulated in the lens capsule, this opaque lens material is referred to as Soemmerring's ring. On occasion, regenerating lens material may extend into the pupillary opening and obstruct the visual axis (Fig. 6.2). This may occur more frequently when radial tears are present in the anterior lens capsule and after intraocular lens implantation. In both cases, the capsular leaflets may not completely fuse together, thereby creating a conduit through which lens material can extrude into the pupillary space. Surgery during the neonatal period seems to increase the risk of this complication developing [42].

6.2.4
General Anesthesia During the Neonatal Period

A final factor to consider when deciding on an optimal age to perform cataract surgery in an infant is the relative risk of general anesthesia at different ages. The immaturity of an infant's cardiovascular, pulmonary, and gastrointestinal systems, as well as their liver, kidneys, and thermoregulation puts them at increased risk from general anesthesia [32]. The most life-threatening risk to an infant is postoperative apnea, which has been shown to be higher in preterm infants less than 44 postconception weeks of age [45]. For this reason, it has been recommended that all nonessential surgery be delayed for preterm infants until they are 44 postconception weeks of age or older [15]. While an increased risk of postoperative apnea in a full-term infant following general anesthesia has not been established, waiting until an infant is older to perform cataract surgery allows all of their systems to mature further and should therefore be safer.

Summary for the Clinician

- **The optimal time to remove a dense unilateral cataract in an infant and to initiate optical treatment are within the first 6 weeks of life**
- **The optimal time to remove dense bilateral cataracts in an infant and to initiate optical treatment are within the first 10 weeks of life**
- **Removing a cataract before an infant is 4 weeks of age may increase the risk of this eye developing aphakic glaucoma, pupillary membranes, and lens reproliferation into the pupillary opening**
- **General anesthesia is associated with a higher incidence of postoperative apnea in preterm infants younger than 44 postconception weeks of age**
- **In most cases, cataract surgery should be deferred until an infant is 4 weeks of age**

6.3
Visual Rehabilitation in Children with a Unilateral Congenital Cataract

Until the 1970s, it was generally believed that there was no means of restoring vision in an eye with a unilateral congenital cataract (UCC). In 1973, Frey and co-workers [10] reported that a good visual outcome could be achieved on occasion in an infant with a unilateral cataract. Subsequently, Beller and Hoyt [3] demonstrated that excellent visual results could be obtained in selected children with a UCC with early treatment and excellent contact lens (CL) and patching compliance. They emphasized the importance of early treatment. Although case reports have documented excellent visual results in an occasional child with a UCC treated with early surgery, CL correction, and patching of the unaffected eye [7], the majority of these eyes continued to have a poor visual outcome [27]. Obstacles to achieving a good visual outcome include a delay in diagnosis and poor compliance with CL wear and patching therapy.

6.3.1 Visual Rehabilitation in Children with Bilateral Congenital Cataracts

The visual outcome of children with bilateral congenital cataracts has improved dramatically over the past 30 years. For example, while in 1971, 10% of the children enrolled in the Western Pennsylvania School for the Blind had been treated for cataracts, the percentage had dropped to 1% by 1991 [5]. Nevertheless, as many as one-quarter of children in the US with bilateral infantile cataracts still remain legally blind even after cataract surgery and optical correction. The visual outcome is even worse for children with bilateral infantile cataracts in developing countries, primarily due to a delay in the diagnosis and treatment of their cataracts. For example, Jain [18] reported that in India most children with congenital cataracts do not undergo cataract surgery until they are 1–5 years of age.

6.3.2 Contact Lenses

Contact lenses have been the preferred means of optically correcting aphakia in infants because they more closely simulate the optics of the crystalline lens than do spectacles. During the first 4 years of life, an aphakic infantile eye undergoes a mean decrease in its refractive error of 9–15 D [27, 33]. Therefore, the ability to easily change the power of a CL as refractive needs change is a significant advantage. Excellent visual acuities have been obtained in infants with bilateral aphakia using CLs, with up to two-thirds of these children achieving 20/40 or better visual acuity in at least one eye [11, 29]. Contact lens compliance is usually good for children with bilateral aphakia and if they become CL intolerant, they can be treated with spectacles.

The treatment of monocular aphakia during infancy with CLs has been less successful. In published series, only 8–24% of these eyes achieved 20/40 or better visual acuity and the majority saw 20/200 or worse [29, 34]. These poor visual outcomes largely arise from poor CL and patching compliance. The poor visual acuity in the aphakic eye then makes it more difficult to patch the fellow eye, which then causes further visual deterioration. Ultimately, many parents abandon patching and CL treatment for their child due to the difficulty and time demands of this treatment regimen. Assaf and co-workers [2] reported that only 44% of children with unilateral aphakia were wearing their CL when they returned for follow-up. Poor compliance in these patients is multifactorial but lens loss, difficulty inserting and removing CLs in a small child, and the absence of a discernible visual benefit – since the fellow eye has normal vision – all contribute to poor CL compliance. The resulting poor vision in the aphakic eye then creates a number of problems. First, there is a greater risk of the normal eye being injured [38]. Second, if their fellow eye becomes blind secondary to injury or disease later in life they do not have a back-up eye with useful vision. Lastly, many of these patients develop a sensory strabismus, which often must be corrected surgically.

6.3.3 Intraocular Lenses

IOLs are now the standard optical treatment for older children with aphakia, but their use during infancy is still controversial because of concerns regarding their safety in a growing eye with an anticipated large myopic shift. However, a growing body of literature describes favorable

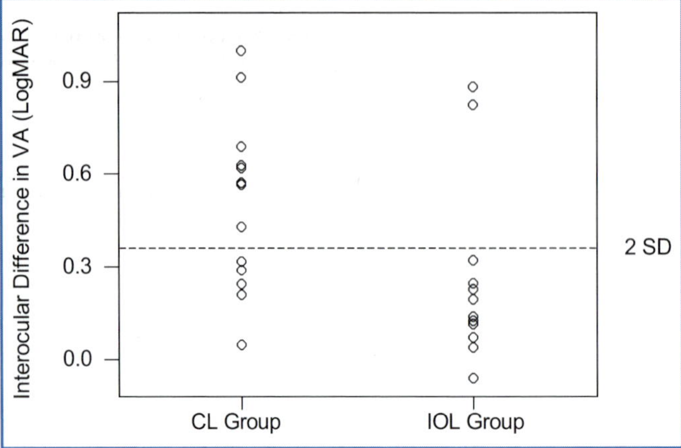

Fig. 6.3. The difference in grating visual acuity (LogMAR) between the affected and unaffected eyes according to treatment group. The line labeled 2 SD is 2 standard deviations beyond the mean normal for interocular acuity differences at 12 months of age (0.36). The mean interocular difference in grating acuity for the patients in the IOL group (0.26) is significantly lower than the mean for the patients in the CL group (0.50) (p=0.048)

outcomes achieved with IOL implantation in infants with UCCs. After a 17-year follow-up, Ben Ezra [4] reported 20/60 visual acuity and a myopic shift from +2.5 D to −4.75 D in the pseudophakic eye of a patient who underwent a unilateral lensectomy, posterior capsulotomy, and anterior vitrectomy when 10 weeks of age. Dahan [9] implanted an IOL in 17 infants after unilateral cataract surgery. After a mean follow-up of 7.5 years (range, 2–11.5 years), the pseudophakic eyes in these 17 children had a mean visual acuity of 20/60 (range, 20/30–20/200). The mean initial postoperative refractive error in these pseudophakic eyes was +6.4 D (range, +3 to +9 D); and the mean last refractive error was −1.0 D (range, +3.50 to −8.0 D). The mean myopic shift was −7.4 D (range, −2.50 to −12.75 D), slightly less than the 9–15 D, which has been reported in monocularly aphakic children corrected with CLs [33].

A retrospective study in the US evaluated 39 infants at five clinical centers who underwent cataract surgery with or without the implantation of an IOL [23]. After surgery, the aphakic patients wore aphakic CLs while the pseudophakic patients had their residual refractive error corrected with spectacles. Traveling testers then assessed grating acuity, ocular alignment, and reoperation rates for 25 of these patients.

The mean age at the time of surgery for the 13 aphakic children tested by the traveling testers was 9 weeks (range, 2–21 weeks) compared to 11 weeks (range, 3–22 weeks) for the 12 pseudophakic children (p=0.5). The mean length of follow-up for the aphakic children was 18 months (range, 7–27 months) vs 15 months (range, 4–27 months) for the pseudophakic children (p=0.3). The median LogMar grating acuity of the pseudophakic eyes was 0.60 (range, 0.32–1.31) compared to 0.73 (range, 0.53–1.44) for the CL treated aphakic eyes (p=0.09). The median LogMar grating acuity for the fellow eyes of the pseudophakic children was 0.40 (range, 0.26–0.73) compared to 0.32 for the fellow eyes of the aphakic children (range, 0.02–0.75, p=0.33). The median interocular difference between pseudophakic and aphakic children was statistically significant (0.17 vs 0.57, p=0.03). Figure 6.3 displays the interocular difference between affected and unaffected eyes for the two groups. The line labeled 2 SD shows two standard deviations beyond mean normal interocular difference.

Eight (67%) of the pseudophakic patients underwent reoperations 2–20 weeks following cataract surgery. None of the aphakic patients required a reoperation. In two pseudophakic patients, a reoperation was performed to free iris that was adherent to the cataract incision site causing corectopia. Two pseudophakic patients underwent reoperations to aspirate regenerated lens material that extended into the visual axis. Two eyes underwent pars plana vitrectomies to excise pupillary membranes; in one of these patients, the membrane recurred, necessitating a second reoperation. Two eyes

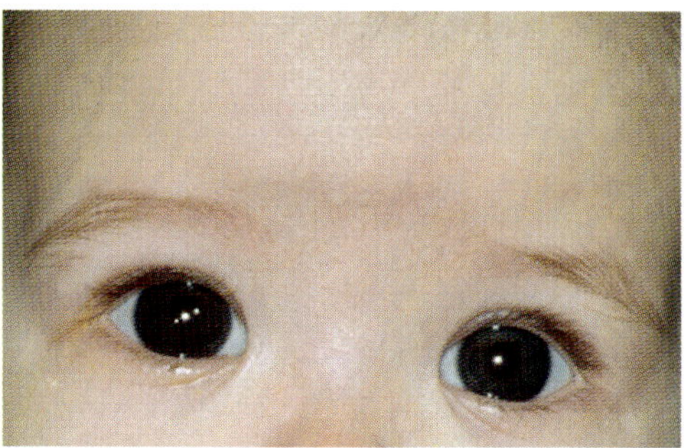

Fig. 6.4. Buphthalmos secondary to glaucoma in a 3-month-old child who underwent cataract surgery and the primary implantation of an IOL in the right eye when 3 weeks of age. The glaucoma was treated with a suture trabeculotomy. The intraocular pressure has remained in the normal range off all medication for the past 4 years

underwent posterior synechiolysis while undergoing other procedures. Finally, two pseudophakic patients underwent a reoperations to treat open angle glaucoma. Both of these patients presented with buphthalmos, corneal edema, and raised IOP (35 and 30 mmHg) (Fig. 6.4). They were initially treated with medical therapy; surgery was performed when medical treatment was inadequate. In both cases, the children had undergone cataract surgery and IOL implantation when less than 4 weeks of age. Patient 1 underwent a 270° trabeculotomy using a 6-0 Prolene suture when 11 weeks of age. At the time of surgery, gonioscopy revealed that the angle was open except for two peripheral anterior synechiae along the cataract incision site. The intraocular pressure has remained in the normal range in this eye off all mediations after a 4-year follow-up. Patient 10 had a Baerveldt implant placed when 6.3 months of age.

The pseudophakic eyes (n=11) had a mean refractive error of +6.81 ± 4.35 D (range, +2 to +12.75 D) 4 weeks following cataract surgery. After a mean follow-up of 13 ± 6 months (range, 5–22 months), their mean refractive error was +1.32 ± 3.94 D (range, –6.0 to +5.5 D).

The Snellen acuities and reoperation rates were then evaluated for 22 of these 25 children at a mean age of 4.3 years (IOL group, n=10; CL group, n=12) [25]. The visual acuity results were similar in the two treatment groups (p=0.99); however, two of the four (50 %) children in the IOL group compared with two of the seven (28 %) children in the CL group undergoing surgery during the first 6 weeks of life had 20/40 or better visual acuity. None of the children in either treatment group had visual acuity of 20/40 or better when cataract surgery was performed after the child was 7 weeks of age or older. Three (27 %) patients in the CL group and two (25 %) patients in the IOL group had a visual acuity worse than 20/400. The children in the IOL group had a mean of 1.1 reoperations (range, 1–2), whereas the children in the CL group had a mean of 0.36 reoperations (p=0.09). The most common reoperation in the IOL group were membranectomies (n=8) whereas the most common reoperation in the CL was the implantation of a secondary IOL (n=4). In addition, four (40 %) children in the IOL group and six (55 %) children in the CL group underwent strabismus surgery.

Summary for the Clinician (Table 6.2)

- **Small noncontrolled studies suggest that infants undergoing cataract surgery coupled with primary IOL implantation**
  - **Will require more reoperations**
  - **A higher percentage of them will have excellent visual acuity (20/40 or better)**
  - **A similar percentage of them will have a poor visual outcome (<20/400) as aphakic children treated with contact lenses**

6.3.4 Surveys of North American Pediatric Ophthalmologists

In August 1997, the North American members of the American Association of Pediatric Ophthalmology and Strabismus (AAPOS) were surveyed to determine the number of infants they had treated with a unilateral cataract, the frequency of IOL implantation in infants with a unilateral cataract, and the youngest age of a child when they had implanted an IOL [24]. Most respondents (89 %) reported treating at least one infant with a unilateral cataract during the previous year. However, relatively few report-

Table 6.2. Pros and cons of intraocular lens vs contact lens correction of unilateral infantile aphakia

Intraocular lenses	Contact lenses
Arguments for:	
1. Closely approximates the optics of the crystalline lens	1. Power can easily be changed as the eye grows
2. Full-time partial optical correction is guaranteed	2. Secondary IOL can be implanted when the child is older when the refractive error of the eye is stable
3. Limited human data show better visual outcome than CL correction	
Arguments against:	
1. Their long-term safety in a growing eye has not been established	1. Two-thirds or more of patients with this treatment have visual outcome <20/80
2. The surgery required to implant an IOL is technically more difficult	2. Poor CL adherence may reduce patching adherence
3. An overcorrection with spectacles or CLs is needed initially or after the eye if fully grown	3. CLs are frequently lost and there may be a delay in their replacement
4. Limited human data show higher complication rate	4. Ongoing maintenance takes time each day and can be stressful for patients and parents

ed treating many cases (e.g., more than two-thirds reported treating fewer than three cases per year). Only 3.5% of pediatric ophthalmologists had ever implanted an IOL in a child less than 6 months of age. More than one-half (52%) of the respondents expressed a willingness to participate in a clinical trial comparing IOLs and CLs as a means of optically correcting aphakia in infants following unilateral cataract surgery.

In June 2001, the membership of AAPOS was again surveyed to ascertain (a) their relative preference for CL vs IOLs to optically correct infants with unilateral aphakia, (b) their concerns regarding the implantation of an IOL or the use of a CL during infancy, (c) their usage of an IOL to optically correct the last three infants they had treated with cataract surgery, and (d) their willingness to randomize an infant with a unilateral cataract to a clinical trial comparing treatment with an IOL vs a CL. On a scale of 1 to 10 with 1 strongly favoring an IOL and 10 strongly favoring a CL, the median score was 7.5, suggesting that CLs are still the preferred treatment for most pediatric ophthalmologists in North America. Their major concerns with IOL implantation were poor predictability of power changes, surgical complications, inflammation, and the technical difficulty of surgery. The main concerns with CL correction were poor compliance, the high loss rate, high cost, and keratitis. Twenty percent of the respondents had implanted in an infant ≤6 months of age; a sixfold increase since our 1997 survey. The percentage of the respondents who indicated that they would be willing to randomize an infant with a unilateral cataract to treatment with a CL vs an IOL has increased from 52% in 1997 to 61% in 2001.

Summary for the Clinician

- **Most AAPOS members still favor optically correcting infants with contact lenses following cataract surgery**
- **There was a sixfold increase in the number of AAPOS members who had implanted an IOL in an infant's eye between 1997 and 2001**
- **The majority of AAPOS members expressed a willingness to participate in a clinical trial comparing IOLs and contact lenses for the treatment of infants with unilateral cataracts**

6.4 Infant Aphakia Treatment Study

The Infant Aphakia Treatment Study (IATS) is a multicenter randomized clinical trial comparing IOL and CL correction for monocular aphakia. Infants will be eligible for the study who are less than 7 months of age and have a visually significant cataract in one eye. Cataract surgery will be performed in a standardized fashion by a surgeon who has been certified for the study. All patients will undergo a lensectomy, posterior capsulotomy, and anterior vitrectomy. Infants will be randomized at the time of surgery to either IOL implantation or CL correction. Infants randomized to the IOL group will have an IOL implanted into the capsular bag. Spectacles will be used to correct the residual refractive error. Infants randomized to the CL group will be fit with a CL immediately after surgery. All children will be examined by investigators at fixed intervals using standard protocols with the primary outcome being resolution acuity using Teller acuity card, assessed at 12 months of age by a traveling tester. It is anticipated that a second primary outcome examination will be performed on these children when they are 4 years of age using optotype visual acuity. Secondary outcomes will include the number of complications requiring reoperations, the incidence of cosmetically significant strabismus, the magnitude of the myopic shift, and the stress experienced by the parents of these children.

6.4.1 Eligibility Criteria

Eligible patients will have a visually significant unilateral cataract (3 mm dense central opacity) and will be 28–210 days of age at the time of cataract surgery. Patients will be excluded who have an acquired cataract, microphthalmos (corneal diameter <9 mm), glaucoma, anterior persistent fetal vasculature causing stretching of the ciliary processes, uveitis, optic nerve disease, retinal disease, prematurity (<36 gestational weeks), or ocular disease in the fellow eye.

6.4.2 Surgical Procedure for Infants Randomized to Contact Lenses

A lensectomy will be performed by making two stab incisions in the eye. An infusion cannula will be placed in one stab incision. A vitreous-cutting instrument will be inserted through the second incision through which a mechanized anterior capsulotomy, lens aspiration, posterior capsulotomy, and anterior vitrectomy will be performed.

6.4.3 Surgical Procedure for Infants Randomized to IOL

A 3-mm scleral tunnel incision will be created superiorly. An infusion cannula will then be placed in a limbal stab incision lateral to the scleral tunnel incision. A stab incision will then be created in the center of the scleral tunnel incision through which the vitreous cutting instrument will be inserted. An anterior capsulotomy and lens aspiration will be performed in a similar fashion as in the eyes randomized to CL correction. The scleral tunnel incision will then be enlarged and an IOL will be implanted into the capsular bag. A primary posterior capsulotomy and anterior vitrectomy will be created in a standardized fashion through the pars plana. Three approaches have been used to create a primary posterior capsulotomy: (a) a limbal incision prior to IOL implantation, (b) a limbal incision after IOL implantation, and (c) a pars plana incision. Creating a posterior capsulotomy through the limbal incision obviates the need for a second incision, but it makes it more difficult to implant the IOL into the capsular bag, which is believed to enhance the long-term safety of IOL implantation [1]. Implanting the IOL first and then creating a primary capsulotomy through the pars plana simplifies the placement of the IOL into the capsular bag, but increases the risk of long-term retinal complications stemming from an iatrogenic retinal break or vitreous incarcerated in the pars plana incision site [8]. Performing the posterior capsulotomy and vitrectomy through the limbal incision after implanting the IOL offers the benefits of both approaches but can be technically challenging. Gimbel [12] advocated performing a posterior capsulorrhexis and then prolapsing the optic through the posterior capsulotomy without performing an anterior vitrectomy, but this surgical technique has only been performed on older children and the anterior hyaloid face frequently opacifies after this procedure, necessitating reoperation [27].

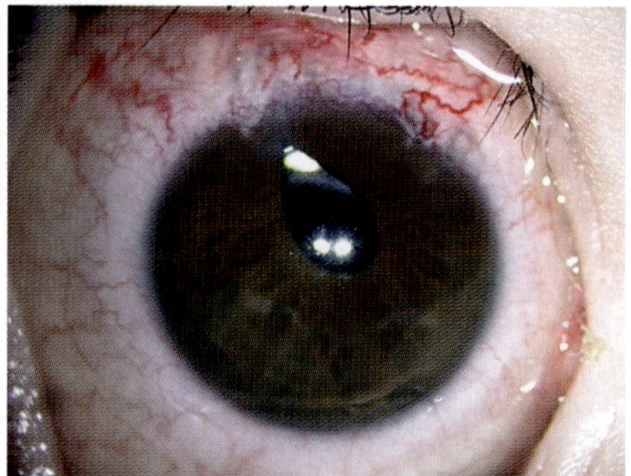

Fig. 6.5. Corectopia in a 12-month-old child who was hit in the eye 4 days following the implantation of a secondary IOL. The child had had a unilateral cataract in this eye and underwent a lensectomy when 4 weeks of age. After losing multiple contact lenses, her parents requested a secondary IOL. An acrylic IOL was implanted into the capsular bag through a 3.2-mm scleral tunnel incision after opening the anterior and posterior capsular leaflets. When the corectopia was repaired, it was noted that there was vitreous to the wound, but the IOL remained centered in the capsular bag

6.4.4 Type of IOL

The design of and materials used for IOLs continue to evolve. Improvements in lens construction and the use of more stable polymers have led to less postoperative inflammation, lens deposits, and capsular opacification. Many newer lenses can be folded, making it possible to implant them through smaller incisions, which reduces the risk of wound dehiscence and makes it possible to achieve a stable refractive error more rapidly following cataract surgery (Fig. 6.5). However, none of these newer lens designs and materials have been used over a long period of time; therefore, their long-term safety is unknown. The current lens material with the longest safety record is polymethylmethacrylate (PMMA), a polymer with over 30 years of use. The safety record of PMMA is excellent, with no reports of problems due to degradation or structural failure. One-piece PMMA lenses have been advocated for use in children because of their long-term record of safety [9]. IOLs made of acrylic have recently gained popularity because they can be folded and inserted through smaller incisions. Acrylic IOLs have become the most commonly implanted IOLs in adults by cataract surgeons. Acrylic lenses also decrease the incidence of posterior capsule opacification, which has decreased the need for subsequent capsular opening procedures. Because of these advantages, the implantation of acrylic IOLs in children is increasing rapidly [48]. Although the long-term safety of acrylic lenses is unknown, no structural or material failures in children have been reported. It is anticipated that in the near future, PMMA lenses will be phased out of routine use in adults and will be reserved only for unusual circumstances. Indications are that this trend is also occurring in the pediatric age group. One-piece all acrylic lenses will be used exclusively in the IATS.

6.4.5 IOL Power

Our targeted postoperative refraction will be an undercorrection of 8 D in children undergoing cataract surgery when 4–6 weeks of age and 6 D for children over 6 weeks of age but under 7 months of age. In our pilot study, we implanted IOLs ranging in power from 24 to 30 D (mean, 26.2 ± 2.3 D); actual mean postoperative refractive error 4 weeks after surgery was +6.81 ± 4.35 D. Mean postoperative myopic shift was 5.49 D after a 1-year follow-up. Initial axial length (p=0.70) or type of IOL implanted (p=1.0) did not correlate with the magnitude of the myopic shift.

McClatchey [31] created a logarithmic model to analyze the rate of refractive growth of 100 pseudophakic and 106 aphakic eyes of children followed longitudinally for 3 or more years. Pseudophakic eyes had a lower rate of refractive growth than the aphakic eyes (–4.6 vs –5.7, p=0.03). These growth rates were then used to create an algorithm to predict the myopic shift that will be experienced by eyes undergoing IOL implantation during the first 6 months of life. It is hoped that the children in IATS will be emmetropic when 2–3 years of age and low myopes later in childhood. By initially undercorrecting these children, we hope to minimize their need for a spectacle overcorrection during much of their childhood.

Summary for the Clinician

- The Infant Aphakia Treatment Study is a multicenter clinical trial comparing IOLs and contact lenses for the treatment of infants with a unilateral cataract
- The primary outcome will be grating acuity at 12 months of age
- Secondary outcomes will be the number of postoperative complications, the magnitude of the myopic shift, the incidence of strabismus and parenting stress

6.5 Bilateral Simultaneous Surgery

While most pediatric ophthalmologists advocate removing bilateral cataracts as two separate procedures to minimize the risk of bilateral endophthalmitis, others favor bilateral simultaneous surgery in selected patients in order to decrease the number of times general anesthesia will be required, to rehabilitate both eyes simultaneously and to reduce the cost of the procedures [16]. Bilateral simultaneous cataract surgery has also been advocated in adults requiring general anesthesia [17]. In children, it has been proposed that bilateral simultaneous surgery be reserved for children who are at increased risk of complications with general anesthesia (Fig. 6.6) [50]. Extra precautions should be taken to minimize the risk of endophthalmitis such as using a different set of surgical instruments for each eye.

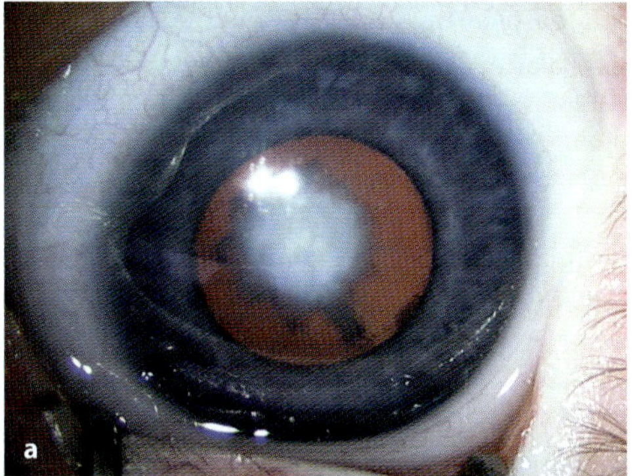

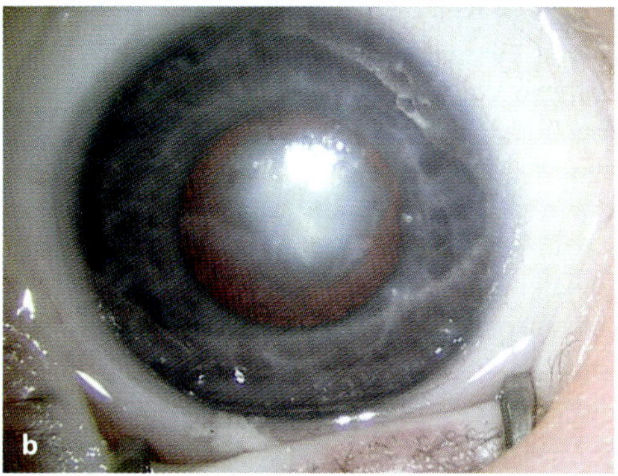

Fig. 6.6 a, b. Bilateral nuclear cataracts in a 4-week-old boy with Lowe syndrome and renal dysfunction. Bilateral simultaneous lensectomies were performed to obviate the need for multiple sessions of general anesthesia. Postoperatively the child was fit with rigid gas permeable contact lenses

6.5.1 Endophthalmitis

Endophthalmitis is one of the most serious complications that can occur following infantile cataract surgery [46]. It has been reported to have a prevalence of 7/10,000 surgeries, which is similar to the prevalence reported following cataract surgery in adults [20]. In most cases, it is diagnosed within several days of cataract surgery. It is most frequently caused by *Staphylococcus aureus*, *Staphylococcus epidermidis*, *Streptococcus pneumoniae*, and *Streptococcus viridans*. Nasolacrimal duct obstruction, periorbital eczema, and upper respiratory infection are important risk factors for the development of postoperative endophthalmitis. For this reason, nasolacrimal duct obstructions should be treated prior to cataract surgery, and cataract surgery should be postponed if an infant has an upper respiratory infection. Most children have a poor visual outcome following endophthalmitis [13]. In one series, 65 % of the eyes developing postoperative endophthalmitis had a final visual acuity of no light perception.

6.5.2 Visual Rehabilitation

The visual rehabilitation of children with bilateral congenital cataracts is facilitated by removing both cataracts simultaneously since both eyes are more likely to have the same visual experience. Wright [49] has advocated bilateral patching for up to 2 weeks for infants with both unilateral and bilateral congenital cataracts to prevent amblyopia from developing. By performing simultaneous cataract surgery, the risk of unequal visual input to either eye can be minimized.

Summary for the Clinician

- **Bilateral simultaneous cataract surgery may be preferable in infants at increased risk of complications with general anesthesia**
- **The risk of endophthalmitis should be minimized by taking special precautions such as using a separate instrument tray for each eye**

References

1. Ahmadieh H, Javadi MA, Ahmady M et al (1999) Primary capsulotomy, anterior vitrectomy, lensectomy, and posterior chamber lens implantation in children: limbal versus pars plana. J Cataract Refract Surg 25:768–775
2. Assaf AA, Wiggins R, Engel K et al (1994) Compliance with prescribed optical correction in cases of monocular aphakia in children. Saudi J Ophthalmol 8:15–22
3. Beller R, Hoyt CS, Marg E et al (1981) Good visual function after neonatal surgery for congenital monocular cataracts. Am J Ophthalmol 91:559–565
4. Ben Ezra D (1996) Cataract surgery and intraocular lens implantation in children. Am J Ophthalmol 121:224–225
5. Biglan AW (1992) Outcome of treatment for bilateral congenital cataracts. Discussion. Trans Am Ophthalmol Strabismus 90:194–197
6. Birch EE, Stager DR (1996) The critical period for surgical treatment of dense congenital unilateral cataract. Invest Ophthalmol Vis Sci 37:1532–1538
7. Birch EE, Swanson WH, Stager DR et al (1993) Outcome after very early treatment of dense congenital unilateral cataract. Invest Ophthalmol Vis Sci 34:3687–3698
8. Buckley EG, Klombers LA, Seaber JH et al (1993) Management of the posterior capsule during pediatric intraocular lens implantation. Am J Ophthalmol 115:722–728
9. Dahan E, Drusedau MUH (1997) Choice of lens and dioptric power in pediatric pseudophakia. J Cataract Refract Surg 23:618–623
10. Frey T, Friendly D, Wyatt D (1973) Re-evaluation of monocular cataracts in children. Am J Ophthalmol 76:381–388
11. Gelbart SS, Hoyt CS, Jastrebeski G et al (1982) Long-term results in bilateral congenital cataracts. Am J Ophthalmol 93:615–621
12. Gimbel HV (1996) Posterior capsulorhexis with optic capture in pediatric cataract and intraocular lens surgery. Ophthalmology 103:1871–1875
13. Good WV, Hing S, Irvine AR et al (1990) Postoperative endophthalmitis in children following cataract surgery. J Pediatr Ophthalmol Strabismus 27:283–285
14. Gregg FM, Parks MM (1992) Stereopsis after congenital monocular cataract extraction. Am J Ophthalmol 114:314–317
15. Gregory GA, Steward DJ (1983) Life-threatening perioperative apnea in the ex "premie" (editorial). Anesthesiology 59:495
16. Guo S, Nelson LB, Calhoun J et al (1990) Simultaneous surgery for bilateral congenital cataracts. J Pediatr Ophthalmol Strabismus 27:23–25
17. Hug NR, Sturmer J (2003) Simultaneous bilateral cataract extraction – a retrospective study. Klin Monatsbl Augenheilkd 220:106–110
18. Jain IS, Pillay P, Gangwar DN et al (1983) Congenital cataract: etiology and morphology. J Pediatr Ophthalmol Strabismus 20:238–246
19. James LM, McClearon AB, Waters GD (1993) Congenital malformation surveillance. Data for birth defects prevention: Metropolitan Atlanta Congenital Defects Program (MACDP) 1968–1991 and Birth Defects Monitoring Program (BDMP) 1970–1991. Teratology 48:545–709
20. Katan HM, Flynn HW, Pflugfeler SC et al (1991) Nosocomial endophthalmitis surgery. Ophthalmology 98:227–238

21. Koch DD, Kohnen T (1997) Retrospective comparison of techniques to prevent secondary cataract formation after posterior chamber intraocular lens implantation in infants and children. J Cataract Refract Surg 23:657–663
22. Lambert SR, Buckley EG, Plager DA et al (1999) Unilateral intraocular lens implantation during the first six months of life. J AAPOS 3:344–349
23. Lambert SR, Lynn M, Drews-Botsch C et al (2001) A comparison of grating acuity visual acuity, strabismus, and reoperation outcomes among children with aphakia and pseudophakia after unilateral cataract surgery during the first six months of life. J AAPOS 5:70–75
24. Lambert SR, Lynn M, Drews-Botsch C et al (2003) Intraocular lens implantation during infancy: perceptions of parents and the American Association for Pediatric Ophthalmology and Strabismus members. J AAPOS 3:344–349
25. Lambert SR, Lynn M, Drews-Botsch C et al (2004) Optotype acuity and re-operation rate after unilateral cataract surgery during the first 6 months of life with or without IOL implantation. Br J Ophthalmol 88:1387–1390
26. Lambert SR, Lynn M, Reeves R et al: Is there a latent period for the surgical treatment of children with dense bilateral congenital cataracts. J AAPOS (in press)
27. Lorenz B, Wörle J (1991) Visual results in congenital cataract with the use of contact lenses. Graefes Arch Clin Exp Ophthalmol 229:123–132
28. Lorenz B, Wörle J, Friedl N et al (1993) Ocular growth in infant aphakia. Bilateral versus unilateral congenital cataracts. Ophthalmic Paediatr Genet 14:177–178
29. Lorenz B, Wörle J, Friedl N et al (1994) Monocular and binocular functional results in cases of contact lens corrected infant aphakia. In: Cotlier E, Lambert SR, Taylor D (eds) Congenital cataracts. RG Landes/CRC Press, Boca Raton, FL, pp 151–162
30. Lundvall A, Kugelberg U (2002) Outcome after treatment of congenital bilateral cataract. Acta Ophthalmol Scand 80:593–597
31. McClatchey SK, Dahan E, Maselli E et al (2000) A comparison of the rate of refractive growth in pediatric aphakic and pseudophakic eyes. Ophthalmology 107:118–122
32. Miller RD (2000) Developmental physiology of the infant. In: Anesthesia, 5th edn. Churchill Livingstone, Edinburgh, pp 2089–2092
33. Moore BD (1993) Pediatric aphakic contact lens wear: rates of successful wear. J Pediatr Ophthalmol Strabismus 30:253–258
34. Neumann D, Weissman BA, Isenberg SJ et al (1993) The effectiveness of daily wear contact lenses for the correction of infantile aphakia. Arch Ophthalmol 111:927–930
35. Parks MM, Johnson DA, Reed GW (1993) Long-term visual results and complications in children with aphakia. A function of cataract type. Ophthalmology 100:826–841
36. Rabiah PK (2004) Frequency and predictors of glaucoma after pediatric cataract surgery. Am J Ophthalmol 137:30–37
37. Rahi JS, Dezateux on behalf on the British Congenital Cataract Interest Group (1999) National cross-sectional study of detection of congenital and infantile cataract in the United Kingdom: role of childhood screening and surveillance. BMJ 318:362–365
38. Rahi JS, Logan S, Timms C et al (2002) Risk, causes, and outcomes of visual impairment after loss of vision in the non-amblyopic eye: a population-based study. The Lancet 360:597–602
39. Sheppard RW, Crawford JS (1973) The treatment of congenital cataracts. Surv Ophthalmol 17:340–347
40. Stayte JM, Reeves B, Wortham C (1993) Ocular and vision defects in preschool children. Br J Ophthalmol 77:228–232
41. Stewart-Brown SL, Haslum MN (1988) Partial sight and blindness in children of the 1970 birth cohort at 10 years of age. J Epidemiol Community Health 42:17–23
42. Trivedi RH, Eilson ME Jr, Bartholomew LR et al (2004) Opacification of the visual axis after cataract surgery and single acrylic intraocular lens implantation in the first year of life. J AAPOS 8:156–164
43. Vishwanath M, Cheong-Leen R, Taylor D et al (2004) Is early surgery for congenital cataract a risk factor for glaucoma? Br J Ophthalmol 88: 905–910
44. Watts P, Abdolell M, Levin AV (2003) Complications in infants undergoing surgery for congenital cataract in the first 12 weeks of life. Is early surgery better? J AAPOS 7:81–85
45. Welborn LG, Ramirez N, Oh TH et al (1986) Postanesthetic apnea and periodic breathing in infants. Anesthesiology 65:658–661
46. Wheeler DT, Stager DR, Weakley DR Jr (1992) Endophthalmitis following pediatric intraocular surgery for congenital cataracts and congenital glaucoma. J Pediatr Ophthalmol Strabismus 29: 139–141
47. Wiesel TN, Hubel DH (1965) Comparison of the effects of unilateral and bilateral eye closure on cortical unit responses in kittens. J Neurophysiol 28:1029–1040
48. Wilson ME, Elliott L, Johnson B et al (2001) AcrySof acrylic intraocular lens implantation in children: clinical indications of biocompatibility. J AAPOS 5:377–380

49. Wright KW, Spiegel PH (2003) Lens abnormalities. In: Wright KW, Spiegel PH, Pediatric Ophthalmology and Strabismus Springer-Verlag, New York, pp 467–468

50. Zwaan J (1996) Simultaneous surgery for bilateral pediatric cataracts. Ophthalmic Surg Lasers 27:15–20

Management of Infantile Glaucoma

Thomas S. Dietlein, Guenter K. Krieglstein

Core Messages

- Treatment patterns and prognosis of infantile glaucomas are very heterogeneous depending on the underlying pathomechanism of glaucoma
- Glaucoma surgery is the primary option in treatment of infantile glaucoma except when the prognosis for the child's life or that of the eye is very poor or when multiple previous glaucoma surgeries have achieved only limited success
- Several restrictions for medical treatment in infantile glaucoma need to be considered. Brimonidine can cause severe systemic side-effects in children younger than 8 years
- First-line interventions in primary congenital glaucoma are trabeculotomy or trabeculectomy or a combination of both. In cases with a sufficiently clear cornea and good gonioscopic view, goniotomy is also a first-line option
- Second-line interventions in congenital glaucoma are tube implants, which lead to a high rate of reintervention
- In refractory cases or complex malformations with high intra- and postoperative risks, cyclodestructive methods may be an alternative, achieving moderate success in long-term IOP control
- The inflammatory and aphakic glaucomas represent a special group with limited results from any form of surgery. The prognosis of infantile glaucoma surgery in chronic uveitis associated with autoimmune diseases may be influenced by systemic immunomodulative therapy

7.1 Classification

In the ophthalmic literature the term "infantile glaucoma" has been used for a broad and heterogeneous spectrum of glaucoma in childhood. Manifest glaucoma in children younger than 3 years usually causes visible distension of the eye globe (Fig. 7.1), leading to the historical term "buphthalmia" (ox eye). In order to achieve accurate diagnoses and to subdivide this huge disease entity, several authors have proposed classifications of the glaucomas in childhood according to age, morphology of the anterior segment, and the presence of further ocular or systemic abnormalities (Table 7.1). Tomey [54] has presented a very helpful overview of these classifications. Nevertheless, the terms "infantile glaucoma," "congenital glaucoma," and "developmental glaucoma" are frequently used in the literature as synonyms without consideration of

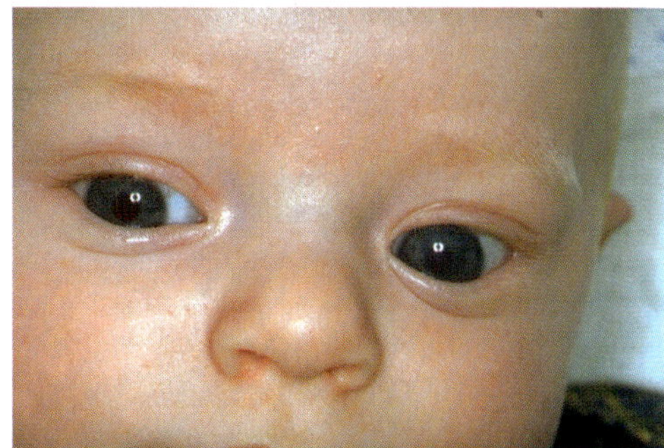

Fig. 7.1. Eleven-month-old boy with primary congenital glaucoma showing enlarged horizontal corneal diameter and slight corneal cloudiness in the left eye

Table 7.1. Classifications of the glaucomas in childhood

Age	Congenital glaucoma	Manifestation at birth or thereafter
	Infantile glaucoma	Manifestation between 1st and 4th year
	Juvenile glaucoma	Manifestation after the 4th year
Associated pathologies	Primary glaucoma	Isolated dysgenesis of the TM
	Secondary glaucomas	Associated ocular or systemic pathology
Morphology of the anterior segment	Trabeculodysgenesis	(e.g., primary congenital glaucoma)
	Iridotrabeculodysgenesis	(e.g., Riegers syndrome)
	Iridocorneotrabeculodysgenesis	(e.g., Peter's anomaly)

exact age. When comparing the outcome of different treatment patterns, it is now mandatory to accurately differentiate the age distribution and the subdiagnoses of the patient group treated.

7.2 Diagnostic Aspects

7.2.1 Clinical Background

Glaucoma in childhood is a relatively rare disease with an incidence of 1 in 10,000 live births [15], which requires special knowledge in management owing to the very heterogeneous pathomechanisms and prognosis of the subgroups. There are some reports of a self-limiting congenital glaucoma [27], but also many papers focusing on the refractory congenital glaucomas, especially if associated with other ocular malformations, such as chronic uveitis, aniridia or Peters anomaly [2, 3, 15, 30]. Consequently, it is crucial to differentiate between individual prognoses before determining therapy.

As the characteristic symptoms of blepharospasm, photophobia, and epiphora in congenital glaucoma are reported with very high frequency by parents, the individual anamnesis is an important and reliable clinical parameter. The early onset of these suspicious symptoms seems helpful in congenital glaucoma as manifest clinical symptoms are mostly seen during the first 3 months of life [15, 17].

Table 7.2. Work-up of clinical examination in congenital/infantile glaucoma

Careful individual anamnesis
Skiascopy (Myopia? Anisometropia?)
Biomicroscopy of the anterior and posterior segment (Haab striae? Distension of the superior limbal region? Glaucomatous excavation?)
Measurement of the horizontal corneal diameters
Hand-held tonometry
Gonioscopy (Iris insertion? Synechiae?)
A-scan sonography (Deviation from age-related growth?)
B-scan sonography (Retinoblastoma?)
Ultrasound biomicroscopy (completely opaque cornea)

Sometimes, in very young children, megalocornea, chronic conjunctivitis, and lacrimal stenosis can imitate the classical features of congenital glaucoma. In order to avoid the risk of treating a nonglaucomatous eye for glaucoma, the exact diagnosis of congenital glaucoma often needs to be confirmed by an examination under general anesthesia as cooperation in the young child may be lacking. If possible, examination for congenital glaucoma should include tonometry, skiascopy, biomicroscopy of the anterior and posterior segment, gonioscopy, and sonographic measurement of the axial length (Table 7.2). Under certain circumstances or with increasing age, visual field testing, laser scanning optic disc morphometry, or ultrasound biomicroscopy may be possible and helpful.

7.2.2 Tonometry

It is important to consider that normal intraocular pressure (IOP) in children ranges from 9–12 mmHg under general anesthesia. IOP measurements of 16–18 mm Hg under general anesthesia already require cautious interpretation. Intraocular pressure measurement in children under general anesthesia should not be performed in the initial phase but during deep anesthesia, in order to avoid the massive fluctuations occurring in the initial phase of general anesthesia [26]. Several studies have demonstrated that intraocular pressure is lowered under general anesthesia, especially halothane anesthesia [4]. Chloral hydrate or ketamine sedation seems to avoid a considerable decrease of IOP, but also requires meticulous monitoring and supervision during and after a child's sedation [28, 54].

Tonometry in general anesthesia has to be performed using hand-held devices, e.g., the Schiötz, Perkins, or Tonopen tonometer. Any form of tonometry in the awake child is relatively unreliable owing to unpredictable factors such as pressure of the eye lids or increased episcleral pressure in the crying child. Tonometry in the young child is usually performed with devices designed for adult patients, thus introducing the risk of systematic measurement errors. Experimental and clinical studies have shown that pathological conditions of the sclera and cornea can lead to considerable tonometric measurement errors. In buphthalmic eyes with corneal scars and opacifications, significantly higher values are obtained with indentation tonometry than with applanation tonometry. As the diameter of the cornea and axial length of the eye are increased in children with congenital glaucoma, the central cornea is significantly thinner in these children than those with nonglaucomatous eyes. [29] This may also contribute to a considerable underestimation of the actual intraocular pressure in buphthalmic eyes.

7.2.3 Optic Disc Evaluation

Glaucomatous optic disc cupping is seen in the majority of children with infantile glaucoma, as far as limited corneal clarity allows visualization of the optic disc. The degree of optic disc excavation depends on the size of the optic disc, the pressure level, and the duration of increased intraocular pressure.

A reversal of optic disc cupping after pressure-reducing surgery can be observed at an early stage of primary congenital glaucoma. This phenomenon of an "improved" cup disc ratio occurs if intraocular pressure is successfully reduced, especially during the 1st year of life. Between the 2nd and 5th years of life, unchanged cupping is more frequent following successful glaucoma surgery [57]. In older children, optic disc cupping is considered to be the safest parameter to indicate the stage of glaucomatous damage.

Little information is available on the clinical potential of optic disc morphometry by laser scanning tomography in children with congenital glaucoma. Compliance in children of 4 or 5 years is often already sufficiently good to perform laser scanning tomography of the optic

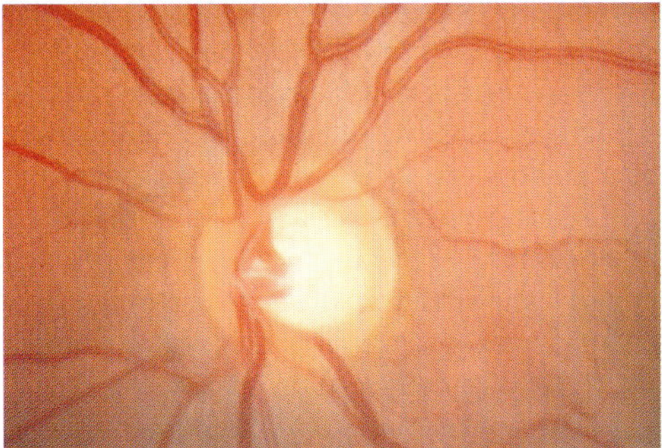

Fig. 7.2. Macroexcavation in a large optic disc (>4 mm^2). This healthy 6-year-old boy was suspected of having childhood glaucoma. Follow-up revealed no change of the macroexcavation

disc and this is extremely helpful to rule out or to clearly quantify a macroexcavation in a very large optic disc (Fig. 7.2) and to avoid unnecessary treatment.

7.2.4 Sonography

7.2.4.1 A-Scan

The pathological increase of the axial length leading to the typical buphthalmic configuration of the eye is an extremely frequent sign in congenital glaucoma during the 1st years of life. Beyond the 4th year of life, the onset of glaucoma is usually not associated with buphthalmic growth of the eye owing to age-dependent changes in the sclera architecture. In contrast to tonometry, which offers only a snapshot of intraocular pressure fluctuations, the pathologically increased axial length in congenital glaucoma reflects the long-term level of intraocular pressure.

Preoperative axial length and age are basic factors in the interpretation of ocular growth following glaucoma surgery in primary congenital glaucoma. Temporary cessation of ocular growth is a frequent finding after successful pressure-reducing surgery in eyes with an axial length greater than 22 mm and in children aged 3 months or older.

7.2.4.2 B-Scan

B-scan sonography – wherever available – should be obligatory in buphthalmic eyes with severe opacities of cornea, lens, or vitreous to rule out secondary glaucoma owing to retinoblastoma, other tumor-like lesions, or persistent primary hyperplastic vitreous. Although rare, these secondary glaucomas require different treatment strategies with their own prognosis.

Follow-up examination of buphthalmic eyes with opaque optical media should also include B-scan sonography, because of the relatively high incidence of retinal detachment following any kind of antiglaucomatous surgery.

7.2.4.3 Ultrasound Biomicroscopy

Ultrasound biomicroscopy is a useful diagnostic tool in cases of complete corneal opacification hindering clear identification of anterior chamber structures. Iris adhesions to the cornea can be visualized by ultrasound biomicroscopy, allowing diagnoses such as Peters anomaly or iris tamponade following perforation [21]. Such information can be helpful in determining subsequent treatment strategies if glaucoma surgery or keratoplasty is planned.

7.2.5 Corneal Morphology

7.2.5.1 Corneal Opacifications

Much attention is focused on the cornea in the diagnosis of congenital glaucoma. There are several typical signs that can be observed such as a stretched superior limbal region (Fig. 7.3), tears in the Descemet membrane, the so-called Haab striae (Fig. 7.4), and corneal opacifications (Fig. 7.5). Corneal opacities are frequent in infantile glaucoma, occurring in up to 75% of glaucomatous eyes [17]. Corneal clouding as an isolated ocular symptom (without Haab striae and limbal stretching) in infants is a suspect sign of a genetic (congenital hereditary endothelial dystrophy, Turner or Noonan syndrome)

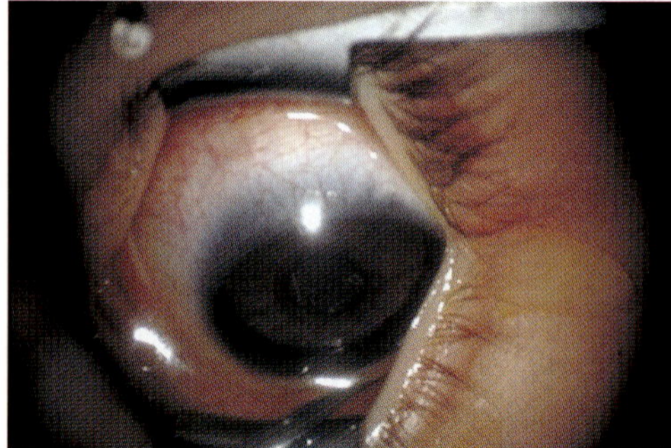

Fig. 7.3. Primary congenital glaucoma in 14-month-old girl showing massive distension and stretching of the superior limbus region

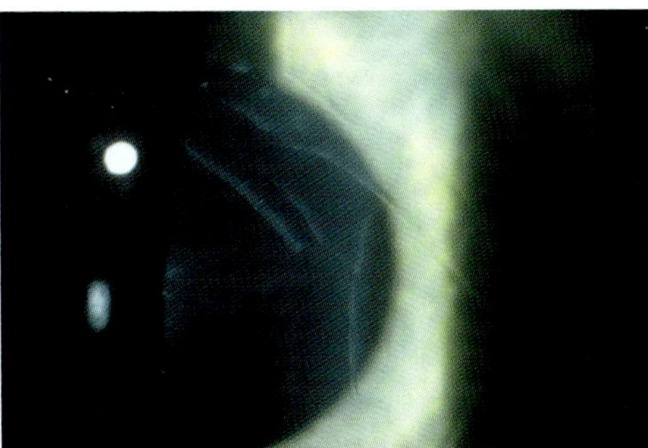

Fig. 7.4. Haab striae (endothelial tears) in a adult patient who had undergone glaucoma surgery for congenital glaucoma in his first year of life

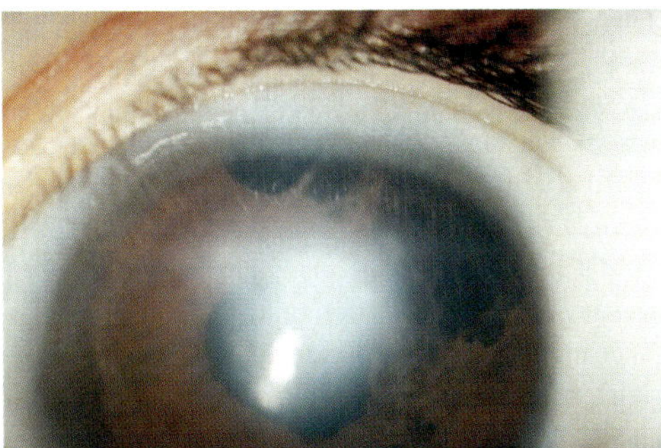

Fig. 7.5. Iridocorneotrabeculodysgenesis with glaucoma in a 3-year-old girl

or metabolic (mucopolysaccharidoses, cystinosis) disease, sometimes imitating congenital glaucoma. Even where meticulous examination is not possible, such as in a crying or restless, awake child, the degree of corneal clarity should always be observed. Even the smallest corneal opacity can be symptomatic of a severe ophthalmological disease such as congenital glaucoma or anterior-dysgenesis syndrome.

7.2.5.2 Corneal Diameters

Owing to the extremely stretched superior limbal region in buphthalmic eyes, it seems reasonable to measure corneal diameters horizontally rather than vertically. Enlarged corneal diameters of more than 12 mm during the 1st year of life are highly indicative of buphthalmia. Average horizontal corneal diameters in the newborn are between 9.5 and 10 mm. In the 1st year of life, corneal diameters reach 10.5–12.0 mm. Corneal diameters are accepted as a diagnostic criterion of high sensitivity for congenital glaucoma. However, as a factor for monitoring the long-term progression of glaucoma, the measurement of the corneal diameters seems inappropriate in most cases, although no larger reliable studies exist on changes in buphthalmic corneal diameter following pressure-reducing surgery.

Megalocornea has been reported as a developmental, nonprogressive anomaly with corneal diameters of at least 12 mm in the newborn. In contrast to congenital glaucoma, the limbal region is not stretched in megalocornea, and ruptures of the Descemet membrane with edema and opacities are also absent. However, associations between megalocornea and congenital glaucoma have been described in one family. All patterns of inheritance have been reported.

7.2.6 Visual Field Testing

Visual field testing requires a minimum of compliance and understanding from the patient. This kind of examination is therefore rarely feasible in children younger than 8 years. Conventional kinetic manual perimetry has been shown to be of use in detecting localized visual field defects in children between 4 and 14 years of age [16].

7.2.7 Objective Refraction

Determination of objective ocular refraction is extraordinarily important in the management of infantile glaucoma in order to protect against amblyopia. Reliable skiascopy is frequently hindered by corneal clouding or endothelial scars. The majority of glaucomatous eyes are myopic beyond the first months of life even when pressure-reducing surgery has been successfully performed [38]. In 65–100% of patients, amblyopia due to ametropia or anisometropia threatens visual acuity in later life, even in pressure-controlled buphthalmic eyes [15].

Summary for the Clinician

Typical clinical signs of congenital glaucoma occurring in the first 2 years of life:

- History of epiphora, photophobia and blepharospasm during the first months of life
- Corneal opacities, tears of the Descemet membrane (Haab striae), an overstretched superior limbal region and large corneal diameters
- In contrast to management in adult glaucoma, several specifications have to be considered in the diagnostic work-up:
- Abnormally increased ocular axial length (in comparison to the normal age-correlated growth curve) is a common feature of congenital glaucoma. However, if onset of glaucoma occurs after 3 years of age the typical stretching of the globe is usually absent
- Despite manifest congenital glaucoma the intraocular pressure may be normal under deep general anesthesia. Several sources of error may confuse intraocular pressure measurements in buphthalmic eyes
- Glaucomatous excavation of the optic disc is usually present, but evaluation of the optic disc is often impossible owing to corneal opacities. Glaucomatous excavation can be reversible in very young children following IOP control
- Visual field testing is usually impossible in children younger than 6–8 years. Optic disc morphometry can be performed even in younger children from 4 years of age
- Skiascopy, or another method of determining the objective ocular refraction, should be performed regularly, because refractive problems such as ametropia and anisometropia are very common in buphthalmic eyes and may also contribute to amblyopia

7.3 Medical Treatment

Medical treatment is usually a treatment option of second choice in young children if surgery has to be postponed for certain reasons: if life expectancy is undoubtedly limited owing to a complex syndrome or severe, life-threatening disease or, exceptionally, if multiple previous antiglaucomatous surgical interventions have achieved only limited success requiring further pressure-reducing treatment with poor surgical prognosis.

Fundamental problems connected with medical treatment of children with congenital glaucoma include an understandable poor compliance on instillation of drops. Topical and systemic side effects can also arise, owing to the relatively high concentration of pharmaceutical agents, originally designed for adults, in the child's body, and on long-term application of preservatives such as benzalkonium chloride.

For all new medications introduced into glaucoma management over the last 15 years, knowledge of long-term side-effects (>20 years) of their use in early childhood is naturally lacking. This may be of particular importance for iris pigmentation after use of latanoprost.

7.3.1 Miotics

Pilocarpine and other miotics are often used postoperatively to prevent the formation of anterior synechiae (e.g., following goniotomy, trabeculotomy, or cyclodialysis). Changing pupil size and disturbed accommodation limit the use of this agent in long-term treatment of infantile glaucoma.

Another concern may be the use of strong-acting miotics in highly myopic eyes, since an association has been described between miotics use and retinal detachment in highly myopic eyes with glaucoma.

7.3.2 Beta-Blockers

Topical beta-blockers are the best documented antiglaucomatous agents with regard to efficacy and side effects. Owing to systemic resorption, topical timolol can cause bradycardia, arterial hypotension and pulmonary problems in children, especially when drops are instilled bilaterally with no interval between applications to the two eyes. These side effects will undoubtedly occur more often in very young children than in older patients.

7.3.3 Carbonic Anhydrase Inhibitors

Systemic acetazolamide may cause severe systemic side effects including metabolic acidosis, renal problems, and hepatic necrosis. Owing to its chemical structure, acetazolamide should not be given in cases with a sulfonamide allergy. Under controlled circumstances, acetazolamide is sometimes used for short periods, preferably in older children. Topical carbonic anhydrase inhibitors, such as dorzolamide and brinzolamide, are less likely to cause side effects than oral acetazolamide, but seem to be less effective in pressure reduction [45]. Little is known about the disturbance of endothelial function in buphthalmic eyes with extensive Haab striae on treatment with topical carbonic anhydrase inhibitors.

7.3.4 Prostaglandins

The use of latanoprost in pediatric glaucoma has been described [23]. Mean IOP reduction after addition of latanoprost in 48 pediatric patients was relatively small. Pressure-reducing efficacy, especially in young patients with infantile glaucoma, seems to be more limited than in older patients with juvenile glaucoma.

The special use of latanoprost as an additional antiglaucomatous medication has been studied in children with port wine stain-related pediatric glaucoma. Nearly half of the patients had controlled IOP at 1 year follow-up [44].

Little is known, however, about the long-term changes in iris pigmentation and the clinical importance of this for children. As in adults, the application of latanoprost in uveitic glaucoma should be avoided. Latanoprost was suspected of having caused heavy sweat secretion over the entire body 1–2 h after local administration in a child with aniridia [51].

7.3.5 Alpha-2 Agonists

Brimonidine is a topical alpha-2 agonist that is widely used as a hypotensive drug in adults. In a retrospective analysis six out of 22 children between the ages of 0 and 14 years had to stop local administration of brimonidine 0.2%. Reasons for terminating treatment were fainting attacks in two children, tiredness in another two, and local irritations in a further two patients [10]. A considerable proportion of young children suffer from systemic side effects following brimonidine 0.2% drops [9, 22], leading to the recommendation not to use this medication in young children.

Severe systemic problems such as bradycardia and hypothermia have been described following topical application not only of brimonidine but also of apraclonidine in children.

7.4 Surgical Therapy

Owing to the rarity of congenital glaucoma and the unusual tissue consistency of buphthalmic sclera and cornea, any glaucoma surgery in buphthalmia (Table 7.3) requires special equipment, knowledge, skill, and experience.

Prospective randomized clinical studies of surgical strategies in congenital glaucoma are extremely rare. The reasons for this could be the low incidence of the disease or the uncertainty of randomization, to which many parents will not consent. Thus, most data are taken from retrospective studies in large tertiary glaucoma centers, reflecting the surgical experience and

Table 7.3. Surgical treatment options in congenital and infantile glaucoma

Primary congenital glaucoma
Goniotomy
Trabeculotomy
Combined trabeculotomy-trabeculectomy
Trabeculectomy
Refractory congenital glaucomas
Glaucoma implants (Ahmed valve, Baerveldt and Molteno implant)
Laser cyclophotocoagulation (cyclocryocoagulation)
Adjunctive antimetabolites in filtration surgery
Cyclodialysis

preferences of some very highly skilled glaucoma surgeons but also regional differences between patient groups with regard to ethnic origin, type of glaucoma, and patient compliance.

Another well-known problem is the discrepancy between success criteria used in different studies, which can range from the simple statement "no further re-surgery required" to attainment of certain intraocular pressure measurements after a given period or satisfactory values for a combination of clinical parameters such as clinical symptomatology, corneal clearness, intraocular pressure, A-scan sonography, and optic disc morphology.

7.4.1 Goniotomy

The technique of goniotomy was introduced clinically by Barkan in the early 1940s. Goniotomy involves incision of the thickened trabecular beams and disconnection of the abnormally forward insertion of the iris. However, a clear cornea and highly specialized surgical experience are required for this delicate surgery. Especially in the intraoperatively flattened anterior chamber of newborns with leaking corneal incisions, maneuvers with the goniotomy knife carry certain risks, even when high-viscosity viscoelastics are used.

Success rates of 60–90% have been reported following goniotomy in childhood glaucoma [15, 41, 46, 49]. However, re-goniotomies have to be performed in up to one-third of patients. In order to perform this kind of surgery in eyes with a cloudy cornea, endoscopic approaches have been described [33]. To guarantee a stable anterior chamber, endoscopic goniotomy has also been performed using an anterior chamber maintainer. With this technique, a 240° goniotomy can be performed with no major complications [7].

Retrospective studies in juvenile uveitis patients around 10 years of age have also revealed relatively good results for conventional goniotomy in experienced hands. The overall success rate after goniotomies (54 in 40 eyes) was 72% with a postoperative IOP of 14–16 mmHg. Kaplan-Meier survival probabilities were 0.81 at 5 years and 0.71 at 10 years. The most frequent complication was hyphema in 80% of the goniotomies. Prognosis for the outcome was better in eyes with fewer anterior synechiae, in phakic eyes, in eyes without prior surgery, and in patients younger than 10 years [30].

If the surgeon has sufficient experience with this technique and clinical results are comparable to ab-externo approaches in his hands, it is reasonable to perform goniotomy or similar pressure-reducing ab-interno surgery (e.g., endoscopically guided goniotomy) as a primary intervention, because the conjunctiva will not be damaged and thus future surgery is not prejudiced.

7.4.2 Trabeculotomy

As with goniotomy, success rates of around 70–90% have been reported within a period of 2–9 years following trabeculotomy [14, 15, 31, 41]. However, one-third of the eyes operated on required a second or tertiary trabeculotomy. This ab-externo method is not dependent on the visibility of the chamber angle structures through an often cloudy cornea. However, abnormal anatomy of the limbus in congenital glaucoma makes it difficult to clearly identify the lumen of Schlemm's canal that should be cannulated by a trabeculotome. In these cases, trabeculotomy might be changed into a trabeculectomy by excising a small block of scleral tissue as for routine trabeculectomy. This externalization of trabeculotomy is also performed as a planned procedure in developmental glaucoma (see Sect. 7.4.3).

A 360° trabeculotomy has been proposed by threading a polypropylene suture into Schlemm's canal for the whole circumference and tearing the meshwork with the suture. The pressure-reducing potential of this procedure has been demonstrated in a retrospective study of 24 eyes, achieving success rates of more than 90% [40]. However, massive ocular hypotony has also been described in a small series following 360° suture trabeculotomy [25].

7.4.3 Trabeculotomy Combined with Trabeculectomy

Trabeculectomy has been combined with trabeculotomy as a primary intervention achieving comparable or better success rates to trabeculotomy alone.

In the difficult group of very young patients undergoing glaucoma surgery within the 1st month of life, an Indian retrospective study revealed success rates of 89% after 1 year and 72% after 3 years for the combined trabeculotomy–trabeculectomy approach. No essential intra- and postoperative complications were seen in any patient though anesthesia-related problems occurred in two patients [37].

Elder [20], who exclusively studied Palestinian patients younger than 1 year, showed better results for combined trabeculotomy–trabeculectomy procedures (93.5%) after 2 years than for trabeculectomy (72%), although the incidence of corneal haze in the trabeculectomy group was obviously higher (82% vs 56%), whereas other preoperative parameters (e.g., age, intraocular pressure, corneal diameters) were similar in the two groups. The author explained the superior outcome of the combined procedure by establishing two different new ways of facility improvement (through the trabecular meshwork and through the sclera).

Slightly worse results for combined trabeculotomy–trabeculectomy (72% success rates) were noted for primary congenital glaucoma in a retrospective study in Saudi Arabian patients. In this study, outcome was much worse for eyes with associated ocular malformations (45% success rate) although mitomycin C was additively used in 87% of the eyes [43].

7.4.4 Trabeculectomy

Depending on follow-up and risk profile in the study patients, the success rates published in the literature for primary trabeculectomy alone range from 50% to over 90% in congenital glaucoma [18, 20, 24]. Burke [11] reported surgical success in 18 of 21 eyes (86%) with congenital glaucoma after a mean follow-up of nearly 4 years. In the same patient group, Fulcher [24] even observed a 5-year success rate of 92% after the first trabeculectomy in 13 eyes with primary congenital glaucoma, although no patients younger than 4 months of life or with a corneal diameter larger than 13.5 mm were treated in this study.

Debnath et al. [14], who clearly described the distribution of risk factors in their Saudi Arabian study group, found a 1-year success rate of 54% for trabeculectomy. The authors concluded that their high failure rate might be influenced by an ethnic factor. Furthermore, the proportion of patients manifesting glaucoma soon after birth was relatively high in this study and obviously predisposed the group to poor results for both procedures. Trabeculectomy was rarely followed by cataract, endophthalmitis, or vitreous loss.

In another retrospective study comparing the outcomes of trabeculotomy, trabeculectomy and combined trabeculotomy–trabeculectomy, there was no significant difference between outcome for the surgical techniques after 5 years. [18]

Several authors do not recommend trabeculectomy as a primary procedure in congenital glaucoma, as they have attained only moderate success rates associated with severe intra- and postoperative complications such as vitreous loss, endophthalmitis, retinal detachment, scleral collapse, subluxation of the lens, and uveitis as possible risks. Shallow anterior chamber and hyphema are the most common postoperative complications and these usually resolve spontaneously.

The rate of resurgery (1/3) after initial trabeculectomy is comparable to that after trabeculotomy or goniotomy, but prognosis is particularly poor for neonatal forms of congenital glaucoma and highly myopic eyes. Secondary trabeculectomy in primary congenital glaucoma achieves significantly worse results than primary trabeculectomy [18].

7.4.5 Use of Antifibrotic Agents

Intra- or postoperative application of topical mitomycin C or 5-fluorouracile in young children with a long life expectancy is associated with the risk of late toxicity and potential mutagenicity of these antimetabolites, even though the filtering procedures combined with the use of mitomycin are becoming increasingly routine in antiglaucomatous surgery. Further possible deleterious complications of filtering procedures with mitomycin C are rupture of thin-walled blebs, wound leakage, late endophthalmitis, and long-standing hypotony. Owing to extreme scleral thinning in buphthalmia, the potential risk of localized retinal necrosis has also to be considered. However, in refractory cases the use of antimetabolites or other methods to prevent scarring seems unavoidable where goniosurgery and ab-externo procedures without antimetabolites have failed.

The intraoperative use of mitomycin C (MMC) during trabeculectomy and its long-term effectiveness in congenital glaucoma have been investigated in several retrospective studies, with the general conclusion that there are significantly more complications associated with the use of MMC in infantile glaucomas [38, 48]. Incidence and frequency of postoperative complications (thin avascular filtering blebs, choroidal detachment, wound leakage) following combined trabeculotomy–trabeculectomy were found to depend on the concentration of mitomycin C used (0.2 mg/ml vs 0.4 mg/ml) [1]. A higher concentration of mitomycin C (0.5 mg/ml) administered intraoperatively for 3–4 min during trabeculectomy produced a considerable rate of late bleb-related infection (17%) at an average follow-up of 28 months [50]. The success rate in this study was 59% after 3 years for primary and secondary pediatric glaucomas.

Another retrospective study investigated the outcome of trabeculectomy with and without MMC in aphakic and pseudophakic eyes in children. Neither IOP levels nor success rates after 2 years differed significantly between the two groups. In the MMC group, one patient developed bleb-related endophthalmitis in both eyes underlining the relatively high risk of bleb infection after MMC administration [38].

7.4.6 Glaucoma Implants

The most frequently used glaucoma shunt implants are the Molteno, Ahmed, and Baerveldt implants [8, 42]. They are used following failed prior surgery, in aphakia and in different types of anterior segment anomalies. Several retrospective studies have proven the pressure-reducing potential of drainage devices in infantile glaucoma. The Ahmed valve was implanted in a consecutive series of 60 eyes in 44 patients (mean age, 6 years). More than two-thirds of the patients attained IOP control 2 years following the procedure with reduction of pressure-lowering eye drops from 4 to 2 medications. However, complications occurred in 30 eyes (50%), leading to severe visual loss in four patients. Interestingly, uveitic glaucoma was a risk factor for tube extrusion in this study [42].

A shallow anterior chamber is a frequently seen complication (25%) in the early postoperative period following Ahmed implant surgery. Prognosis of glaucoma implant surgery seems to be partially influenced by the surgeon's experience [19].

In a retrospective comparison between trabeculectomy with mitomycin C (MMC) and Ahmed/Baerveldt implants in children younger than 3 years, postoperative complications requiring surgical revision were more common in the implant group (45.7%) than in the MMC group (12.5%), but success rates (IOP

<23 mmHg with maximum medication) were also higher in the implant group after 1 (87%) and after 6 years (53%) than in the MMC group (36% and 19%) [8]. The most common post-operative intervention in the implant group was tube repositioning.

In eight eyes of five patients with aniridia (mean age, 92 months) a glaucoma drainage device achieved intraocular pressure reduction from 35 mmHg to 15 mmHg with a follow-up of 19 months. The success rate after 1 year was 88% in this retrospective study. One eye lost light perception owing to postoperative retinal detachment [3].

Simultaneous use of an Ahmed glaucoma valve implant and penetrating keratoplasty in refractory congenital glaucoma with corneal opacities has limited long-term efficacy. IOP control was achieved in one-third of eyes after 4 years, and graft success in only 17% of eyes [2]. Complications included conjunctival scarring, corneal graft failure, and corneal ulcerations (*Streptococcus pneumoniae*).

Systemic immunomodulation seems to have a favorable influence on the outcome of glaucoma implant surgery in patients with uveitic glaucoma and autoimmune disease (e.g., juvenile rheumatoid arthritis) [13].

7.4.7 Nonperforating Glaucoma Surgery

Nonperforating glaucoma surgery, such as deep sclerectomy or viscocanalostomy, has been performed in infantile glaucoma as a primary and secondary intervention. The efficacy and surgical risks of this surgery are a matter of controversy. While some authors report good success rates of 75% without essential surgical side effects, others emphasize the problems and risks of these procedures in refractory congenital glaucoma leading to a further thinning of the scleral envelope [36, 53].

Nonperforating glaucoma surgery has been proposed as a safe and promising approach in episcleral venous pressure glaucoma (e.g., Sturge-Weber-Krabbe syndrome), as surgical risks are minimized and late goniopuncture can produce a late and "controlled" filtration [36].

7.4.8 Cyclodialysis

Cyclodialysis was abandoned long ago owing to the unpredictability of the surgical outcome. With the increasing use of viscoelastics, cyclodialysis has become more and more attractive as an ab-interno technique, alone in refractory aphakic glaucoma or in combination with goniotomy in the developmental glaucomas [34]. If successful, the uveoscleral outflow can be greatly increased. However, long-standing ocular hypotony can result from cyclodialysis.

7.4.9 Cyclodestructive Procedures

Over the last decade, laser destruction of the ciliary body has gradually replaced cryodestruction as the cyclodestructive procedure of choice in refractory congenital glaucoma, since the ocular side effects are less severe after laser surgery. Owing to the anomalous limbal anatomy of buphthalmic eyes, it is feasible to perform transscleral laser coagulation of the ciliary body with the aid of transscleral illumination in order to determine the exact localization of the ciliary body and to identify areas of previous destruction.

The most frequent method used to destroy the nonpigmented ciliary body in pediatric glaucoma is contact-diode transscleral cyclophotocoagulation (TSCPC). Most retrospective studies reveal that this laser procedure is generally applied more than once in each patient. Although IOP reduction can be achieved by TSCPC after 1 year, the success rates are not always completely convincing, ranging between 27% and 79% [5, 28, 35] depending on the success criteria used and the number of laser interventions. The results following contact-diode transscleral laser cyclophotocoagulation seem to be worse in congenital or juvenile glaucoma compared than in older patients with primary open-angle glaucoma [50]. Possibly, regenerative mechanisms of the infantile ciliary epithelium contribute to this finding.

The postoperative risk of phthisis seems relatively low, around 3.5% [28]. Signs of intraocular inflammation are relatively frequent, around 25%. Especially in aphakic eyes, severe vision-threatening postoperative complications including retinal and choroidal detachment have been described in children. [5]

7.4.10 Surgical Iridectomy (Laser Iridotomy)

Iridectomy is the treatment of choice in certain cases of angle-closure glaucoma. Pupillary block that should be treated by iridectomy may be present in spherophakia (e.g., Weill-Marchesani syndrome), in uveitic glaucoma with 360° posterior synechiae, and in nanophthalmic eyes. Pupillary block mechanisms due to lens dislocation (e.g., in Marfan's syndrome) should be primarily treated by lens extraction rather than by iridectomy. Other reasons for angle-closure glaucoma in children may be iridociliary cysts, hyperplastic primary vitreous, and retinopathy of prematurity [47].

7.4.11 Special Aspects

7.4.11.1 Secondary Glaucoma in Pediatric Uveitis

Secondary glaucoma is observed in nearly 30% of children with chronic uveitis. Owing to the high rate of band keratopathy, the visual prognosis is still poor today for every third child. In older children with glaucoma and arthritis, the medical treatment option is effective in 30–50% of cases, thus avoiding glaucoma surgery with unpredictable prognosis.

A few studies have reported good surgical results following glaucoma implant surgery combined with systemic immunomodulation in children with uveitis, but also following goniotomy and trabeculodialysis.

7.4.11.2 Aphakic Glaucoma

In contrast to primary congenital glaucoma, some standard techniques, including filtering surgery with antimetabolites [6, 38] or goniosurgery [56], reveal unsatisfactory results in aphakic glaucoma in children. Acceptable long-term results have been reported – albeit with a considerable rate of postoperative complications – for glaucoma implant surgery [12] and with temporarily limited success for cyclodiode laser treatment [32].

A recent study has raised the question of whether delayed surgery in congenital cataract might reduce the risk of glaucoma. In this retrospective analysis, early cataract surgery during the 1st month of life increased the 5-year risk of secondary glaucoma (50%) compared to those eyes that underwent cataract surgery later (15%). Corrected visual acuity did not differ between eyes operated before and after 1 month of age. The 5-year risk of glaucoma in at least one eye was 25% following bilateral limbal lensectomy, with anterior vitrectomy remaining at a constant level for the first 5 years [55]. From these data, glaucoma risk in modern surgery of congenital cataract by a limbal approach must still be considered relatively high.

7.5 Surgical Complications

7.5.1 Intraoperative Complications

Chamber angle bleeding with small hyphema occurs in two-thirds of eyes during trabeculotomy and in a quarter of eyes undergoing primary trabeculectomy. The blood is usually absorbed during the 1st postoperative day. A frequent intraoperative complication (>5%) of trabeculotomy is early perforation of the anterior chamber by the trabeculotomy probe. Further, relatively rare, instrumentally induced intraoperative complications of trabeculotomy are cyclodialysis with postoperative hypotony, iris damage, and lens subluxation [31]. Although trabeculectomy is widely performed by many ophthalmic surgeons, this procedure remains technically challenging in congenital glaucoma, as the limbal anatomy is usually distorted and the sclera extraordinarily thin. This can lead to inadvertent scleral perforation during preparation of the scleral flap. Another potential risk can be prolapse of the vitreous or ciliary body through the peripheral iridectomy into the trabeculectomy opening, especially in the case of a primarily dislocated lens. Typical intraoperative problems of goniotomy may be touching of the lens, with subsequent cataract formation and leaking corneal incisions. Intraoperative complications of cyclodialysis ab-interno also include massive hemorrhage.

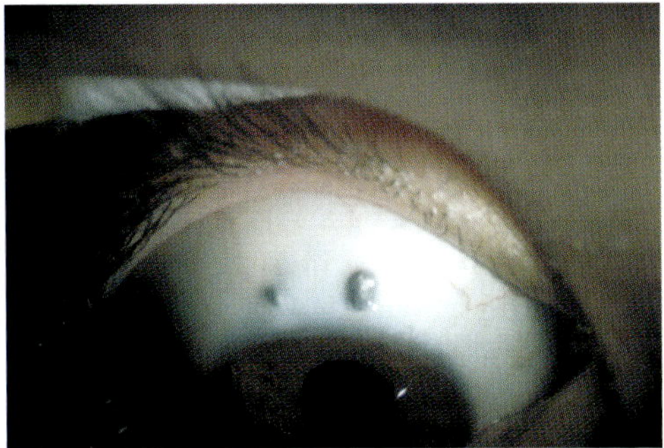

Fig. 7.6. Slit-lamp photography in a 4-year-old girl 2 years following primary trabeculectomy because of primary congenital glaucoma. Uveal prolapse at the edges of the scleral flap has occurred, but is covered by conjunctiva. The intraocular pressure has been normal following surgery

7.5.2 Postoperative Complications

Retinal detachment in buphthalmic eyes following trabeculotomy has been reported with a frequency of 3% over a mean follow-up period of 9 years [31]. This demonstrates the general susceptibility to retinal tears in the stretched and highly myopic buphthalmic eye rather than a special postoperative risk of any one surgical method. Even after goniotomy, Rice [46] reported several cases of retinal detachment with congenital glaucoma. Long-standing postoperative hypotony may sometimes lead to retinal detachment.

Prolapse of the elongated ciliary processes and iris incarceration in the trabeculectomy opening are not infrequent findings after trabeculectomy (Fig. 7.6) and do not therefore necessarily reflect surgical failure. Scleral incisions performed during scleral flap dissection in trabeculectomy or deep sclerectomy increase the risk of scleral rupture in case of subsequent blunt trauma to the buphthalmic eye (Fig. 7.7).

Further severe postoperative complications comprise subluxation of the crystalline and cataract formation, typically following trabeculectomy, but also following trabeculotomy or goniotomy. The risk of blebitis and endophthalmitis should be borne in mind, especially after filtering surgery with mitomycin C, but also after glaucoma implant surgery if conjunctival erosion occurs.

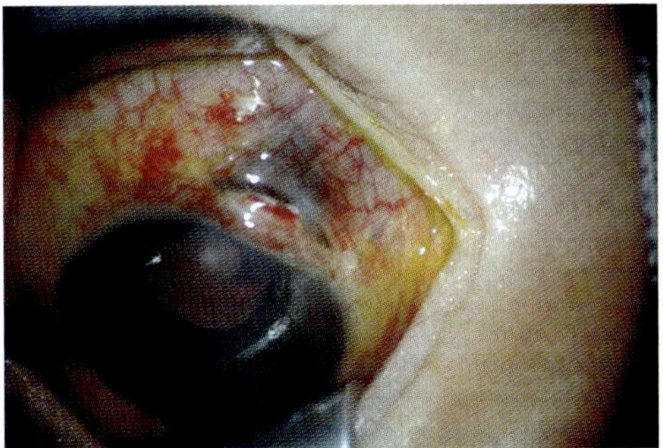

Fig. 7.7. Eight-month-old girl with primary congenital glaucoma that had a blunt trauma to the eye 2 weeks following uncomplicated trabeculectomy, resulting in a broad uveal prolapse along the scleral flap

In eyes with Peters anomaly, the risk of postoperative complications is especially high. In a retrospective study of 34 eyes in 19 patients who had undergone trabeculectomy, trabeculotomy, goniotomy, Molteno shunt implantation, cyclodialysis, or cyclocryotherapy, a graft failure was observed in 26 eyes (76%), cataract in six eyes (18%), inoperable retinal detachment with phthisis in 12 eyes (35%), and phthisis alone in six (18%). Finally, there was no light perception in 12 eyes (35%), light perception alone in seven eyes (12%), and vision between 20/400 and hand motion in 12 eyes (35%) [58].

7.6 Prognosis

Although the main pathological feature reported in primary congenital glaucoma is trabeculodysgenesis, resulting in outflow obstruction and a rise in intraocular pressure, the starting point for pressure-reducing surgery varies from patient to patient and prognosis of any surgery seems to be largely governed by the underlying nature of dysgenesis. Any association with other ocular or systemic abnormalities evidently reduces the long-term prognosis. Early and severe manifestation of buphthalmia (axial length >24 mm) seems to be a limiting factor for individual prognosis in trabeculotomy and trabeculectomy, but also in glaucoma implant surgery. Russell-Eggitt also reported a poor outcome for goniotomy in very young patients with congenital glaucoma, thereby confirming the importance of age for individual prognosis, whatever form of pressure-reducing surgery is used [49]. The limited prognostic power of preoperative intraocular pressure can mainly be attributed to the many sources of error in tonometry in buphthalmic eyes.

7.7 Concluding Remarks

For many reasons, information on surgical treatment in congenital glaucoma is based almost exclusively on retrospective studies. Retrospective studies comparing the outcome of different strategies have to be evaluated with caution, especially if the decision to operate in a certain way follows regional and historical trends or individual preferences and experience, as is obvious in the treatment of congenital glaucoma. Furthermore, the small number of patients treated by each particular surgical strategy limits the statistical significance of most retrospective studies.

Summary for the Clinician

- **Pressure-reducing surgery is considered the treatment of choice in congenital glaucoma, as medical options, such as the use of brimonidine, are limited owing to systemic side effects**
- **First-line surgical interventions in primary congenital glaucoma are goniotomy, trabeculotomy, combined trabeculotomy–trabeculectomy or trabeculectomy**
- **Prognoses for all surgical interventions are strongly linked to the child's age, the preoperative distension of the eye, and further concomitant ocular and systemic pathologies**
- **Severe postoperative complications in buphthalmic eyes include retinal detachment, lens dislocation, cataract, and endophthalmitis following application of mitomycin C**
- **Amblyopia may develop as a result of corneal opacities and refractive problems (e.g., ametropia, anisometropia)**

References

1. Agarwal HC, Sood NN, Sihota R, Sansa L, Honavar SG (1997) Mitomycin-C in congenital glaucoma. Ophthalmic Surg Lasers 28:979–985
2. Al-Torbak AA (2004) Outcome of combined Ahmed glaucoma valve implant and penetrating keratoplasty in refractory congenital glaucoma with corneal opacity. Cornea 23:554–559
3. Arroyave CP, Scott IU, Gedde SJ, Parrish RK 2nd, Feuer WJ (2003) Use of glaucoma drainage devices in the management of glaucoma associated with aniridia. Am J Ophthalmol 135:155–159
4. Ausinsch B, Munson ES, Levy NS (1978) Intraocular pressure in children with glaucoma during halothane anesthesia. Ann Ophthalmol 9:1391–1394
5. Autrata R, Rehurek J (2003) Long-term results of transscleral cyclophotocoagulation in refractory pediatric glaucoma patients. Ophthalmologica 217:393–400
6. Azuara-Blanco A, Wilson RP, Spaeth GL, Schmidt CM, Augsburger JJ (1999) Filtration procedures supplemented with mitomycin C in the management of childhood glaucoma. Br J Ophthalmol 83:151–156

7. Bayraktar S, Koseoglu T (2001) Endoscopic goniotomy with anterior chamber maintainer: surgical technique and one-year results. Ophthalmic Surg Lasers 32:496–502
8. Beck AD, Freedman S, Kammer J, Jin J (2003) Aqueous shunt devices compared with trabeculectomy with mitomycin-C for children in the first two years of life. Am J Ophthalmol 136:994–1000
9. Berlin RJ, Lee UT, Samples JR, Rich LF, Tang-Liu DD, Sing KA, Steiner RD (2001) Ophthalmic drops causing coma in an infant. J Pediatr 138: 441–443
10. Bowman RJ, Cope J, Nischal KK (2004) Ocular and systemic side effects of brimonidine 0.2% eye drops (Alphagan) in children. Eye 18:24–26
11. Burke JP, Bowell R (1989) Primary trabeculectomy in congenital glaucoma. Br J Ophthalmol 73: 186–190
12. Cunliffe IA, Molteno ACB (1998) Long-term follow-up of Molteno drains used in the treatment of glaucoma presenting in childhood. Eye 12:379–385
13. DaMata A, Burk SE, Netland PA et al (1999) Management of uveitic glaucoma with Ahmed glaucoma valve implantation. Ophthalmology 106:2168–2172
14. Debnath SC, Teichmann KD, Salamah K (1989) Trabeculectomy versus trabeculotomy in congenital glaucoma. Br J Ophthalmol 73:608–611
15. DeLuise VP, Anderson DR (1983) Primary infantile glaucoma (congenital glaucoma). Surv Ophthalmol 28:1–19
16. DeSouza EC, Berezovsky A, Morales PH, de Arruda Mello PA, de Oliveira Bonomo PP, Salomao SR (2000) Visual field defects in children with congenital glaucoma. J Pediatr Ophthalmol Strabismus 37:266–272
17. Dietlein TS, Jacobi PC, Krieglstein GK (1996) Assessment of diagnostic criteria in management of infantile glaucoma. An analysis of tonometry, optic disc cup, corneal diameter and axial length. Int Ophthalmol 20:21–27
18. Dietlein TS, Jacobi PC, Krieglstein GK (1999) Prognosis of ab-externo surgery for primary congenital glaucoma. Br J Ophthalmol 83:317–322
19. Djodeyre MR, Peralta Calvo J, Abelairas Gomez J (2001) Clinical evaluation and risk factors of time to failure of Ahmed Glaucoma Valve implant in pediatric patients. Ophthalmology 108:614–620
20. Elder MJ (1994) Combined trabeculotomy-trabeculectomy compared with primary trabeculectomy for congenital glaucoma. Br J Ophthalmology 78:745–748
21. Engels BF, Dietlein TS, Jacobi PC, Krieglstein GK (1999) Ultrasound biomicroscopy diagnosis of congenital glaucoma. Klin Monatsbl Augenheilkd 215:338–341
22. Enyedi LB, Freedman SF (2001) Safety and efficacy of brimonidine in children with glaucoma. J AAPOS 5:281–284
23. Enyedi LB, Freedman SF, Buckley EG (1999) The effectiveness of latanoprost for the treatment of pediatric glaucoma. J AAPOS 3:33–39
24. Fulcher T, Chan J, Lanigan B, Bowell R, O'Keefe M (1996) Long-term follow-up of primary trabeculectomy for infantile glaucoma. Br J Ophthalmol 80:499–502
25. Gloor BR (1998) Risks of 360° suture trabeculotomy. Ophthalmologe 95:100–103
26. Goethals M, Missotten L (1983) Intraocular pressure in children up to five years of age. J Pediatr Ophthalmol Strab 20:49–51
27. Grehn F, Mackensen G (1982) Rieger's anomaly with signs of hydrophthalmia and spontaneous pressure regulation. Klin Monatsbl Augenheilkd 181:197–201
28. Hamard P, May F, Quesnot S, Hamard H (2000) Trans-scleral diode laser cyclophotocoagulation for the treatment of refractory pediatric glaucoma. J Fr Ophthalmol 23:773–780
29. Henriques MJ, Vessani RM, Reis FA, de Almeida GV, Betinjane AJ, Susanna R Jr (2004) Corneal thickness in congenital glaucoma. J Glaucoma 13:185–188
30. Ho CL, Wong EYM, Walton DS (2004) Goniosurgery for glaucoma complicating chronic childhood uveitis. Arch Ophthalmol 122:838–844
31. Ikeda H, Ishigooka H, Muto T, Tanihara H, Nagata M (2004) Long-term outcome of trabeculotomy for the treatment of developmental glaucoma. Arch Ophthalmol 122:1122–1128
32. Jacobi PC, Dietlein TS, Krieglstein GK (1999) Microendoscopic trabecular surgery in glaucoma management. Ophthalmology 105:538–544
33. Kirwan JF, Shah P, Khaw PT (2002) Diode laser cyclophotocoagulation: role in the management of refractory pediatric glaucomas. Ophthalmology 109:316–323
34. Klemm M, Schwartz R, Niefer H, Wiezorrek R, Draeger J (1995) Results of cyclodialysis combined goniotomy in treatment of dysgenetic glaucoma. Ophthalmologe 92:531–535
35. Klimczak-Slaczka D, Prost ME (2000) Use of cyclophotocoagulation with diode laser in treatment of secondary glaucoma in children. Klin Oczna 102:345–348
36. Libre PE (2003) Nonpenetrating filtering surgery and goniopuncture (staged trabeculectomy) for episcleral venous pressure glaucoma. Am J Ophthalmol 136:1172–1174
37. Lueke C, Dietlein TS, Jacobi PC, Konen W, Krieglstein GK (2002) Risk profile of deep sclerectomy for treatment of refractory congenital glaucomas. Ophthalmology 109:1066–1071

38. Mandal AK, Walton DS, John T, Jayagandan A (1997) Mitomycin-C augmented trabeculectomy in refractory congenital glaucoma. Ophthalmology 104:996–1001
39. Mandal AK, Gothwal VK, Bagga H, Nutheti R, Mansoori T (2003) Outcome of surgery on infants younger than 1 month with congenital glaucoma. Ophthalmology 110:1909–1915
40. Mendicino ME, Lynch MG, Drack A, Beck AD, Harbin T, Pollard Z, Vela MA, Lynn MJ (2000) Long-term surgical and visual outcomes in primary congenital glaucoma: 360° trabeculotomy versus goniotomy. J AAPOS 4:205–210
41. Meyer G, Schwenn O, Grehn F (2000) Trabeculotomy in congenital glaucoma: comparison to goniotomy. Ophthalmologe 97:623–628
42. Morad Y, Donaldson CE, Kim YM, Abdolell M, Levin AV (2003) The Ahmed drainage implant in the treatment of pediatric glaucoma. Am J Ophthalmol 135:821–829
43. Mullaney PB, Selleck C, Al-Awad A, Al-Mesfer S, Zwann J (1999) Combined trabeculotomy and trabeculectomy as an initial procedure in uncomplicated congenital glaucoma. Arch Ophthalmol 117:457–460
44. Ong T, Chia A, Nischal KK (2003) Latanoprost in port wine stain related paediatric glaucoma. Br J Ophthalmol 87:1091–1093
45. Portellos M, Buckley EG, Freedman SF (1998) Topical versus oral carbonic anhydrase inhibitor therapy for pediatric glaucoma. J AAPOS 2:43–47
46. Rice NSC (1977) The surgical management of the congenital glaucomas. Aust J Ophthalmol 5:174–179
47. Ritch R, Chang BM, Liebmann JM (2003) Angle closure in younger patients. Ophthalmology 110:1880–1889
48. Rodrigues AM, Junior AP, Montezano FT, de Arruda Melo PA, Junior JP (2004) Comparison between results of trabeculectomy in primary congenital glaucoma with and without the use of mitomycin C. J Glaucoma 13:228–232
49. Russell-Eggitt IM, Rice NSC, Jay B, Wyse RKH (1992) Relapse following goniotomy for congenital glaucoma due to trabecular dysgenesis. Eye 6:197–200
50. Schlote T, Derse M, Rassmann K, Nicaeus T, Dietz K, Thiel HJ (2001) Efficacy and safety of contact transscleral diode laser cyclophotocoagulation for advanced glaucoma. J Glaucoma 10:294–301
51. Schmidtborn F (1998) Systemic side-effects of latanoprost in a child with aniridia and glaucoma. Ophthalmologe 95:633–634
52. Sidoti RA, Belmonte SJ, Liebmann JM, Ritch R (2000) Trabeculectomy with mitomycin C in the treatment of pediatric glaucomas. Ophthalmology 107:422–429
53. Tixier J, Dureau P, Becquet F, Dufier JL (1999) Deep sclerectomy in congenital glaucoma. Preliminary results. J Fr Ophthalmol 22:545–548
54. Tomey KF (2004) Childhood glaucoma and amblyopia. In: Grehn F, Stamper RL (eds) Essentials in ophthalmology: glaucoma. Springer, Berlin Heidelberg New York, pp 105–124
55. Vishwanath M, Cheong-Leen R, Taylor D, Russell-Eggitt I, Rahi J (2004) Is early surgery for congenital cataract a risk factor for glaucoma? Br J Ophthalmol 88:905–910
56. Walton DS (1995) Pediatric aphakic glaucoma. A study of 65 patients. Trans Am Ophthalmol Soc 93:403–413
57. Wu SC, Huang SC, Kuo CL, Lin KK, Lin SM (2002) Reversal of optic disc cupping after trabeculotomy in primary congenital glaucoma. Can J Ophthalmol 37:337–341
58. Yang LL, Lambert SR, Lynn MJ, Stulting RD (2004) Surgical management of glaucoma in infants and children with Peters anomaly: long-term structural and functional outcome. Ophthalmology 111:112–117

Pediatric Ocular Oncology

8

Carol L. Shields, Jerry A. Shields

Core Messages

- There are numerous benign and malignant tumors in the pediatric ocular region
- Capillary hemangioma of the eyelid is one of the most common eyelid tumors in neonates and toddlers and it is generally managed conservatively with observation unless there is strabismus or amblyopia. Oral or injection steroids can be used to reduce the tumor size
- Eyelid nevus tends to occur in the late childhood years, similar to cutaneous nevi elsewhere on the body
- The most common conjunctival tumor in childhood is the nevus. The nevus is often pigmented and cystic. In some instances it is completely clear (amelanotic). It rarely evolves into melanoma
- There are several benign and malignant intraocular tumors of childhood
- The benign intraocular tumors include retinal astrocytic hamartoma, retinal hemangioma (capillary, cavernous, and racemose hemangioma), vasoproliferative tumor, choroidal hemangioma, choroidal nevus, and many others. Intraocular medulloepithelioma can be either benign or malignant
- The malignant intraocular tumors include retinoblastoma and choroidal melanoma as well as a few other rarer conditions
- Retinoblastoma is the most common intraocular malignancy of childhood. With proper management, life prognosis is excellent
- Chemoreduction and thermotherapy is most often employed for bilateral retinoblastoma management
- Enucleation is most often employed for unilateral retinoblastoma management, but chemoreduction with globe salvage can be achieved in some cases
- Most orbital tumors in childhood are benign
- The most common benign orbital tumor in childhood is the dermoid cyst
- Rhabdomyosarcoma is a malignant orbital tumor in childhood, requiring systemic chemotherapy and orbital radiotherapy once the diagnosis is established on biopsy

8.1 General Considerations

Several benign and malignant ocular tumors can occur in childhood. Tumors in the ocular region can lead to loss of vision, loss of the eye and, in the case of malignant neoplasms, to loss of life. Therefore, it is important for the clinician to recognize childhood ocular tumors and to refer affected patients for further diagnostic studies and appropriate management. Based on our extensive clinical experience with ocular tumors over the last 30 years, we review some general concepts of childhood eye tumors and discuss the clinical manifestations of selected specific tumors of the eyelid, conjunctiva, intraocular structures, and orbit in children. For more detailed information, the reader is encouraged to consult the references cited at the end of this article [28–32].

8.1.1 Clinical Signs of Childhood Ocular Tumors

The clinical characteristics of childhood ocular tumors vary with whether the tumor is located in the eyelids, conjunctiva, intraocular tissues, or the orbit. Eyelid and conjunctival tumors are generally quite evident, prompting an early visit to a physician. Since most tumors in the ocular area have characteristic features, an accurate diagnosis of eyelid and conjunctival tumors can usually be made with inspection alone. Therefore, additional diagnostic studies are often unnecessary. Unlike tumors of the eyelids and conjunctiva, intraocular tumors are not readily visible. Infants and very young children do not complain of visual loss and their visual acuity is difficult to assess. However, there are several features that should alert the pediatrician to consider the possibility of an intraocular tumor and prompt a timely referral.

One of the more important signs of an intraocular tumor in children is leukocoria, or a white pupillary reflex (Fig. 8.1). There are many causes of leukocoria in children [33–35]. The more common ones include congenital cataract, retinal detachment due to retinopathy of prematurity, persistent hyperplastic primary vitreous, and congenital retinal telangiectasia with exudation (Coats disease). Retinoblastoma is probably the most serious condition to cause leukocoria in children. Any child with leukocoria should be referred promptly to an ophthalmologist for further diagnostic evaluation.

Most children with strabismus do not have an intraocular tumor. However, about 30% of patients with retinoblastoma present initially with either esotropia or exotropia, due to the tumor location in the macular area, which disrupts the child's fixation. It is important that a retinal examination using the indirect ophthalmoscope be performed on every child with strabismus to exclude an underlying tumor.

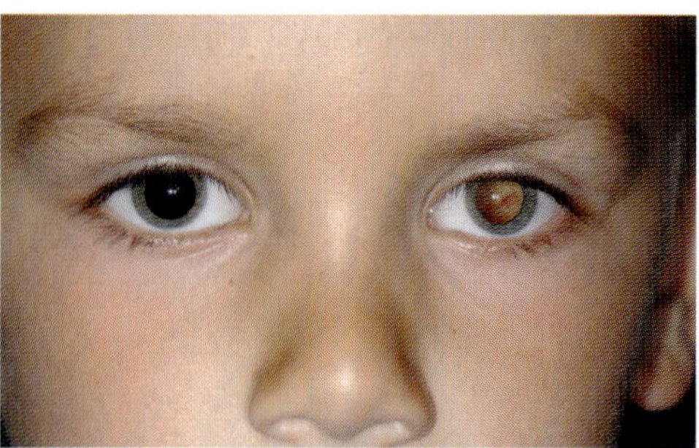

Fig. 8.1. Leukocoria secondary to retinoblastoma

An older child with an intraocular tumor may complain of visual impairment or may be found to have decreased vision on visual testing in school. This usually occurs from destruction of the central retina by the tumor or by the presence of vitreous hemorrhage, hyphema, or secondary cataract formation.

Unlike tumors of the eyelid and conjunctiva, orbital tumors cannot be directly visualized. Therefore, they often attain a relatively large size before becoming clinically evident. They generally present with proptosis or displacement of the eye. Pain, diplopia, and conjunctiva edema may also be early clinical features of an orbital tumor. Computed tomography (CT) and magnetic resonance imaging (MRI) have revolutionized the diagnosis and treatment of orbital tumors [1].

8.1.2 Diagnostic Approaches

Although some atypical tumors can defy clinical diagnosis, most ophthalmic tumors in children can be accurately diagnosed by a competent ophthalmologist or ocular oncologist.

8.1.2.1 Eyelid and Conjunctiva

Most eyelid and conjunctival tumors are recognized by their typical clinical features, and special diagnostic studies are of little additional help. Smaller suspicious tumors in these tissues can be removed by excisional biopsy and the diagnosis established histopathologically. Larger tumors where the resulting defect cannot be repaired primarily are best diagnosed by incisional biopsy and definitive treatment is withheld until a definite diagnosis is established.

8.1.2.2 Intraocular Tumors

Concerning intraocular tumors, lesions of the iris can often be recognized with external ocular examination or slit-lamp biomicroscopy. Tumors of the retina and choroid can be visualized with ophthalmoscopy, which often reveals typical features depending on the type of tumor. Many small tumors are difficult to visualize and may only be detected by an experienced ophthalmologist using binocular indirect ophthalmoscopy. Ancillary studies such as fundus photography, fluorescein angiography, indocyanine green angiography, ocular ultrasonography, and occasionally CT or MRI are of supplemental value in establishing the diagnosis. Optical coherence tomography (OCT) is a newer fundus scanning method using a rapid, noncontact technique with color-coded images in about 5 min. Children comfortably tolerate this technique [10]. OCT can provide in vivo, high-resolution information of the retina to the 10-µm level. Fine-needle aspiration biopsy (FNAB) has recently been employed in selected intraocular tumors of children. Such procedures in children often require general anesthesia.

8.1.2.3 Orbital Tumors

Some orbital tumors occur in an anterior location and can be recognized by their extension into the conjunctiva and eyelid area. This is particularly true of childhood vascular tumors such as capillary hemangioma and lymphangioma. Other tumors reside in the deeper orbital tissues and are less accessible to inspection, palpation, and biopsy. Orbital ultrasonography can be performed quickly in many ophthalmologists' offices and can sometimes provide useful diagnostic information in cases of anterior orbital tumors. As mentioned earlier, CT and MRI have revolutionized orbital tumor diagnosis in children and have greatly improved the management of such cases [1]. These imaging techniques can accurately localize and diagnosis orbital masses and assist in proper management. Hence, exploratory orbitotomy is almost never necessary today.

8.1.3 Therapeutic Approaches

The treatment of an ocular tumor in a child also depends on the location of the tumor and the size of the lesion.

8.1.3.1 Eyelid and Conjunctiva

True neoplasms of the eyelid and conjunctiva can be removed surgically by a qualified ophthalmologist or ocular oncologist. Inflammatory lesions that simulate neoplasia can be managed by antibiotics or corticosteroids, depending on the diagnosis. Some malignant neoplasms such as leukemias and lymphomas are best managed with a limited diagnostic biopsy followed by irradiation and/or chemotherapy.

8.1.3.2 Intraocular Tumors

The management of intraocular tumors is more complex. Certain benign intraocular tumors that are asymptomatic are usually managed by serial observation. Some symptomatic benign tumors can be treated with laser or cryotherapy depending on the mechanism of visual impairment. Malignant tumors, such as retinoblastoma, sometimes require enucleation of the eye. In recent years, however, there has been a trend away from enucleation for retinoblastoma, with the increasing use of more conservative methods of management, such as laser photocoagulation, cryotherapy, and various techniques of radiotherapy [2, 29, 36]. Even more recently, there has been a trend toward using chemoreduction to reduce the tumor(s) to a small size so that enucleation and irradiation can be avoided [2].

8.1.3.3 Orbital Tumors

The treatment of an orbital tumor varies greatly with the clinical or histopathologic diagnosis. Benign vascular tumors, such as capillary hemangioma and lymphangioma, can be managed by serial observation or patching treatment of the opposite eye to decrease the severity of associated amblyopia. Circumscribed tumors in the anterior orbit may be managed by excisional biopsy. Many malignant tumors, such as rhabdomyosarcoma and orbital leukemia, may require limited biopsy to establish he diagnosis, followed by irradiation or chemotherapy [28].

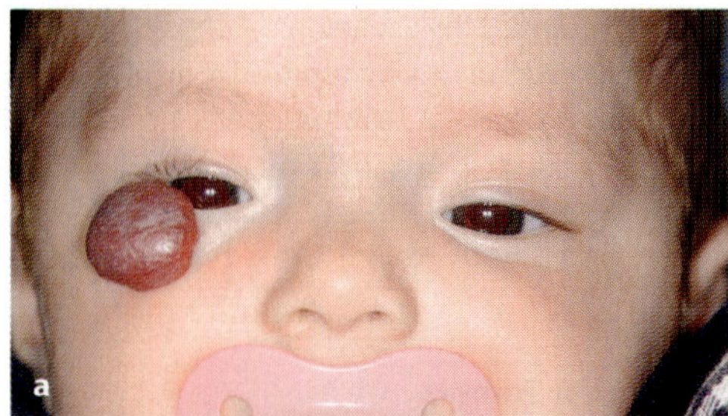

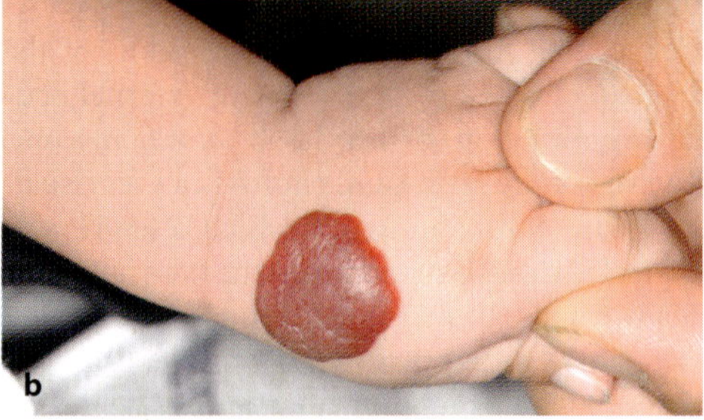

Fig. 8.2 a, b. Capillary hemangioma of the eyelid. **a** Eyelid hemangioma in an infant twin #1 managed with observation as it did not obstruct visual acuity. **b** Cutaneous hemangioma in twin #2 on the hand

8.2 Eyelid Tumors

There is a large number of pediatric cutaneous tumors that can affect the skin of the eyelids [9]. Only the more important ones will be considered here.

8.2.1 Capillary Hemangioma

The capillary hemangioma or strawberry hemangioma can occur on skin in 10% of infants and is recognized to be more common in premature infants and twins (Figs. 8.2–8.4). Capillary hemangioma of the eyelids can be a reddish, diffuse or circumscribed mass [5] (Figs. 8.2–8.4). It usually has clinical onset at birth, or shortly thereafter, tends to enlarge for a few months, and then slowly regress. The main complications of this benign tumor are strabismus and amblyopia. In recent years, the most frequently used treatment has been refraction, glasses for refractive error, patching of the opposite eye, and close follow-up. More recently, there has been a trend toward corticosteroids or complete surgical excision of those lesions that are relatively small and localized. Intralesional or oral corticosteroids may hasten regression of the tumor in some cases (Fig. 8.4). Radiotherapy is almost never used today.

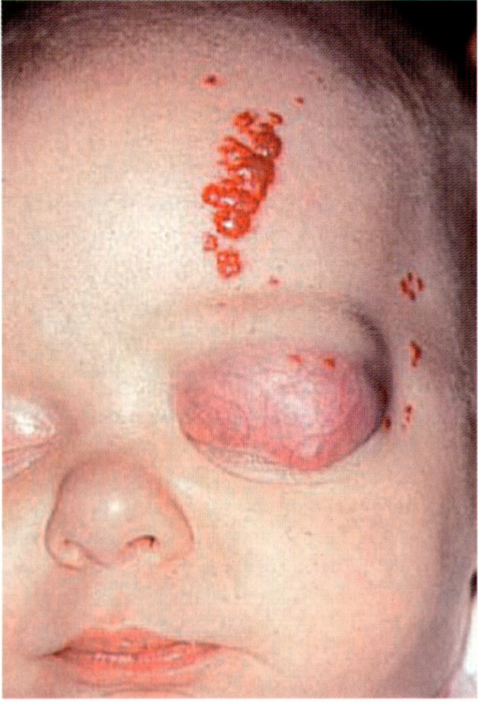

Fig. 8.3. Extensive capillary hemangioma of the eyelid, facial skin, and orbit

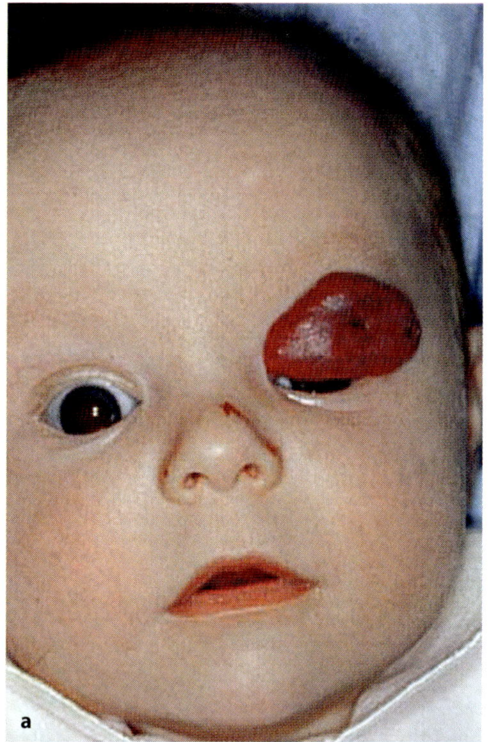

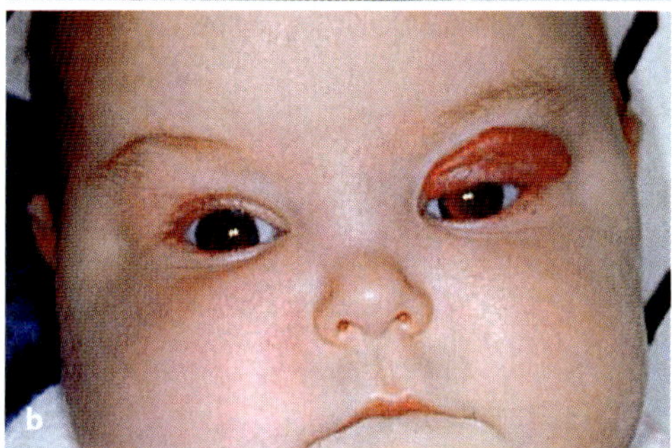

Fig. 8.4 a, b. Large capillary hemangioma of the eyelid obstructing vision. **a** Before treatment. **b** After 2 months of oral corticosteroids. Note the tumor reduction and facial weight gain

8.2.2 Facial Nevus Flammeus

Facial nevus flammeus is a congenital cutaneous vascular lesion that occurs in the distribution of the Vth cranial nerve (Fig. 8.5). It may be an isolated entity or it may occur with variations of the Sturge-Weber syndrome. Infants

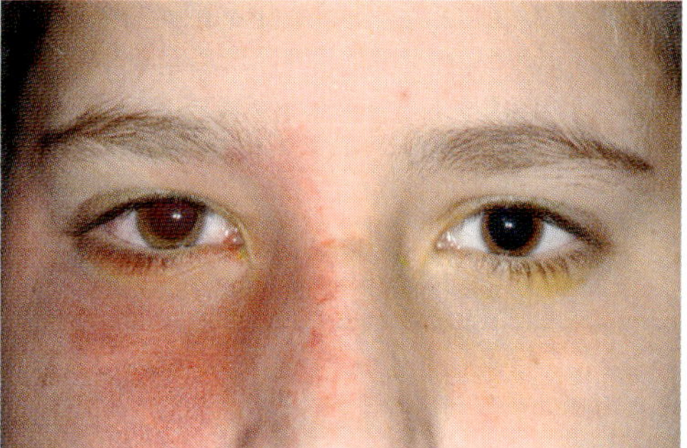

Fig. 8.5. Nevus flammeus of the face in a child with Sturge Weber syndrome

with this lesion have a higher incidence of ipsilateral glaucoma, diffuse choroidal hemangioma, and secondary retinal detachment. Affected infants should be referred to an ophthalmologist as early as possible in order to diagnosis and treat these serious ocular conditions. Management of the cutaneous lesion includes observation, cosmetic make-up, or laser treatment.

8.2.3 Kaposi's Sarcoma

With the increasing incidence of the acquired immune deficiency syndrome in children, opportunistic neoplasms such as Kaposi's sarcoma, are being diagnosed more frequently. Although the affected patient may have cutaneous lesions elsewhere, the eyelid can occasionally be the initial site of involvement. The lesion appears as a reddish-blue subcutaneous mass near the eyelid margin. It generally responds best to chemotherapy and radiotherapy.

8.2.4 Basal Cell Carcinoma

Although basal cell carcinoma is primarily a disease of adults, it is occasionally seen in younger patients, particularly if there is a family history of the basal cell carcinoma syndrome. It generally occurs on the lower eyelid as a slowly progressive mass that frequently develops a central ulcer (rodent ulcer). Lesions near the eyelid margin often develop loss of eyelashes in the area of involvement. Treatment is local excision using frozen section control and eyelid reconstruction.

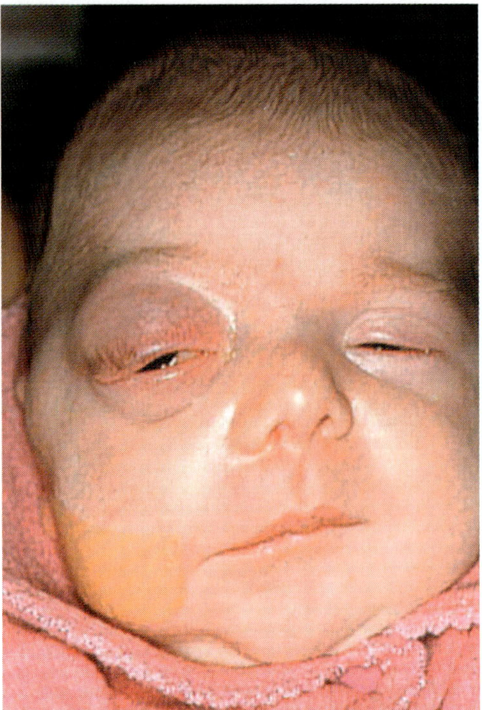

Fig. 8.6. Neurofibroma of the eyelid and orbit in an infant. Note the café au lait spot on the cheek

8.2.5 Melanocytic Nevus

A melanocytic nevus is a tumor composed of benign melanocytes. It can occur on the eyelid as a variably pigmented well-circumscribed lesion, identical to those that occur elsewhere on the skin. It does not usually cause loss of cilia. The blue nevus is often apparent at birth, whereas the junctional or compound nevus may not become clinically apparent until puberty. Transformation into malignant melanoma is rare and usually occurs later in life. Although most eyelid nevi in children can be safely observed, they are occasionally excised because cosmetic considerations or because of fear of malignant transformation.

8.2.6 Neurofibroma

A neurofibroma can occur on the eyelid as a diffuse or plexiform lesion that is often associated with von Recklinghausen's neurofibromatosis. In the earliest stages the lesion produces a characteristic S-shaped curve to the upper lid. Larger lesions produce thickening of the eyelid with secondary blepharoptosis (Fig. 8.6). Since these diffuse tumors are often difficult or impossible to completely excise, they should be managed by periodic observation or surgical debulking if they cause a major cosmetic problem.

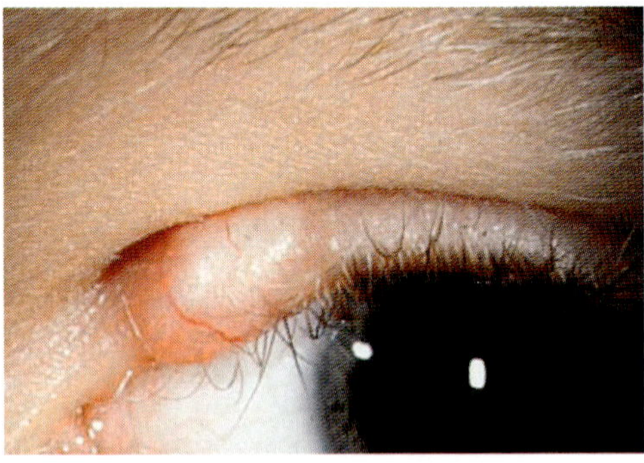

Fig. 8.7. Neurilemoma in a 9-year-old boy

8.2.7 Neurilemoma (Schwannoma)

Neurilemoma is a benign peripheral nerve sheath tumor that is composed purely of Schwann cells of peripheral nerves. It more commonly occurs in the orbit of young adults, but it can appear as a solitary eyelid lesion in children [37]. It often occurs as a circumscribed solitary lesion (Fig. 8.7) unassociated with neurofibromatosis. It is a benign tumor that can be excised surgically.

Summary for the Clinician

- Most eyelid tumors in children are benign
- Capillary hemangioma of the eyelid presents a few days to a few weeks after birth
- Capillary hemangioma of the eyelid requires treatment if there is threat of visual compromise. Treatment with oral or injection steroids or even with surgical resection can be successful
- Eyelid nevus generally presents in the preteen years or later and can be safely observed

8.3 Conjunctival Tumors

There are many pediatric conjunctival tumors and these have been well described in the literature [19, 20]. Only the most important ones will be considered here.

8.3.1 Dermoid

The conjunctival dermoid is a congenital solid mass that occurs most often at the corneoscleral limbus inferotemporally (Fig. 8.8). It can occasionally be found over the central portion of the cornea. The round, yellow-white tumor often has fine hairs on its surface. Histopathologically, it is a choristomatous mass lined by keratinizing stratified squamous epithelium and containing dermal elements. The conjunctival dermoid is often a part of Goldenhar's syndrome, a nonhereditary condition that is characterized by preauricular appendages, deafness, and vertebral anomalies.

8.3.2 Epibulbar Osseous Choristoma

Epibulbar osseous choristoma is a choristomatous malformation consisting of a focal deposit of mature bone on the sclera beneath the conjunctiva. It most often occurs superotemporally as a hard fixed mass. This stationary lesion can be observed if it is asymptomatic or locally excised if it is symptomatic.

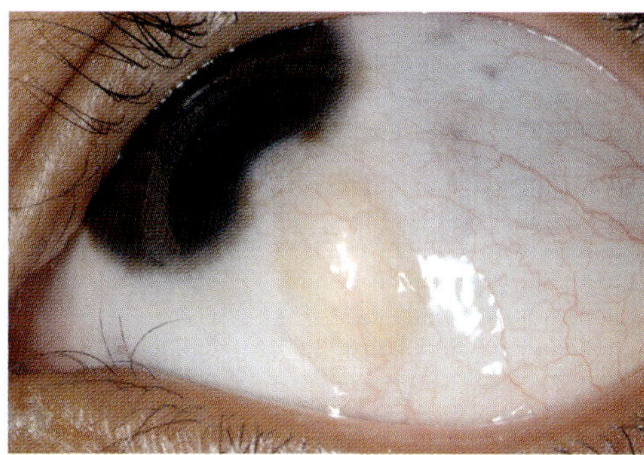

Fig. 8.8. Conjunctival dermoid

8.3.3 Complex Choristoma

A complex choristoma is a mass composed of a variety of ectopic tissues such as cartilage, lacrimal gland adipose tissue, and smooth muscle. It may assume a variety of clinical appearances on the conjunctiva but it generally appears as a diffuse, fleshy thickening of the epibulbar tissues. It is often seen in association with the nevus sebaceous of Jadassohn and arachnoid cysts as a part of the organoid nevus syndrome [38].

8.3.4 Papilloma

Squamous papilloma can occur on the conjunctiva of young children as either a sessile vascular lesion or as a fleshy papillomatous mass (Fig. 8.9). It is believed to be induced by human papillomavirus. If a conjunctival papilloma is not responsive to topical corticosteroids, then surgical excision and conjunctival cryotherapy is prudent. In recalcitrant or multiply recurrent cases, topical mitomycin C, 5 fluorouracil, or interferon can be employed. In recurrent cases, oral cimetidine can be of benefit [20].

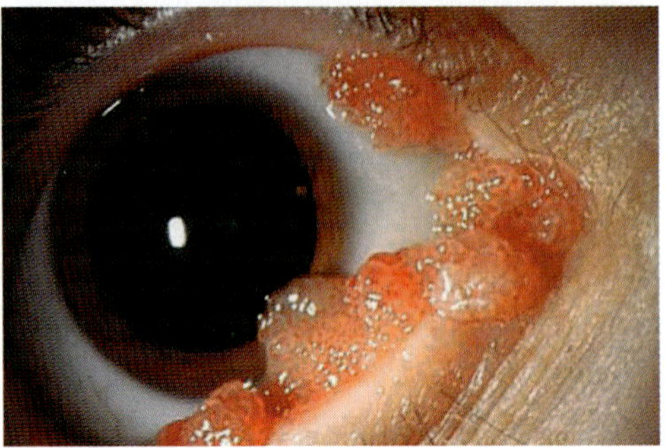

Fig. 8.9. Conjunctival papilloma

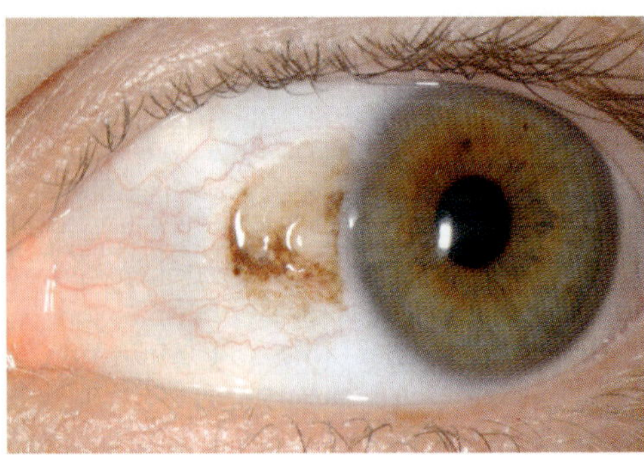

Fig. 8.10. Conjunctival nevus with cysts

8.3.5 Nevus

Conjunctival nevus is a variably pigmented, cystic mass that occurs on the bulbar conjunctiva usually in the interpalpebral area (Fig. 8.10) [20]. It usually becomes clinically apparent in the preteen or teenage years and generally remains stable throughout life. A review of 410 consecutive patients with conjunctival nevus revealed that 89% of patients were Caucasian, and the tumor was located in the bulbar conjunctiva (72%), caruncle (15%), plica semilunaris (11%), fornix (1%), tarsus (1%), and cornea (<1%). Additional features included intralesional cysts (65%), feeder vessels (33%), and visible intrinsic vessels (38%).

In rare instances, a conjunctival nevus can undergo malignant transformation into melanoma. Lesions documented to enlarge are best managed by alcohol keratectomy, local excision, and supplemental cryotherapy.

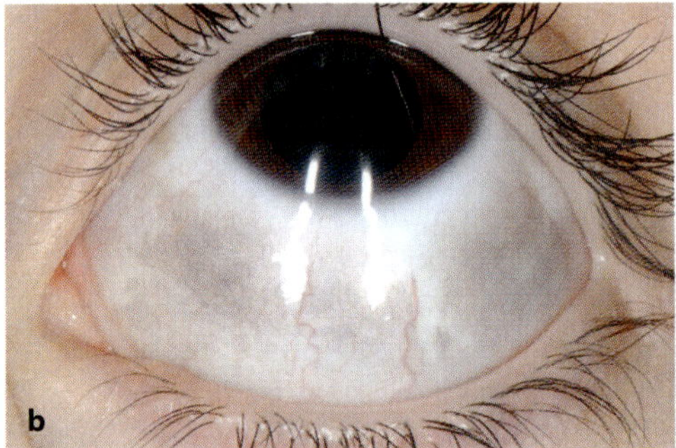

Fig. 8.11 a, b. Ocular melanocytosis. **a** Heterochromia with light brown right iris and dark brown left iris. **b** Episcleral melanocytosis

8.3.6 Congenital Ocular Melanocytosis

Although it is not strictly in the conjunctiva, congenital ocular melanocytosis is included here because it is an important epibulbar lesion of childhood. It is a congenital diffuse, patchy epibulbar pigmentation that is situated deep to the conjunctiva in the sclera (Fig. 8.11). There is usually diffuse pigmentation of the ipsilateral iris, causing heterochromia iridium. If the pigmentation extends onto the surrounding eyelid, it is called oculodermal melanocytosis, or nevus of Ota. Patients with congenital ocular melanocytosis have a higher incidence of malignant melanoma of the uveal tract, usually later in life [48]. Occasionally a uveal melanoma can occur in a child with ocular melanocytosis. It has been estimated that eyes with ocular melanocytosis carry a 1/400 lifetime risk for uveal melanoma [48]. Hence an ophthalmologist should perform a fundus examination every year.

8.3.7 Pyogenic Granuloma

Pyogenic granuloma is fleshy pink mass that can occur anywhere on the conjunctiva. It generally develops fairly rapidly following surgical or nonsurgical trauma. Histopathologically, it consists of a proliferation of small blood vessels with acute and chronic inflammatory cells. It is neither pyogenic nor granulomatous and hence the term "pyogenic granuloma" is a misnomer. It can be treated with topical corticosteroids or surgical resection.

8.3.8 Kaposi's Sarcoma

Kaposi's sarcoma, described above under eyelid tumors, can also occur in the conjunctiva in patients with acquired immune deficiency syndrome. In the conjunctive, it appears as a diffuse red mass that may be mistaken for a hemorrhagic conjunctivitis.

Summary for the Clinician

- Most conjunctival tumors in children are benign
- The majority of conjunctival tumors in children are pigmented or nonpigmented nevi
- Conjunctival nevi often manifest intralesional cysts
- Conjunctival nevi rarely evolve into melanoma (<1%)
- Episcleral melanocytosis is a sign of possible uveal melanocytosis and all affected eyes should be dilated once or twice a year, as there is a small risk for uveal melanoma
- Conjunctival papillomas can be treated with observation, cryotherapy, topical chemotherapy or interferon, and oral cimetidine

8.4 Intraocular Tumors

8.4.1 Retinoblastoma

Retinoblastoma is the most common intraocular malignancy of childhood [29]. Despite its malignant cellularity, only less than 5% of affected children die from this cancer in developed nations [6]. In developing nations, the death rate approaches 50% due to late detection of the disease. Retinoblastoma occurs in hereditary and nonhereditary forms. The hereditary form is usually bilateral and multifocal, whereas the nonhereditary form is unilateral and unifocal. The affected child usually presents with unilateral or bilateral leukocoria (Fig. 8.1), strabismus, or (occasionally) as orbital cellulitis [29, 31, 39]. Although it is usually diagnosed in children under 2 years of age, it can occur in older children [18]. Small fundus tumors are gray-white in color (Fig. 8.12) and often show foci of chalky-colored calcification. Medium-sized tumors are more elevated and have prominent dilated tortuous retinal blood vessels that feed and drain the tumor (Fig. 8.12).

The diagnosis of retinoblastoma is best made by an experienced ophthalmologist using slit lamp biomicroscopy and indirect ophthalmoscopy. Ancillary studies that may provide diagnostic help are ultrasonography and computed tomography.

The management of retinoblastoma is very complex and requires knowledge and experience [2, 7, 8, 22, 23, 26, 27, 29, 31, 36]. Treatment varies depending on number, size, and location of the tumors, and each case must be individualized depending on the clinical circumstances. More advanced tumors are managed by enucleation [2, 23, 36]. The hydroxyapatite implant has been used extensively in children and provides a good cosmetic appearance with fairly good motility of the implant [23]. In recent years, fewer eyes have been enucleated because earlier diagnosis and improvements in conservative methods of management have been refined [2, 8, 36].

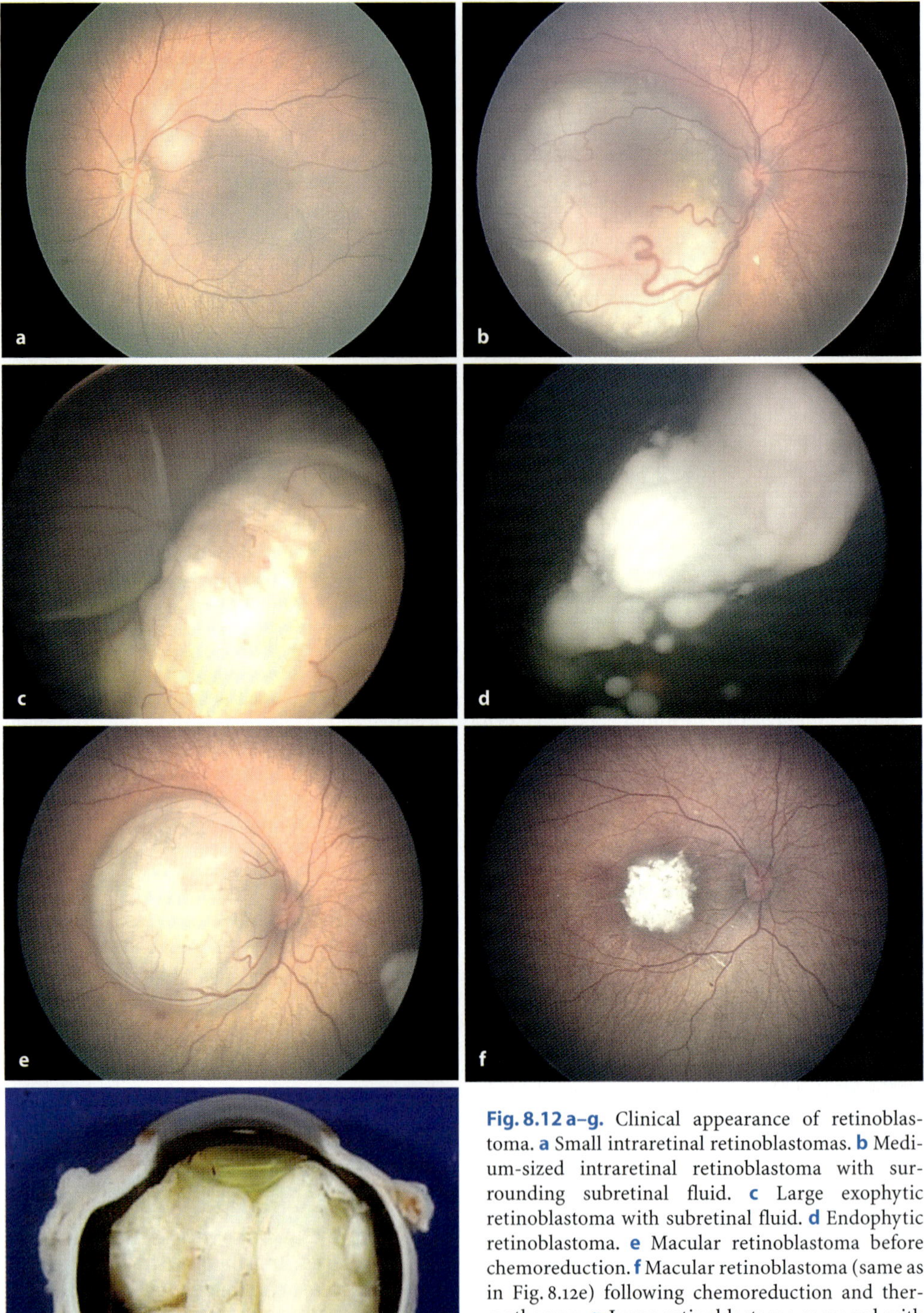

Fig. 8.12 a–g. Clinical appearance of retinoblastoma. **a** Small intraretinal retinoblastomas. **b** Medium-sized intraretinal retinoblastoma with surrounding subretinal fluid. **c** Large exophytic retinoblastoma with subretinal fluid. **d** Endophytic retinoblastoma. **e** Macular retinoblastoma before chemoreduction. **f** Macular retinoblastoma (same as in Fig. 8.12e) following chemoreduction and thermotherapy. **g** Large retinoblastoma managed with enucleation

Less advanced tumors can be treated with chemoreduction and thermotherapy, episcleral plaque brachytherapy, laser photocoagulation, or cryotherapy [2,7,8,22,26,27,29,31] (Fig. 8.12). External beam radiotherapy is typically reserved for eyes that fail the above methods, especially if there is only one remaining eye. With the advent of methods of chemoreduction and chemothermotherapy and improvements in methods of laser photocoagulation and cryotherapy, it is anticipated that fewer eyes will require enucleation or external beam irradiation and that more patients will be managed with conservative methods.

There have been several recent developments related to the genetics of retinoblastoma [24]. The retinoblastoma gene is now recognized to be a recessive suppresser gene located on chromosome 13 at the 13 Q 14 segment and some affected children have other systemic features of the 13 q deletion syndrome. All family members of patients with retinoblastoma should be examined by an ophthalmologist. All patients with retinoblastoma should have DNA analysis to establish the presence or absence of the 13Q mutation and its genetic locus. It is accepted that all bilateral and familial cases of retinoblastoma will manifest a germline mutation, whereas only 10–15% of unilateral sporadic cases will show germline mutation.

8.4.2 Retinal Capillary Hemangioma

Retinal capillary hemangioma is a reddish pink retinal mass that can occur in the peripheral fundus or adjacent to the optic disc [49]. The tumor often has prominent dilated retinal blood vessels that supply and drain the lesion (Fig. 8.13). Untreated lesions can cause intraretinal exudation and retinal detachment. Fluorescein angiography shows rapid filling of the tumor with dye and intense late staining of the mass. Patients with retinal capillary hemangioma should be evaluated for the von Hippel Lindau syndrome, an autosomal dominant condition characterized by cerebellar hemangioblastoma, pheochromocytoma, hypernephroma, and other visceral tumors and cysts. If the tumor produces macular exudation of retinal detachment, it can be treated with methods of laser photocoagulation, cryotherapy, photodynamic therapy, plaque radiotherapy, or external beam radiotherapy. The gene responsible or this syndrome has been localized to the short arm of chromosome 3.

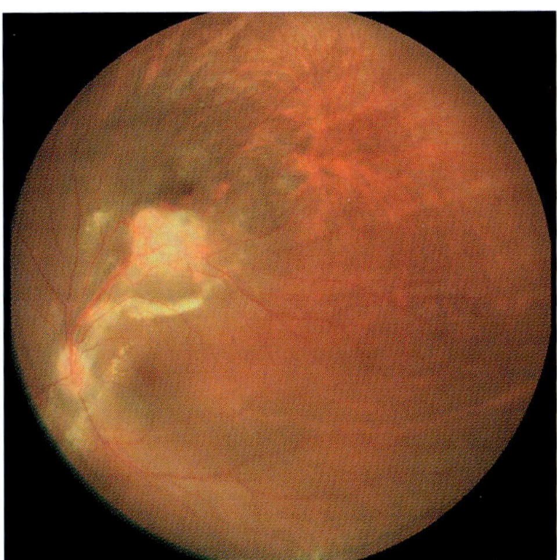

Fig. 8.13. Retinal capillary hemangioma with subretinal fluid and exudation in a child with von Hippel Lindau syndrome

8.4.3 Retinal Cavernous Hemangioma

The retinal cavernous hemangioma typically appears as a globular or sessile intraretinal lesion that is composed of multiple vascular channels that have a reddish-blue color [29]. It may show patches of gray-white fibrous tissue on the surface, but it does not cause the exudation that characterizes the retinal capillary hemangioma. Cavernous hemangioma is a congenital retinal vascular hamartoma that is probably present at birth. This tumor can be associated with similar intracranial and cutaneous vascular hamartomas, but the syndrome does not have the visceral tumors that characterize the von Hippel Lindau syndrome. As a general rule, retinal cavernous hemangioma requires no active treatment. If vitreous hemorrhage should occur, laser or cryotherapy to the tumor can be attempted. If vitreous blood does not resolve, removal by vitrectomy may be necessary.

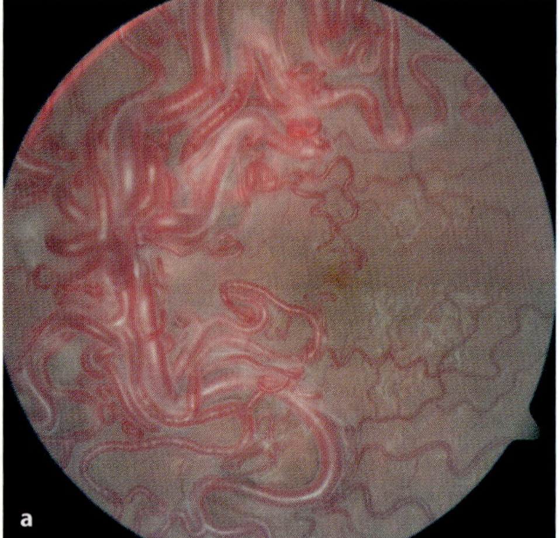

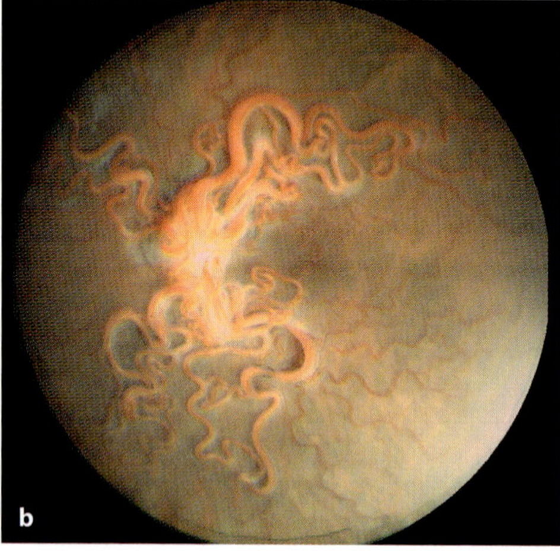

Fig. 8.14 a, b. Retinal racemose hemangioma. **a** Macular image showing the tortuous, dilated vessels. **b** Panoret image showing the entire extent of the hemangioma

8.4.4 Retinal Racemose Hemangioma

The retinal racemose hemangioma is not a true neoplasm but rather a simple or complex arteriovenous communication [29]. It is characterized by a large dilated tortuous retinal artery that passes from the optic disc for a variable distance into the fundus, where it then communicates directly with a similarly dilated retinal vein which passes back to the optic disc (Fig. 8.14). It can occur as a solitary unilateral lesion or it can be part of the Wyburn Mason syndrome, which is characterized by other similar lesions in the midbrain and sometimes the orbit, mandible, and maxilla. It does not appear to have a hereditary tendency.

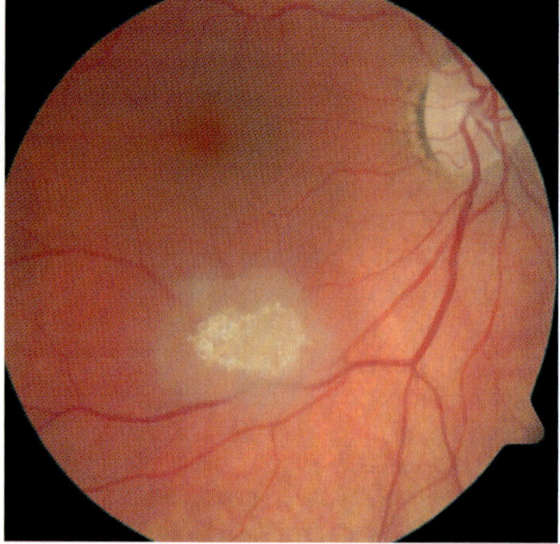

Fig. 8.15. Retinal astrocytic hamartoma with glistening calcification

8.4.5 Astrocytic Hamartoma of Retina

Astrocytic hamartoma of the retina is a yellow white intraretinal lesion that can also occur in the peripheral fundus or in the optic disc region. The lesion may be homogeneous or it may contain glistening foci of calcification (Fig. 8.15). Unlike retinal capillary hemangioma, it does not generally produce significant exudation or retinal detachment. Patients with astrocytic hamartoma of the retina should be evaluated for tuberous sclerosis, characterized by intracranial astrocytoma, cardiac rhabdomyoma, renal angiomyolipoma, pleural cysts, and other tumors and cysts.

8.4.6 Melanocytoma of the Optic Nerve

Melanocytoma of the optic nerve is a deeply pigmented congenital tumor that overlies a portion of the optic disc (Fig. 8.16) [29, 40]. Unlike

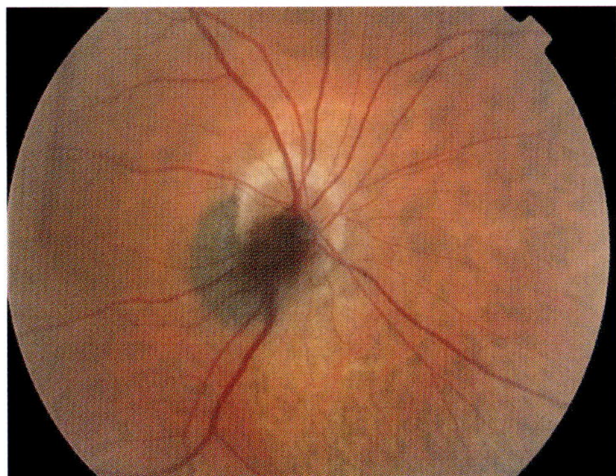

Fig. 8.16. Optic disc melanocytoma with choroidal component

uveal melanoma that occurs predominantly in whites, melanocytoma occurs with equal frequency in all races. It must be differentiated from malignant melanoma.

8.4.7 Intraocular Medulloepithelioma

Medulloepithelioma is an embryonal tumor that arises from the primitive medullary epithelium or the inner layer of the optic cup [29, 41]. It generally becomes clinically apparent in the first decade of life and appears as a fleshy, often cystic mass in the ciliary body (Fig. 8.17). Cataract and secondary glaucoma are frequent complications. Although approximately 60–90% are cytologically malignant, intraocular medulloepithelioma tends to be only locally invasive and distant metastasis is exceedingly rare. Larger tumors generally require enucleation of the affected eye. It is possible that some smaller tumors can be resected locally without enucleation [41].

8.4.8 Choroidal Hemangioma

Choroidal hemangioma is a benign vascular tumor that can occur as a circumscribed lesion in adults or as a diffuse tumor in children [12, 29]. The diffuse choroidal hemangioma usually

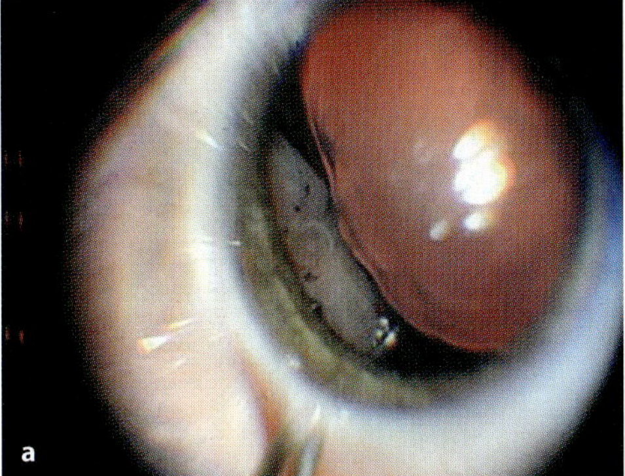

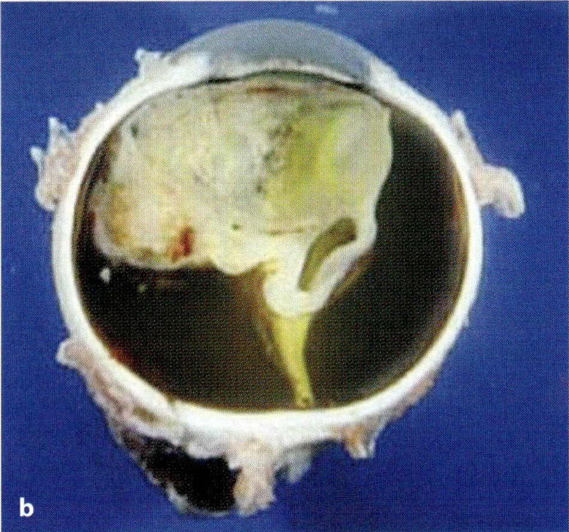

Fig. 8.17 a, b. Medulloepithelioma of the ciliary body. **a** Mass is visible peripheral to the lens on scleral depression. **b** Following enucleation in another case, the mass is seen in the ciliary body with total retinal detachment

occurs in association with ipsilateral facial nevus flammeus or variations of the Sturge-Weber syndrome. Ipsilateral congenital glaucoma is a frequent association. Secondary retinal detachment frequently occurs. Affected children often develop amblyopia in the involved eye.

8.4.9 Choroidal Osteoma

Choroidal osteoma is a benign choroidal tumor that is probably congenital. Although it has been recognized in infancy, it may not be diagnosed clinically until young adulthood [13, 29]. It is

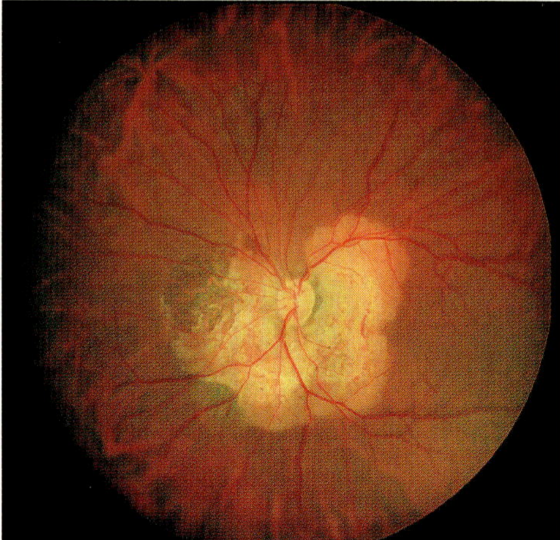

Fig. 8.18. Choroidal osteoma surrounding the optic disc

more common in females. It consists of a plaque of mature bone that generally occurs adjacent to the optic disc (Fig. 8.18). It generally shows slow enlargement and choroidal neovascularization with subretinal hemorrhage as a frequent complication. The pathogenesis is unknown. Serum calcium and phosphorus levels are normal.

8.4.10 Uveal Nevus

Uveal nevus is a flat or minimally elevated, variably pigmented tumor that may occur in the iris (Fig. 8.19) or in the choroid (Fig. 8.20). Although it is most likely congenital, it is usually asymptomatic and not usually recognized until later in life. Although most uveal nevi are stationary and nonprogressive, malignant transformation into melanoma can occur in rare instances [14].

An important variant of iris nevus is the presence of bilateral multiple, slightly elevated melanocytic lesions of the iris, known as Lisch nodules. These lesions become clinically apparent at about age 5 years and are often the first sign of von Recklinghausen's neurofibromatosis.

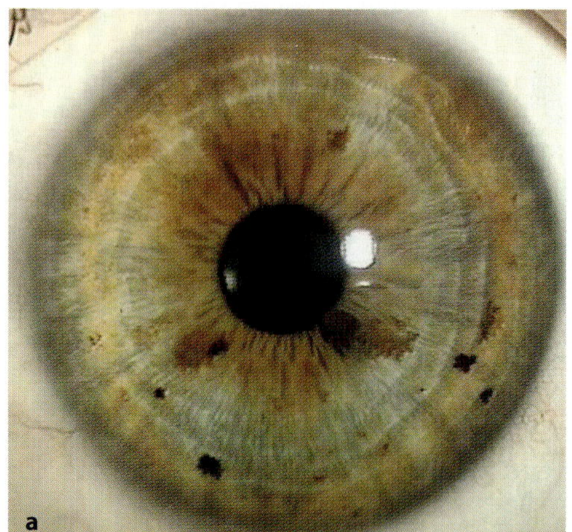

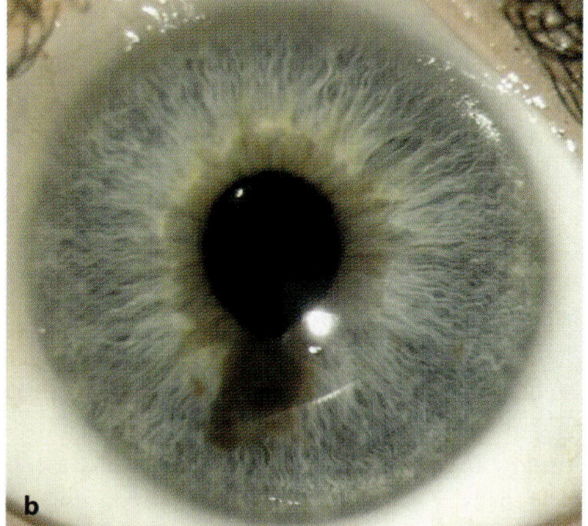

Fig. 8.19 a, b. Iris freckles and nevi. **a** Flat iris freckles on iris surface. **b** Slightly thickened iris nevus distorting the iris stroma and causing corectopia

8.4.11 Uveal Melanoma

Although uveal melanoma is generally a disease of adulthood, it is occasionally diagnosed in children [15]. It is a variably pigmented elevated mass that shows slow progression (Fig. 8.21). If it is not treated early, it has a tendency to metastasize to liver, lung, and other distant sites. Most advanced tumors are treated by enucleation. Radiotherapy of local tumor resection can be employed for less advanced tumors.

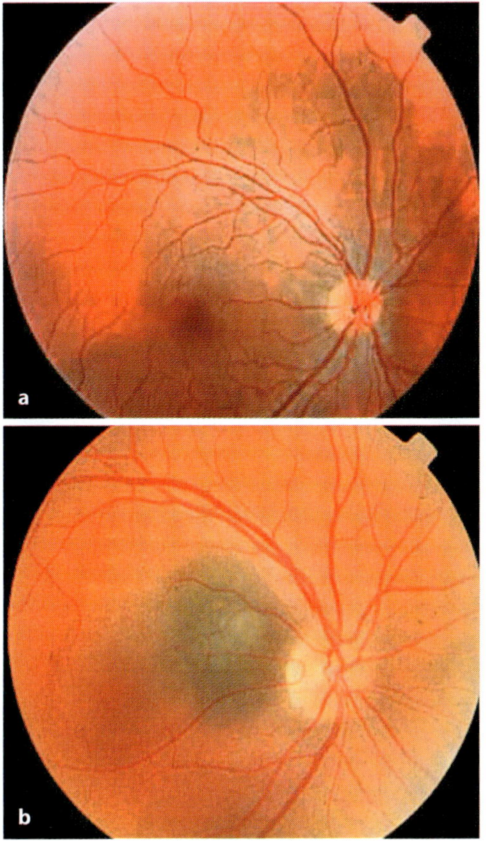

Fig. 8.20 a, b. Choroidal freckles and nevi. **a** Flat macular choroidal freckle. **b** Slightly thickened suspicious choroidal nevus in macular region

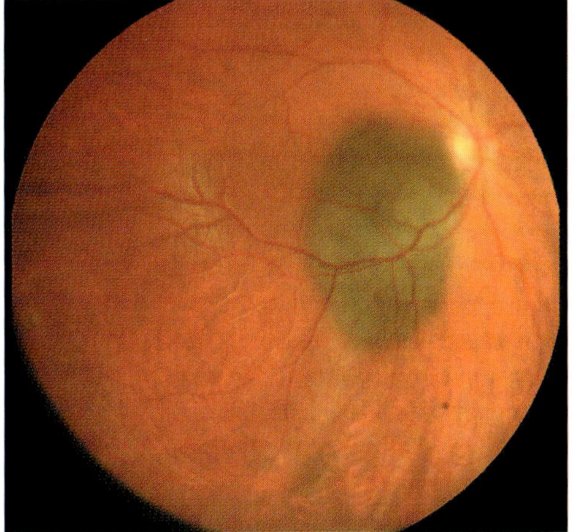

Fig. 8.21. Choroidal melanoma with shallow subretinal fluid and documented growth in a 16-year-old boy

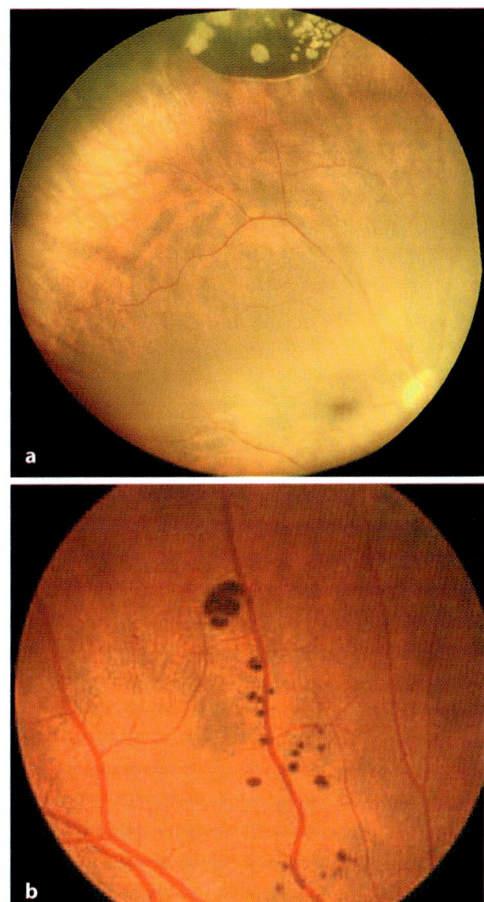

Fig. 8.22 a, b. Congenital hypertrophy of the retinal pigment epithelium (RPE). **a** Solitary type with lacunae and halo. **b** Multifocal type

8.4.12 Congenital Hypertrophy of Retinal Pigment Epithelium

Congenital hypertrophy of the retinal pigment epithelium (CHRPE) is a well circumscribed, flat, pigmented tumor that can occur anywhere in the fundus [16]. It often shows depigmented lacunae within the lesion and a surrounding pale halo. It can occur as a solitary lesion or it can be multiple as part of congenital grouped pigmentation lesion (Fig. 8.22). Similar but distinct multifocal pigmented lesions may be a marker for familial adenomatous polyposis and Gardner's syndrome in which patients have a high likelihood of developing colonic cancer [42].

8.4.13 Leukemia

Childhood leukemias can occasionally exhibit tumor infiltration in the retina, optic disc, and uveal tract. It is characterized by a swollen optic disc and thickening of the retina and choroid, often with hemorrhage and secondary retinal detachment. Intraocular leukemic infiltrates are generally responsive to irradiation and chemotherapy, but they generally portend a poor systemic prognosis.

Summary for the Clinician

- **Retinoblastoma is a highly malignant intraocular tumor of childhood**
- **Most children with unilateral retinoblastoma have the eye enucleated**
- **Most children with bilateral retinoblastoma are treated with chemoreduction and thermotherapy**
- **All children with retinoblastoma should have genetic analysis to establish the presence and site of the 13Q mutation**
- **Benign intraocular tumors of childhood are many and include choroidal nevus, congenital hypertrophy of the RPE, capillary hemangioma of the retina, and others**
- **Young children with retinal capillary hemangioma should be evaluated for von Hippel Lindau syndrome**

8.5 Orbital Tumors

A variety of orbital neoplasms and related space-occupying lesions can affect the orbit [43]. Orbital cellulitis secondary to sinusitis and inflammatory pseudotumors are more common than true neoplasms. Only about 5% of orbital lesions that come to biopsy prove to be malignant [44]. Cystic lesions are the most common group and vascular lesions are the second most common. This section covers orbital tumors and cysts but does not discuss orbital inflammatory or infectious conditions.

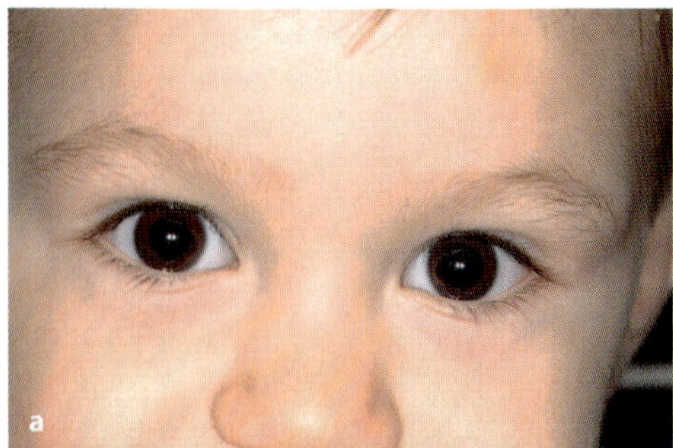

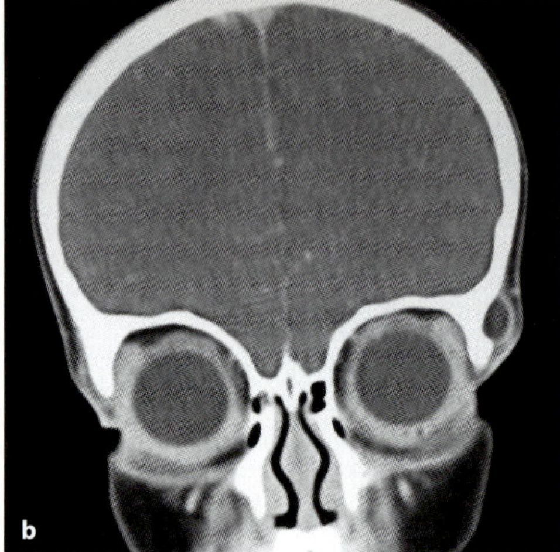

Fig. 8.23 a, b. Dermoid cyst near the lateral orbital rim, barely visible clinically. **a** Slight elevation of lateral orbital skin is shown. **b** Coronal CT showing the cystic mass

8.5.1 Dermoid Cyst

Dermoid cyst is the most common noninflammatory space occupying orbital mass in children [11, 45]. It usually appears in the first decade of life as a fairly firm, fixed, subcutaneous mass at the superotemporal orbital rim near the zygomaticofrontal suture (Fig. 8.23). Occasionally, a dermoid cyst may occur deeper in the orbit unattached to bone. Although it sometimes stationary, it does have a tendency to slowly enlarge. It can occasionally rupture, inciting an intense inflammatory reaction. Management is either serial observation or surgical removal of the mass.

8.5.2 Teratoma

A teratoma is a cystic mass that contains elements of all three embryonic germ layers [28]. An orbital teratoma causes proptosis, which is generally quite apparent at birth. The diagnosis should be suspected by imaging studies. Larger orbital teratomas can destroy the eye. Smaller teratomas can be removed intact without sacrificing the eye, but larger ones that have caused blindness may require orbital exenteration.

8.5.3 Capillary Hemangioma

Capillary hemangioma is the most common orbital vascular tumor of childhood [5, 28].

It usually is clinically apparent at birth or within the first few weeks after birth. It tends to cause progressive proptosis during the first few months of life and then it becomes stable and slowly regresses. Orbital imaging studies show a diffuse, poorly circumscribed, orbital mass that enhances with contrast material. The best management is refraction and treatment of any induced amblyopia with patching of the opposite eye. Local injection of corticosteroids or oral corticosteroids can hasten the regression of the mass and minimize the complications.

8.5.4 Lymphangioma

Lymphangioma is an important vascular tumor of the orbit in children [4, 28, 50]. It tends to become clinically apparent during the first decade of life. It may case abrupt proptosis following orbital trauma, secondary to hemorrhage into the lymphatic channels within the lesion (Fig. 8.24). Such spontaneous hemorrhages, called chocolate cysts, may require aspiration or surgical evacuation to prevent visual loss from compression of the eye.

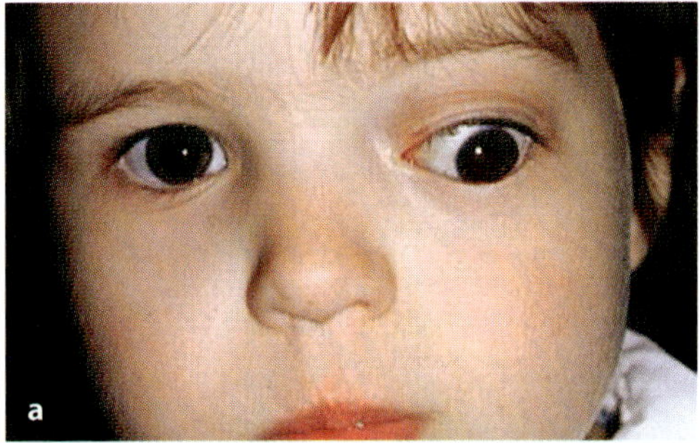

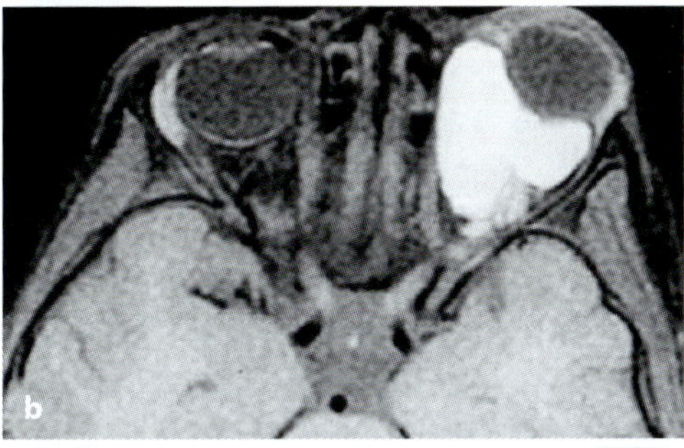

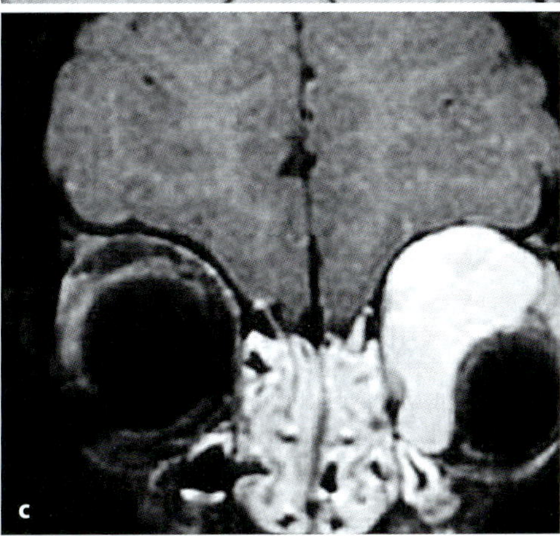

Fig. 8.24 a–c. Orbital lymphangioma producing rapid proptosis in a young child. **a** Downward displacement of the globe is shown. **b** Axial MRI showing bright signal in the blood filled cyst. **c** Coronal MRI showing the mass displacing the globe

8.5.5 Juvenile Pilocytic Astrocytoma

Juvenile pilocytic astrocytoma (optic nerve glioma) is the most common orbital neural tumor of childhood [28]. It is a cytological benign hamartoma that is generally stationary or very

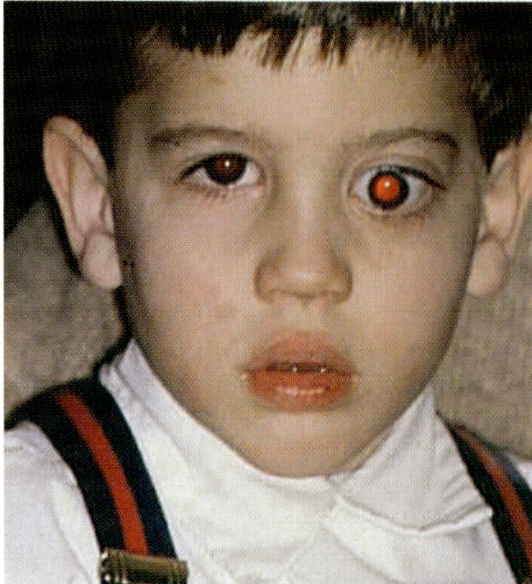

Fig. 8.25. Juvenile pilocytic astrocytoma of optic nerve causing proptosis

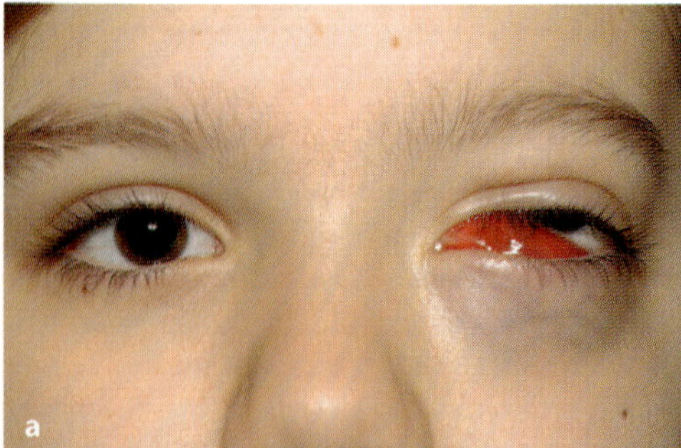

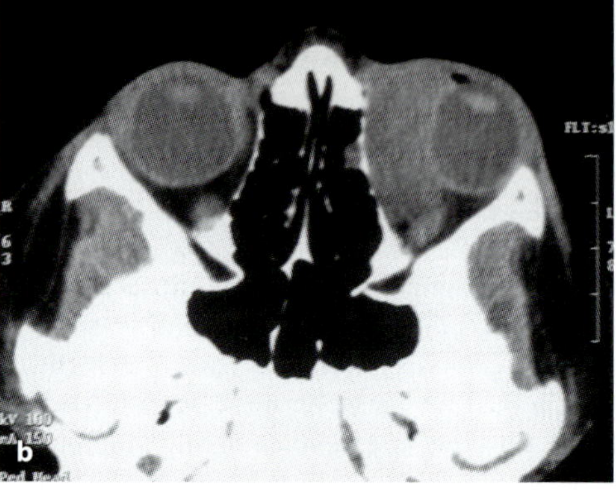

Fig. 8.26 a, b. Orbital rhabdomyosarcoma. **a** Proptosis and tumor involving the inferior fornix is shown. **b** Axial CT showing mass in medial orbit

slowly progressive. The affected child develops ipsilateral visual loss and slowly progressive axial proptosis (Fig. 8.25). Orbital imaging studies show an elongated or oval shaped mass that is well circumscribed because of the overlying dura mater. There is a greater incidence of this tumor in patients with neurofibromatosis. Since surgical excision necessitates blindness, the best management is periodic observation and surgical removal if there is blindness and cosmetically unacceptable proptosis. In cases that extend to the optic chiasm and are surgically unresectable, radiotherapy may be necessary.

8.5.6 Rhabdomyosarcoma

Rhabdomyosarcoma is the most important primary orbital malignant tumor of childhood [17, 28, 46]. It usually occurs in the first decade of life with a mean age of 8 years at the time of diagnosis. It causes fairly rapid proptosis and displacement of the globe, usually without pain or major inflammatory signs (Fig. 8.26). Imaging studies show an irregular but fairly well-circumscribed mass usually in the extraconal anterior orbit. Although orbital exenteration was often employed in the past, more recent experience has suggested that the best cure is obtained by performing a biopsy to confirm the diagnosis and treating with combined irradiation and chemotherapy, using vincristine, Cytoxan and adriamycin [17, 46].

8.5.7 Granulocytic Sarcoma (Chloroma)

Granulocytic sarcoma is the soft tissue infiltration by myelogenous leukemia [3, 28, 47]. Although leukemia usually appears first in the blood and bone marrow, the orbit soft tissues may be the initial site to become clinically apparent. The child presents with a fairly rapid onset of proptosis and displacement of the globe. Confirmation of the orbital lesion can be made by biopsy and the condition treated by chemotherapy or low-dose irradiation.

8.5.8
Lymphoma

The only important lymphoma to affect the orbit of children is Burkitt's lymphoma. Although this tumor was originally recognized exclusively in African tribes, it is being recognized more often in patients with the autoimmune deficiency syndrome (AIDS) and as an American form in otherwise normal children [28].

8.5.9
Langerhans Cell Histiocytosis

Eosinophilic granuloma can affect the orbital bones as an intraosseous bone-destructive inflammatory lesion. Although it can occur anywhere in the orbit, it most often occurs in the anterior portion of the frontal and zygomatic bones. Recent ultrastructural studies have suggested the stem cell in eosinophilic granuloma and certain other tumors in the histiocytic X group is the Langerhans cell. Hence, the term Langerhans cell histiocytosis is becoming preferable [28].

8.5.10
Metastatic Neuroblastoma

Although orbital metastasis in children can occur secondary to Wilms' and Ewing's tumors, metastatic neuroblastoma is the most common metastatic orbital of childhood [28]. The majority of children with orbital metastasis of neuroblastoma have a previously diagnosed primary neoplasm in the adrenal gland. However, the orbital metastasis can be diagnosed before the adrenal primary in about 3% of cases.

Summary for the Clinician

- **Only 5% of orbital tumors in children are malignant**
- **Dermoid cyst is the most common orbital mass in children**
- **Orbital malignancies in children include rhabdomyosarcoma, lymphoma, leukemic infiltrates, and many others**
- **Using accepted chemotherapy protocols, often with nearly 1 year of chemotherapy and a course of radiotherapy, children with orbital rhabdomyosarcoma generally have a favorable life prognosis**

Acknowledgements. Supported by the Eye Tumor Research Foundation, Inc., Philadelphia, PA.

References

1. De Potter P, Shields JA, Shields CL (1994) MRI of the eye and orbit. Lippincott, Philadelphia
2. Epstein J, Shields CL, Shields JA (2003) Trends in the management of retinoblastoma. Evaluation of 1,196 consecutive eyes during 1974–2001. J Pediatr Ophthalmol Strabismus 40:196–203
3. Font RL, Zimmerman LE (1975) Ophthalmologic manifestations of granulocytic sarcoma (myeloid sarcoma or chloroma). Am J Ophthalmol 80:975–990
4. Garrity JA (1997) Orbital venous anomalies. A long-standing dilemma. Ophthalmology 104:903–904
5. Haik BG, Karcioglu ZA, Gordon RA, Pechous BP (1994) Capillary hemangioma (infantile periocular hemangioma). Review. Surv Ophthalmol 38:399–426
6. Hungerford J (1993) Factors influencing metastasis in retinoblastoma. Br J Ophthalmol 77:541
7. Kingston JE, Hungerford JL, Madreperla SA, Plowman PN (1996) Results of combined chemotherapy and radiotherapy for advanced intraocular retinoblastoma. Arch Ophthalmol 114:1339–1343
8. Lee V, Hungerford JL, Bunce C, Ahmed F, Kingston JE, Plowman PN (2003) Globe conserving treatment of the only eye in bilateral retinoblastoma. Br J Ophthalmol 87:1374–1380
9. Marr BP, Shields CL, Shields JA (2005) Neoplastic and inflammatory tumors of the eyelids. In: Tasman WS, Jaeger EA (eds) Duane's foundations of clinical ophthalmology, 3rd edn. Lippincott Williams and Wilkins, Philadelphia (in press)
10. O'Hara BJ, Ehya H, Shields JA, Augsburger JJ, Shields CL, Eagle RC Jr (1993) Fine needle aspiration biopsy in pediatric ophthalmic tumors and pseudotumors. Acta Cytol 37:125–130
11. Sathananthan N, Mosely IF, Rose GE, Wright JE (1993) The frequency and clinical significance of bone involvement in outer canthus dermoid cysts. Br J Ophthalmol 77:789–794

12. Shields CL, Honavar SG, Shields JA, Cater J, Demirci H (2001) Circumscribed choroidal hemangioma. Clinical manifestations and factors predictive of visual outcome in 200 consecutive cases. Ophthalmology 108:2237–2248
13. Shields CL, Shields JA, Augsburger JJ (1988) Review: choroidal osteoma. Surv Ophthalmol 33: 17–27
14. Shields CL, Cater JC, Shields JA, Singh AD, Santos MCM, Carvalho C (2000) Combination of clinical factors predictive of growth of small choroidal melanocytic tumors. Arch Ophthalmol 118:360–364
15. Shields CL, Shields JA, Milite J, De Potter P, Sabbagh R, Menduke H (1991) Uveal melanoma in teenagers and children. A report of 40 cases. Ophthalmology 98:1662–1666
16. Shields CL, Mashayekhi A, Ho T, Cater J, Shields JA (2003) Solitary congenital hypertrophy of the retinal pigment epithelium: clinical features and frequency of enlargement in 330 patients. Ophthalmology 110:1968–1976
17. Shields CL, Shields JA, Honavar SG, Demerci H (2001) The clinical spectrum of primary ophthalmic rhabdomyosarcoma. Ophthalmology 108:2284–2292
18. Shields CL, Shields JA, Shah P (1991) Retinoblastoma in older children. Ophthalmology 98:395–399
19. Shields CL, Shields JA (2004) Tumors of the conjunctiva and cornea. Surv Ophthalmol 49:3–24
20. Shields CL, Fasiudden A, Mashayekhi A, Shields JA (2004) Conjunctival nevi: clinical features and natural course in 410 consecutive patients. Arch Ophthalmol 122:167–175
21. Shields CL, Lally MR, Singh AD, Shields JA, Nowinski T (1999) Oral cimetidine (Tagamet) for recalcitrant, diffuse conjunctival papillomatosis. Am J Ophthalmol 128:362–364
22. Shields CL, Mashayekhi A, Demirci H, Meadows AT, Shields JA (2004) A practical approach to management of retinoblastoma. Arch Ophthalmol 122:729–735
23. Shields CL, Shields JA, De Potter P, Singh AD (1994) Problems with the hydroxyapatite orbital implant: experience with 250 consecutive cases. Br J Ophthalmol 78:702–706
24. Shields CL, Shields JA (2002) Genetics of retinoblastoma. In: Tasman WS, Jaeger EA (eds) Duane's foundations of clinical ophthalmology, 3rd edn. Lippincott Willliams and Wilkins, Philadelphia, pp 1–8
25. Shields CL, Mashayekhi A, Luo CK, Materin MA, Shields JA (2004) Optical coherence tomography in children. Analysis of 44 eyes with intraocular tumors and simulating conditions. J Pediatr Ophthalmol Strabismus 41:338–344
26. Shields CL, De Potter P, Himmelstein B, Shields JA, Meadows AT, Maris J (1996) Chemoreduction in the initial management of intraocular retinoblastoma. Arch Ophthalmol 114:1330–1338
27. Shields CL, Honavar SG Meadows AT, Shields JA, Demirci H, Singh AD, Friedman D, Naduvilaths TJ (2002) Chemoreduction plus focal therapy for retinoblastoma: factors predictive of need for treatment with external beam radiotherapy or enucleation. Am J Ophthalmol 133:657–664
28. Shields JA (1989) Diagnosis and management of orbital tumors. Saunders, Philadelphia
29. Shields JA, Shields CL (1992) Intraocular tumors. A text and atlas. Saunders, Philadelphia
30. Shields JA, Shields CL (1999) Atlas of eyelid and conjunctival tumors. Lippincott Williams and Wilkins, Philadelphia
31. Shields JA, Shields CL (1999) Atlas of intraocular tumors. Lippincott Williams and Wilkins, Philadelphia
32. Shields JA, Shields CL (1999) Atlas of orbital tumors. Lippincott Williams and Wilkins, Philadelphia
33. Shields JA, Parsons HM, Shields CL, Shah P (1991) Lesions simulating retinoblastoma. J. Pediatr Ophthalmol Strabismus 28:338–340
34. Shields JA, Shields CL (2002) Review: Coats disease. The 2001 LuEsther Mertz Lecture. Retina 22:80–91
35. Shields JA (1984) Ocular toxocariasis. A review. Surv Ophthalmol 28:361–381
36. Shields JA, Shields CL, Sivalingam V (1989) Decreasing frequency of enucleation in patients with retinoblastoma. Am J Ophthalmol 108:185–188
37. Shields JA, Kiratli H, Shields CL, Eagle RC Jr, Luo S (1994) Schwannoma of the eyelid in a child. J Pediatr Ophthalmol Strabismus 31:332–333
38. Shields JA, Shields CL, Eagle RC Jr MD, Arevalo F, De Potter P (1997) Ocular manifestations of the organoid nevus syndrome. Ophthalmology 104: 549–557
39. Shields JA, Shields CL, Suvarnamani C, Schroeder RP, DePotter P (1991) Retinoblastoma manifesting as orbital cellulitis. Am J Ophthalmol 112:442–449
40. Shields JA (1978) Melanocytoma of the optic nerve head. A review. Int Ophthalmol 1:31–37
41. Shields JA, Eagle RC Jr, Shields CL, De Potter P (1996) Congenital neoplasms of the nonpigmented ciliary epithelium. (medulloepithelioma). Ophthalmology 103:1998–2006
42. Shields JA, Shields CL, Shah P, Pastore D, Imperiale SM Jr (1992) Lack of association between typical congenital hypertrophy of the retinal pigment epithelium and Gardner's syndrome. Ophthalmology 99:1705–1713

43. Shields JA, Shields CL, Scartozzi R (2004) Survey of 1264 orbital tumors and pseudotumors. The 2002 Montgomery Lecture. Ophthalmology 111: 997–1008
44. Shields JA, Bakewell B, Augsberger JJ, Bernardino V (1988) Space-occupying orbital masses in children: a review of 250 consecutive biopsies. Ophthalmology 93:379–384
45. Shields JA, Kaden IH, Eagle RC Jr, Shields CL (1997) Orbital dermoid cysts. Clinicopathologic correlations, classification, and management. The 1997 Josephine E. Schueler Levture. Ophthal Plast Reconstr Surg 13:265–276
46. Shields JA, Shields CL (2003) Rhabdomyosarcoma: review for the ophthalmologist. Surv Ophthalmol 48:39–57
47. Shields JA, Stopyra GA, Marr BP, Shields CL, Pan W, Eagle RC Jr, Bernstein J (2003) Bilateral orbital myeloid sarcoma as initial sign of acute myeloid leukemia. Arch Ophthalmol 121:138–142
48. Singh AD, DePotter P, Fijal B, Shields CL, Shields JA (1998) Lifetime prevalence of uveal melanoma in white patients with oculo (dermal) melanocytosis. Ophthalmology 105:195–198
49. Singh AD, Shields CL, Shields JA (2001) Major review: Von Hippel-Lindau disease. Surv Ophthalmol 46:117–142
50. Wright JE, Sullivan TJ, Garner A, Wulc AE, Moseley IF (1997) Orbital venous anomalies. Ophthalmology 104:905–913

Paediatric Electrophysiology: A Practical Approach

9

Graham E. Holder, Anthony G. Robson

Core Messages

- Electrophysiological testing provides an objective and noninvasive method for visual pathway evaluation
- Complementary use of different electrophysiological procedures allows accurate characterisation and localisation of dysfunction. EOG: The photoreceptor/RPE interface; ERG: rod and cone photoreceptor and inner retinal function; PERG: macular and retinal ganglion cell function; VEP: intracranial visual pathway function
- Electrophysiology enables distinction between disorders that may present with similar signs and/or symptoms and facilitates differentiation between benign and severe, progressive and stationary disorders
- Invaluable in suspected nonorganic visual loss
- Accurate electrophysiological phenotyping is likely to become increasingly important as genotyping increases and new therapies are developed

9.1 Introduction

The electrophysiological examination of the paediatric patient can be of great clinical importance. In addition to the objective nature of the data provided by electrophysiological testing, the potential inability of a child to describe accurately, if at all, their symptoms places electrophysiology in a privileged position of diagnostic importance. Further, it is noninvasive. A formal clinical audit of the role of electrophysiology in paediatric practice demonstrated a significant influence on management [88]. After an initial description of the available techniques and their uses, the subsequent discussion will adopt a practical approach to diagnosis, based on presenting signs and symptoms, to demonstrate how electrophysiological testing can enable management decisions to be taken with greater confidence.

9.2 Electrophysiological Techniques

9.2.1 Electroretinography

The electroretinogram (ERG) is the mass response of the retina to a luminance stimulus, usually a stroboscopically generated short-duration flash (Fig. 9.1). In adults, ERGs are recorded using corneal electrodes with stimuli delivered via a Ganzfeld bowl. This approach is tenable with older children who are capable of understanding the demands of testing, but there are two distinct schools of thought in relation to the young child or infant. Some adopt the approach that children are simply young adults, and use the same techniques; inevitably this requires either restraint or sedation in some patients. Others adopt the view that the clinical data required in a young child are different to those in an adult population, requiring answers to different, less complex questions, such as "is this baby blind" or "why has this child got nystagmus", and that clinically meaningful and satisfactory data can be obtained using less inva-

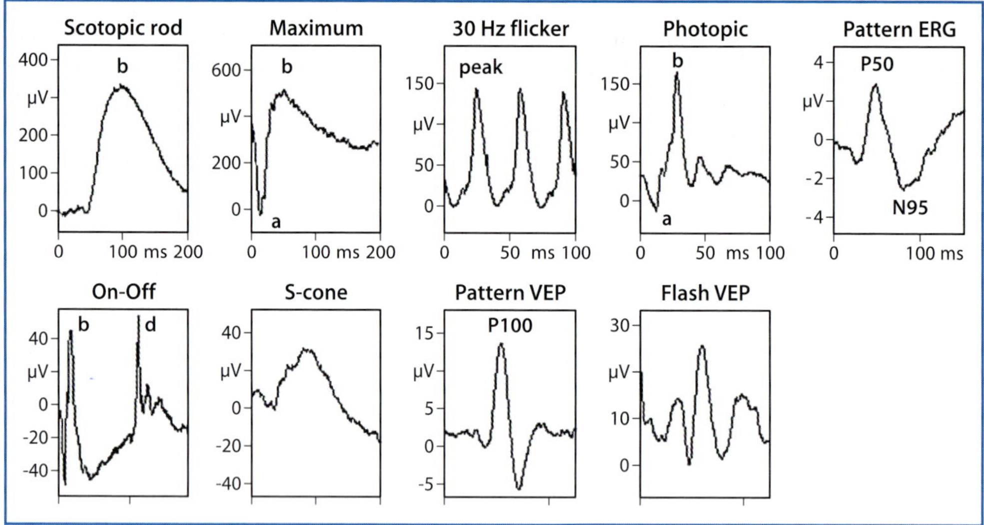

Fig. 9.1. Examples of normal pattern ERG, full-field ERGs, ON-OFF ERGs and S-cone specific ERGs. Major components are labelled. The ON-OFF ERG is recorded to 200 ms orange stimulation with a green photopic background. Normal pattern and flash VEPs are also shown

sive techniques, particularly involving the use of surface recording electrodes [47, 60]. The authors' approach is to adapt procedures according to the ability of the patient to cooperate, using a simplified protocol and surface electrodes in young children and introducing longer procedures, Ganzfeld stimulation, corneal electrodes and mydriasis in those children who are able to tolerate longer, more demanding protocols. The theoretical discussion that follows on the origins of the different ERG components is unaffected by such considerations.

The ERG to a bright flash in a dark-adapted eye consists of two main components, the negative a-wave and the positive b-wave (Fig. 9.1). Approximately the first 10 ms of the a-wave reflects photoreceptor hyperpolarisation, and in general, marked a-wave amplitude reduction reflects photoreceptor loss or dysfunction. The b-wave, which should be of higher amplitude, reflects retinal activity generated post-phototransduction, predominantly in relation to depolarisation of the ON- bipolar cells [76]. An ERG waveform in which the a-wave is spared, but the b-wave shows selective reduction, often such that it is of lower amplitude than the a-wave, is known as a negative or electronegative ERG. A negative ERG does not mean that the ERG is undetectable, merely that the waveform is dominated by the negative a-wave, and as such indicates inner retinal dysfunction. Under photopic conditions, there is a probable contribution from post-receptoral structures to the a-wave, particularly at low luminance levels [15, 76].

Much clinical ERG work is based on the Standards and recommendations of the International Society for Clinical Electrophysiology of Vision (ISCEV). The ISCEV Standard for ERG recording [57] defines a standard flash of 1.5–3.0 $cd.s.m^{-2}$. A response specific for the rod system is obtained using the standard flash attenuated by 2.5 log units in a dark-adapted eye. Dark adaptation, to comply with the ISCEV Standard, requires at least 20 min in complete darkness and maximum mydriasis. The response to the standard flash under dark adaptation is a mixed rod–cone response dominated by rod function. Commencing with the most recent Standard document, ISCEV also suggests the recording of a response to a higher intensity flash (~11.0 $cd.s.m^{-2}$) better to record the a-wave, and thus photoreceptor function. This can be particularly helpful in the young child. Photopic ERGs, in addition to a single flash cone response (with a rod-suppressing background and adequate photopic adaptation), are also recorded to a 30-Hz flicker stimulus (Fig. 9.1); rods have poor temporal resolution and do not contribute significantly to the response at this stimulus rate. The ERG is a mass response, and is normal when dysfunction is confined to small retinal areas. Despite the high photoreceptor density, this also applies to macular dysfunction; an eye with dysfunction confined to the macula does not have a significantly abnormal ERG. Separation of the cone ON (depolarising bipolar cells, DBCs) and OFF (hyperpolarising bipolar cells, HBCs) responses can be performed using long duration stimulation with a photopic background [77], using either a shutter system or light emitting diodes to produce the stimulus.

The above-mentioned techniques can be used in older children. The approach to infants adopted in the authors' laboratories differs. The initial recordings, using surface recording electrodes on the lower eyelids with reference to electrodes at the ipsilateral outer canthi, take place under light-adapted conditions and include the ERGs to single flash and flicker. These determine the presence or absence of cone system function, with the implicit time of the flicker ERG being a particularly good indicator of generalised cone system function. The child is then dark adapted for 5 min, and bright flash stimuli given. These should evoke ERGs of very different waveform and much higher amplitude than the responses to single flashes under light-adapted conditions and allow an estimation of whether there is a functioning scotopic system. For the young infant, the clinical questions are generally (a) is there an ERG? (b) is there generalised cone dysfunction? (c) is there a functioning scotopic system? (d) is there an electronegative ERG? These questions can adequately be answered by such recordings. Typical examples of surface recordings are illustrated in Fig. 9.2. Throughout these recordings, the child is usually sitting on the lap of the mother, and stimulation is applied using a hand-held stroboscopic flash. If the child remains content after 5 min dark adaptation, further recordings, perhaps using rod-specific stimulation, can be used, but the presence or absence of subtle rod system dysfunction is not usually of clinical relevance in a young infant. Mydriasis is not usually used in infants, as the act of instilling mydriatic drops is often sufficient to cause undesired distress.

Childhood ERGs are often prone to the effects of eye movement and eye closure and it is important to demonstrate reproducibility. It is also important to relate the ERGs obtained to the age of the child; the maturation of ERGs in early and late infancy has been extensively and recently reviewed [28, 86].

9.2.2 Pattern Electroretinography

The pattern electroretinogram (PERG) is the response of central retina and is usually measured using a reversing black and white checkerboard. It is important that there is no luminance change during pattern reversal. It allows both a measure of central retinal function and, in relation to its origins, an evaluation of retinal ganglion cell function. It is thus of great value in the electrophysiological differentiation between macular dysfunction and generalised retinal dysfunction or optic nerve dysfunction in the older child with visual acuity loss (see [40] for a comprehensive review). It is important to preserve the optics of the eye for PERG recording, which requires non-contact lens electrodes in contact with the cornea or bulbar conjunctiva to preserve the optics of the eye, and no mydriasis. The gold foil, the DTL and the H-K loop electrode are all suitable. Ipsilateral outer canthus reference electrodes are mandatory; there is contamination from the cortically generated VEP if forehead or ear "reference" electrodes are used [7]. In young children incapable of tolerating corneal electrodes, surface electrodes may be used [14]. The signal:noise ratio is inevitably lower compared with corneal recordings and responses are particularly sensitive to alterations in fixation. Continuous monitoring and "interrupted averaging" [40, 72] during lapses in fixation or to allow blinking is essential in order to optimise the quality of recordings. Surface PERGs may be elicited using large stimulus fields; the use of such stimuli may be beneficial in terms of signal:noise ratio and by encouraging better fixation, but require cautious interpretation and comparison with corresponding normal values. In general, the presence of any PERG excludes severe macular dysfunction.

There are two main components in the so-called transient PERG: P50 at approximately 50 ms and a larger N95 at 95 ms [37] (Fig. 9.1). Assessment concentrates on the amplitude of P50, measured from the trough of the small early negative N35 component; the latency of P50 measured to peak; and the amplitude of N95, measured to trough from the peak of P50. The N95 is a contrast-related component generated in the retinal ganglion cells. Approximately 70 % of P50 appears to be ganglion cell-related, but the remainder is not related to spiking cell function and may be generated more distally in the retina [81]. The exact origins have yet to be ascertained. Although the PERG is generated in inner retina, the P50 component is "driven" by the macular photoreceptors and thus reflects macular function.

For optimal recording of the PERG, an analysis time of 150 ms or greater is usually used. It is a low-amplitude signal and computerised averaging is essential. The necessary stringent technical controls are important and are fully discussed elsewhere [25]. Binocular stimulation and recording is usually preferred so the better eye can maintain fixation and accommodation, but if there is a history of squint it is necessary to use monocular recording. P50 is sensitive to optical blur, and accurate refraction is important. PERG amplitude is related almost linearly to stimulus contrast at low stimulus frequencies. ISCEV recommends a high-contrast black and white reversing checkerboard with approximately 50-min checks in a 10- to 16-degree field.

9.2.3 Cortical Visual Evoked Potentials

Visual evoked potentials (VEPs) are used to assess the integrity and function of the visual pathways, particularly the optic nerves and optic chiasm. Responses are recorded using scalp electrodes placed over the occipital areas. The VEP is a relatively small signal in relation to the background electroencephalographic activity, and computerised signal averaging and repetitive stimulation are used to extract the time-locked VEP. A reversing black and white checkerboard or diffuse flash stimulation is commonly used, but pattern onset/offset is effective in certain conditions (see below) and is less dependent on stable fixation. The checkerboard reversal VEP is usually the most sensitive indicator of optic nerve dysfunction. Monocular stimulation is essential and multi-channel recordings help localisation of dysfunction. Infants and children often require constant encouragement and reassurance and fixation and cooperation should be continuously monitored; averaging may then be suspended during periods of inattention.

The transient (<2/s recommended) checkerboard reversal VEP in adults contains a prominent positive component at approximately 100 ms known as P100 (Fig. 9.1). Stimulus parameters such as contrast, luminance, check size, field size, etc., are important determinants of the waveform, and it is essential for each laboratory to establish its age-matched normal controls. Maturational changes in pattern and flash VEPs have been extensively documented [12, 48, 71].

9.2.4 Electro-oculography

The electro-oculogram (EOG) refers to measurement of the standing potential of the eye. This potential difference is generated across the retinal pigment epithelium and manifests as a dipole between the back of the eye and the electropositive cornea (for a recent review see [25]). The ERG is a global response and allows assessment of the photoreceptor/RPE interface. A normal EOG depends on the integrity of the photoreceptors and a functioning RPE. A reduced EOG is generally accompanied by a reduction in the full-field ERG unless dysfunction is confined to the RPE (see Sect. 9.6.1.2). The ISCEV-standard EOG is measured by recording the potentials generated by fixed excursion eye movements during a standard period of dark adaptation, and then during restoration to full photopic conditions [56]. The eye movement excursions are prompted by alternately flashing lights and accurate testing depends on the child's cooperation and ability to follow these fixation lights; it is rarely possible to test children younger than about 6 years of age. The EOG is usually expressed as a light peak:dark trough ratio, the Arden index.

Accurate diagnosis and phenotyping of retinal dystrophies often relies on the pattern of electrophysiological abnormality. The pattern ERG is used to assess central retinal function and the full-field ERG generalised retinal function. Patients with generalised retinal dysfunction and severe ERG abnormalities can have normal PERGs if the macula is spared. Conversely, patients with disease confined to the macula have normal ERGs, but the PERG P50 may be profoundly abnormal. Thus, optimal phenotyping requires the use of both techniques [40, 25]. The examples that follow are discussed in relation to common presenting symptoms. Such a classification inevitably results in a degree of overlap; selected examples are used here to illustrate this integrated approach to visual electrodiagnosis.

9.3 Investigation of Night Blindness

Correct early diagnosis of night blindness is important because it may be the presenting symptom of a progressive retinal dystrophy with significant implications for vision. However, it may reflect a stationary disorder such as congenital stationary night blindness (CSNB); electrophysiology enables the distinction. Symptoms of night blindness are not always obvious, particularly in infants and young children.

9.3.1 Retinitis Pigmentosa (Rod–Cone Dystrophy)

Retinitis pigmentosa (RP) is a heterogeneous group of disorders characterised by progressive dysfunction affecting the rod more than the cone photoreceptors (a rod–cone dystrophy). Typically patients present with night blindness and visual field constriction. Central vision may or may not be involved. Classical signs include bone-spicule pigmentation, vessel attenuation and disc pallor, but the fundus may be normal in the early stages of disease, and this is often the case in young children. Fundus appearance may be a poor indicator of the severity of dysfunction.

The rod-specific ERG, reflecting rod-system sensitivity, arises in the inner retina and is usually subnormal or undetectable in RP. The most direct ERG measure of rod photoreceptor function is the a-wave of the bright flash (maximal) ERG and in RP this will also be affected with associated reduction of the b-wave (Fig. 9.3). The normal maximal ERG is of high amplitude, usually allowing easy recording. This can be exploited in paediatric cases where surface electrodes may be used effectively to assess rod photoreceptor activity (see below). Photopic cone-mediated ERGs are less severely affected than rod-driven ERGs in RP, but usually show delayed implicit time and amplitude reduction, best seen in the 30-Hz flicker response. The degree of central retinal involvement in RP can be indicated by the PERG; some patients with RP and preserved central vision have an almost undetectable full-field ERG but a normal PERG P50 component (Fig. 9.3) consistent with macular sparing [40, 72, 73]. However, the PERG P50 component can be abnormal in the presence of normal visual acuity [40, 72, 73] and may have some prognostic value in predicting involvement of central vision. Although difficult for young children to perform, multifocal ERG may play a similar role to PERG in the assessment of macular function.

In X-linked RP, accounting for about 5–20% of all familial cases [35], the ERG is usually undetectable or grossly subnormal from an early age (Fig. 9.3D). Asymptomatic female heterozygotes may show a prominent tapetal reflex and there may be intraretinal bone-spicule pigmentation, although the fundus can be normal. The incidence of ERG abnormality in X-linked carriers is high and may involve amplitude or implicit time [3, 9] in both rod and/or cone ERGs. The ERG findings in heterozygotes may show significant interocular asymmetry, unlike

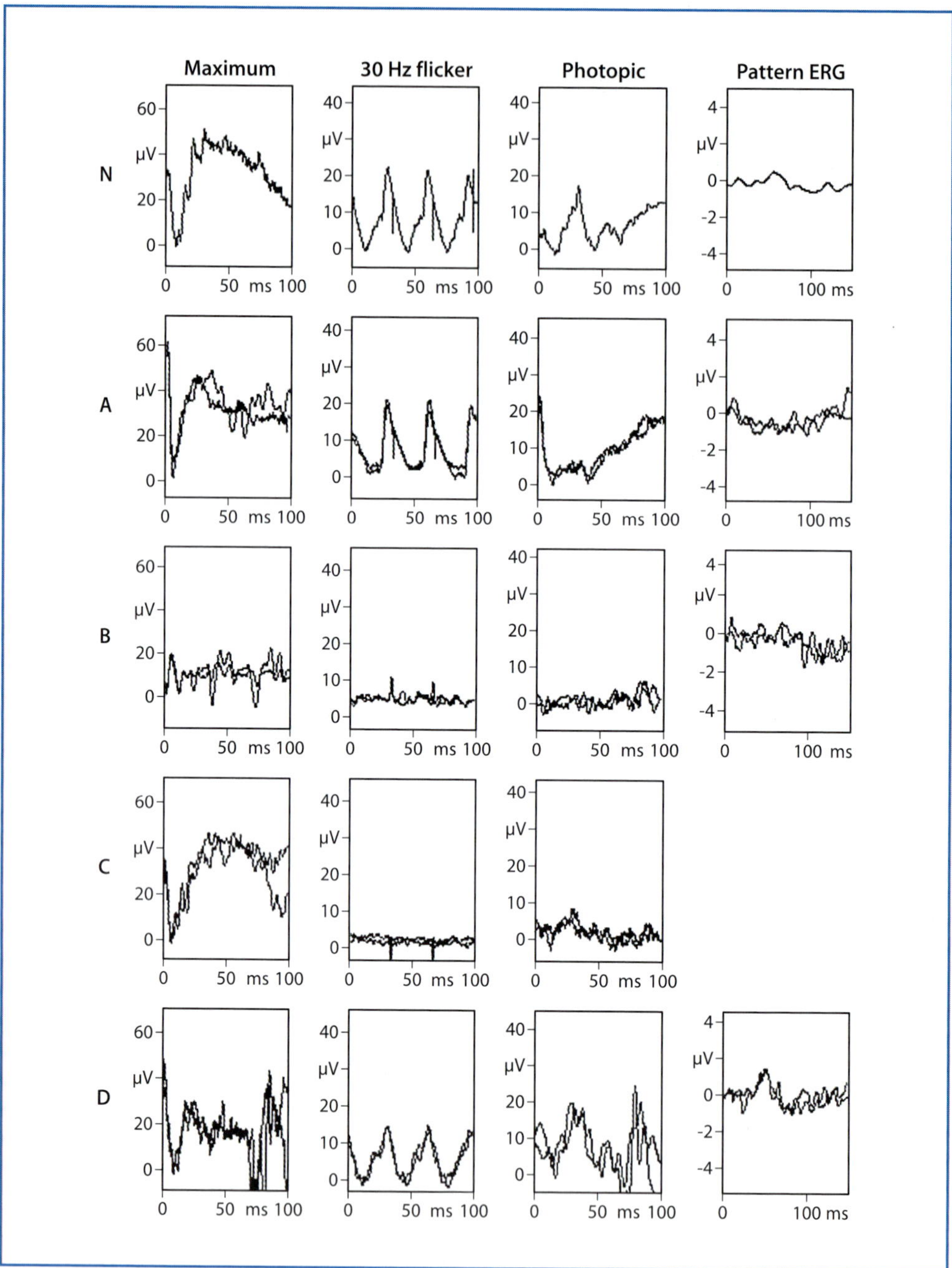

Fig. 9.2. Pattern and flash ERGs in a normal subject (*N*), in a 2-year-old patient with complete CSNB (*A*), in a 6-year-old patient with Leber congenital amaurosis (*B*), in a 1-year-old monochromat (*C*) and in a 7-year old patient with X-linked retinoschisis (*D*). All recordings were taken with surface eyelid electrodes apart from the PERG in patient D, which was obtained using gold foil corneal electrodes. Comparison of A with Fig. 9.4A and C with Fig. 9.5C demonstrates the qualitative similarity of surface and corneal recordings. See text for details

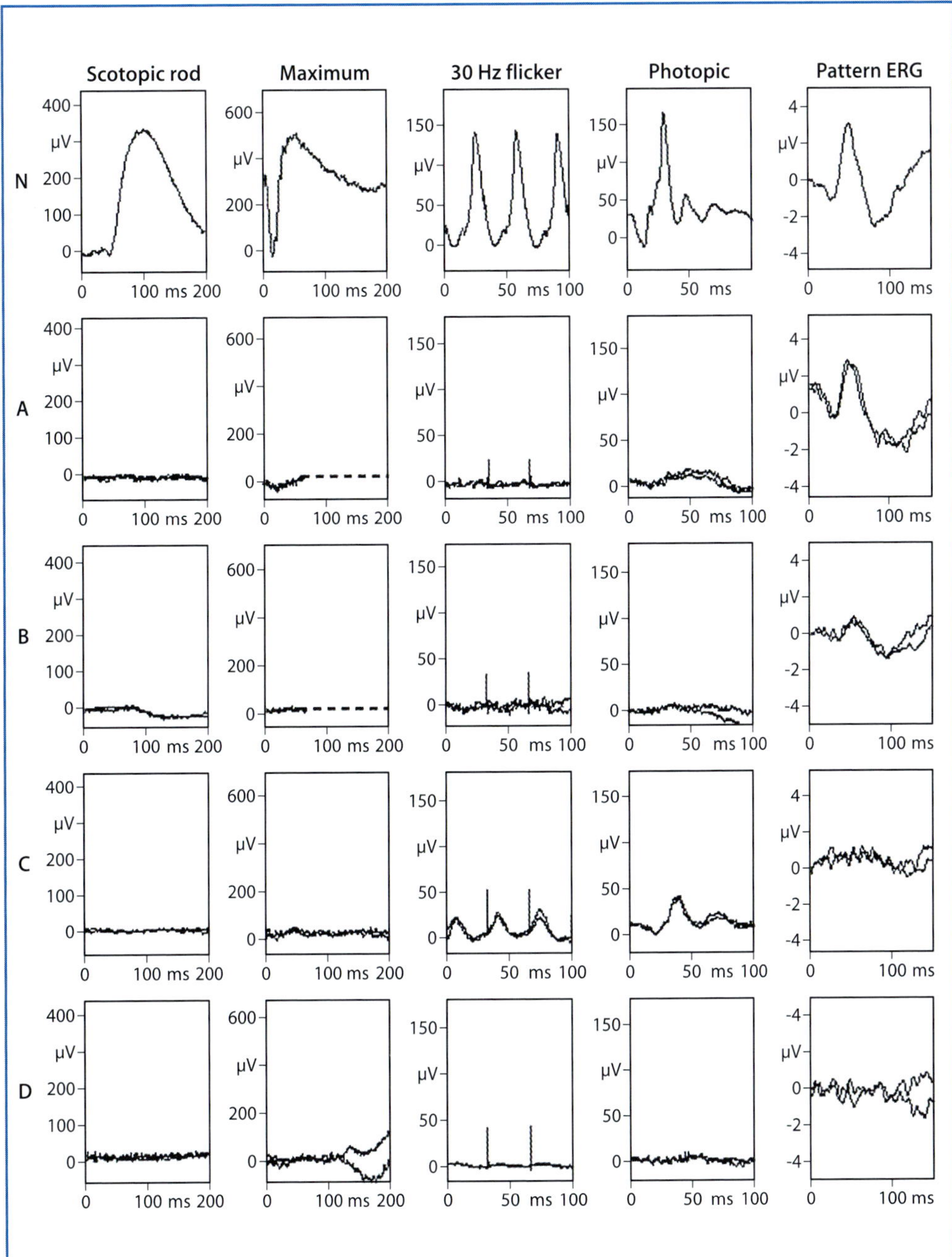

Fig. 9.3. Typical findings in a normal subject (*N*) and in four patients with rod–cone dystrophy. Maximum ERG a-waves are reduced, consistent with rod photoreceptor dysfunction. Photopic ERGs are reduced and delayed, indicating significant but less severe cone system dysfunction. Pattern ERGs in patient A (aged 9 years) are normal, in keeping with macular sparing and normal visual acuity (6/9). In patient B (aged 11 years), PERG P50 component and visual acuity are mildly reduced (6/12). In C (aged 10 years) PERG 50 is severely reduced, consistent with severe macular involvement and significant visual acuity impairment (6/60). The ERG findings in patient D (aged 7 years), with X-linked disease, are typically severe

most hemizygotes. ADRP is more often associated with a milder clinical course and less severe ERG changes in affected children. Autosomal recessive RP is very heterogeneous and both severe and mild variants are seen.

RP of varying severity is associated with syndromic disorders such as Bardet-Biedl (BBS) and Usher syndromes, although a cone–rod pattern of dysfunction can occur in BBS [35]. Full-field ERGs in Usher syndrome are typically markedly abnormal [24].

9.3.2 Congenital Stationary Night Blindness

Most forms of CSNB manifest an ERG maximal response with a normal a-wave and selective b-wave reduction, a negative or electronegative ERG, consistent with abnormalities that are post-phototransduction. It is usually best seen in the scotopic rod-dominated maximal ERG, although it may also occur in cone-mediated ERGs under photopic conditions [46, 65]. Rare forms of CSNB manifest ERG maximal response a-wave reduction consistent with disruption of rod photoreceptor dysfunction and are reviewed elsewhere [23]. CSNB is genetically heterogeneous with AD, AR and X-L inheritance reported.

X-linked CSNB usually presents with nystagmus and poor vision in infancy. The night blindness usually only becomes apparent at an older age. Most children are myopic and strabismus is common. X-linked CSNB can be subdivided into complete (cCSNB) and incomplete (iCSNB) forms, a division originally based on electrophysiology and psychophysics [64] and now known to reflect genetically distinct disorders. The gene for cCSNB maps to Xp11.4, and results from mutation in *NYX* which encodes nyctalopin, believed to play a role in the development of retinal interconnections involving the ON-bipolar cells [6]. The gene for iCSNB (*CACNA1F*) maps to Xp11.23 and encodes a pore-forming subunit of an L-type voltage-gated calcium channel believed to modulate glutamate release from photoreceptor presynaptic terminals [5].

Both X-linked forms of CSNB have markedly electronegative maximal ERGs. The cCSNB (Figs. 9.4A, 9.2A) has an undetectable rod-specific ERG. The cone flicker and photopic (single flash) ERGs show distinctive abnormalities. The photopic ERG has a broad a-wave followed by a b-wave lacking photopic oscillatory potentials and showing a low b:a ratio. This appearance is thought to reflect loss of cone ON-bipolar contribution but preservation of the OFF- pathway found in long and medium wavelength cone systems [40]. This is confirmed by the results of long duration ON- OFF- ERGs [65], which reveal a normal a-wave, a selectively diminished ON- b-wave and preservation of the OFF- d-wave, consistent with involvement of the depolarising ON-bipolar cell pathway. S-cone ERGs are also affected, confirming the defect to be post-phototransduction in rods and all cone types (Fig. 9.4A). The electroretinographic changes in cCSNB are identical to those in melanoma-associated retinopathy [40, 46] and although unlikely to be of relevance in paediatric practice, demonstrate the importance of always placing electrophysiological data in clinical context.

Although also showing a profoundly electronegative maximal ERG, iCSNB typically has a detectable, but subnormal or delayed, rod-specific ERG. These are accompanied by a subnormal, delayed 30-Hz flicker ERG that has a typically bifid appearance (Fig. 9.4B). The photopic single flash ERG may be markedly subnormal and occasionally has an electronegative waveform [85]. Overall, the cone-mediated photopic ERG abnormalities in iCSNB are more apparent than those of cCSNB (Fig. 9.4B); both ON- and OFF- responses are affected [65].

Dominant forms of CSNB may also be associated with an electronegative ERG resulting

Fig. 9.4. Pattern ERGs, full-field ERGs, including ON-OFF- and S-cone ERGs in a normal subject (*N*) and in patients with complete CSNB (*A*), incomplete CSNB (*B*) and enhanced S-cone syndrome (*C*). In the latter case, note the S-cone-specific recordings are similar to those of the single flash photopic ERG. See text for details. Eye movement or blink artefacts, commonly present in paediatric ERGs to bright flashes, occur at about 100 ms, most prominently in the maximal ERG of patient B

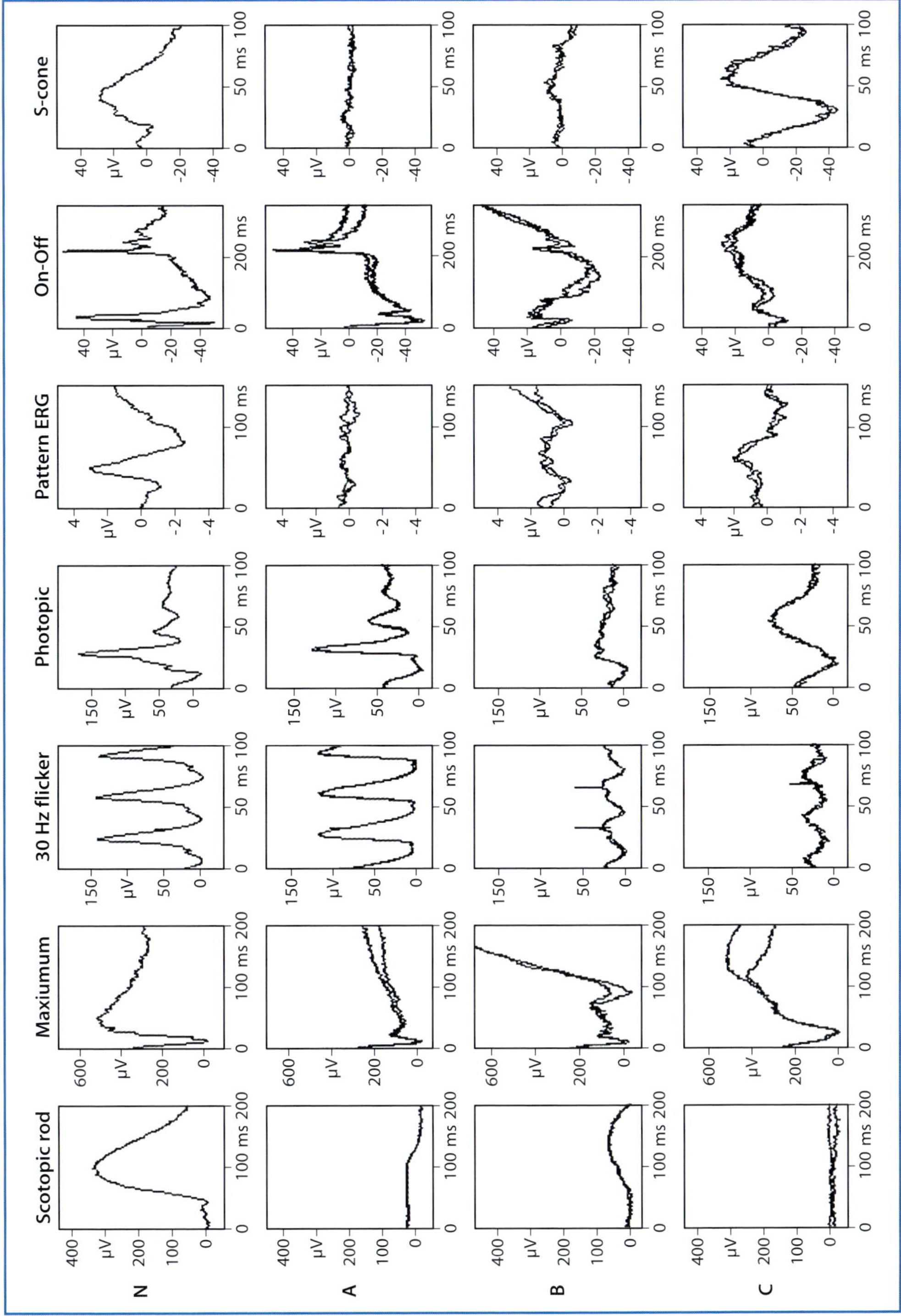
Scotopic rod
Maxiumum
30 Hz flicker
Photopic
Pattern ERG
On-Off
S-cone
N
A
B
C
µV
ms

from post-phototransduction rod system involvement. Some authors report sparing of the cone system [69], but others, using additional short wavelength stimulation, identified involvement of the S-cone system [45]. The PERG is normal in such cases. In some dominant forms of CSNB, there is ERG maximal response a-wave reduction consistent with disruption of phototransduction or rod photoreceptor function (see [23] for a recent review). Patients with recessive CSNB and an electronegative maximal ERG can have other ERG features that may resemble either the complete or incomplete forms of X-linked disease (unpublished data).

Fundus albipunctatus is a recessively inherited, probably stationary disorder of night vision associated with a mutation in RDH5 encoding the RPE enzyme retinol dehydrogenase [23]. The clinical symptoms relate to impaired regeneration of rhodopsin. Funduscopy reveals multiple yellow-white dots located at the level of the RPE in the mid-periphery. The ISCEV standard ERG in such patients shows an undetectable rod-specific ERG and a mildly reduced amplitude a-wave with a lower amplitude b-wave [66]. However, with sufficiently long dark adaptation, usually 2 h or more, rod-derived ERGs become normal. A normal or significantly improved ERG following extended dark adaptation enables fundus albipunctatus to be distinguished from retinitis punctata albescens, a progressive retinal degeneration that also presents with a flecked retinal appearance accompanied by markedly abnormal ERGs that do not normalise following prolonged dark adaptation.

9.3.3 Enhanced S-Cone Syndrome

Enhanced S-cone syndrome (ESCS) is an autosomal recessive trait consequent upon mutation in NR2E3 [30]. A single histological report, in an advanced case, showed an absence of rods and increased numbers of cones, 92% of which were thought to be S-cones, with 15% expressing the L/M cone opsin including some which co-expressed S-cone opsin [63]. Patients typically present with night blindness or maculopathy and may have relatively mild visual field loss. The fundus appearance is characterised in older children and adults by nummular pigment deposition around the arcades at the level of the RPE. They may eventually develop degenerative changes in the region of the vascular arcades. In young children, the fundus changes are very subtle or nonexistent and the ERG is key to making the correct diagnosis.

The ERGs in ESCS are pathognomonic for the disorder (Fig. 9.4C). Full-field ERGs show minimal differences in waveform between photopic and scotopic ERGs elicited by the same intensity stimuli. Flicker ERGs are markedly delayed and subnormal and are distinctive in that the flicker ERG amplitude, which normally lies between that of the photopic a- and b-waves, is of lower amplitude than the photopic a-wave. In ESCS, there is increased sensitivity to short wavelength stimulation. ON-OFF ERGs to longer wavelengths, mediated predominantly by L and M cones, show marked reduction (Fig. 9.4C). Pattern ERG reduction may occur and the P50 component may be markedly delayed.

Summary for the Clinician

RP

- **Patients with RP typically present with progressive night blindness and visual field constriction**
- **Classical signs include bone-spicule pigmentation, vessel attenuation and disc pallor, but the fundus may be normal**
- **Bright flash scotopic ERGs show a reduced a-wave, indicating rod photoreceptor dysfunction with less severe photopic ERG abnormalities**
- **Pattern ERGs can be used to assess the degree of macular involvement**

CSNB

- **Patients typically present with nonprogressive night blindness**
- **X-linked CSNB is characterised by an electronegative maximal scotopic ERG, indicating dysfunction that is post-phototransduction.**
- **Electroretinography enables the distinction between complete and incomplete X-linked and other less common forms (see above)**

ESCS

- **ESCS is a rare recessively inherited disorder characterised by an absence of rods and an abnormally high number of cones sensitive to short wavelength stimulation**
- **Patients typically present with night blindness or maculopathy**
- **ERGs are pathognomonic for the disorder (see above)**

9.4 Early Onset Nystagmus

Early onset nystagmus is seen in three main clinical situations. Firstly, in children with neurological disorders; secondly in children with afferent visual failure; and finally in congenital idiopathic motor nystagmus (CIMN). The main diagnostic dilemma is in differentiating CIMN from sensory forms of nystagmus in a child with nystagmus and a normal fundus [29]. Sensory nystagmus may be associated with a number of disorders including CSNB (Sect. 9.3.2), retinal dystrophies, cone-system dysfunction syndromes, albinism and optic nerve abnormalities. Full-field ERGs can identify a retinal aetiology and, when combined with VEP recordings, may localise dysfunction to the level of the retina or optic pathways or exclude a sensory cause. Equally, exclusion of afferent visual pathway dysfunction may be an important contribution to management.

9.4.1 Cone and Cone–Rod Dystrophy

Patients with cone or cone-rod dystrophy typically present with progressive impairment of central vision, abnormalities of colour vision, photophobia and often nystagmus [78], although there are exceptions [21]. There is wide phenotypic variability and although the fundus may initially appear normal, abnormalities can include peripheral hypopigmentation and/or pigment clumping, disc pallor, macular atrophic changes or bull's eye maculopathy. Interestingly, a recent prospective study identified only a small percentage of patients with bull's eye maculopathy to have cone dystrophy [50]. Visual fields typically reveal central scotomata, although peripheral field loss, depressed sensitivity and ring scotomata may occur. Inheritance may be autosomal recessive, dominant or X-linked (see Ret Net for genetic subtypes).

Strictly, the ERG abnormalities in cone dystrophy are confined to the cone system (Fig. 9.5 A), but mild additional rod involvement may occur in some patients late in the disease. Both cone and rod ERG abnormalities occur in cone–rod dystrophy, with the cone responses being more affected (Fig. 9.5 B). Usually, the 30-Hz flicker response is subnormal and of increased implicit time. For example, the dominant cone–rod dystrophy associated with mutation in *GUCY2D*, (encoding retinal guanylate cyclase) is associated with both with 30-Hz flicker delay and amplitude reduction with milder rod-system dysfunction [22]. Clinically, these patients have poor vision in bright light from childhood, but major reduction in visual acuity occurs after the late teens. Fundus abnormalities are confined to the central macula, and the central atrophy increases with age. PERGs are usually markedly reduced or undetectable.

The macular changes in some patients with cone dystrophy may be absent or subtle, and associated disc pallor may mistakenly be thought to reflect primary optic nerve disease [68, 74]. Pattern VEP delay is common in macular dysfunction [40], and a delayed VEP should not be interpreted as reflecting optic nerve dysfunction without a measure of the retinal response to a similar stimulus. The pattern ERG P50 component is subnormal in macular dysfunction: in mild disease there is P50 reduction with concomitant reduction in N95; in severe disease the PERG is extinguished. These findings are contrasted with those in optic nerve/retinal ganglion cell disease where P50 is usually intact, and the abnormality is confined to the N95 component (see below). The differential effect of ganglion cell dysfunction and macular disease on the PERG facilitates accurate interpretation of a delayed PVEP in the patient with visual symptoms.

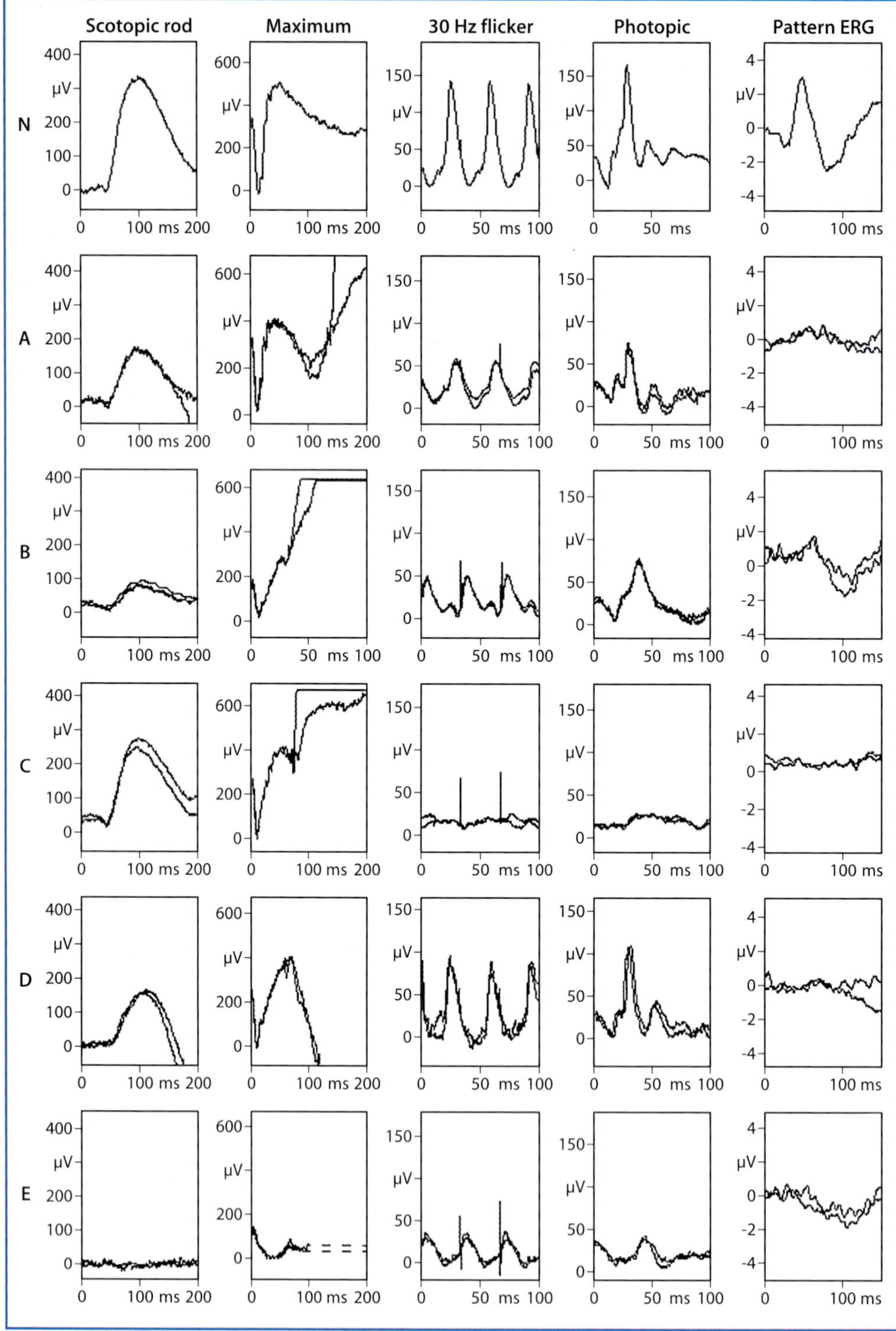
Scotopic rod
Maximum
30 Hz flicker
Photopic
Pattern ERG
N
A
B
C
D
E
µV
ms

Fig. 9.5. Pattern ERGs and full-field ERGs in a normal subject (*N*) and in patients with cone dystrophy (*A*), cone–rod dystrophy (*B*), S-cone monochromatism (*C*), Stargardt fundus flavimaculatus group 1 (*D*) and juvenile onset Batten disease consequent upon *CLN3* (*E*). Prominent blink artefacts occur in maximum ERG waveforms in A, B, C and D at about 100 ms and have been omitted from E for clarity. Patient C had a preserved S-cone ERG (not shown). See text for details

9.4.2 Leber Congenital Amaurosis

Leber congenital amaurosis (LCA) accounts for approximately 15% of congenital blindness. This largely recessively inherited disorder manifests with signs of very poor visual function and roving eye movements or nystagmus. Eye-poking or eye-rubbing, the oculodigital sign, may be present and may eventually lead to sunken orbits, cataract and keratoconus. The majority of patients have normal fundi at presentation, but disc pallor, vessel attenuation and pigmentary changes may follow. The ERG is typically severely reduced or undetectable from early infancy (Fig. 9.2B).

9.4.3 Cone Dysfunction Syndromes

Rod monochromatism is an autosomal recessive disorder characterised by poor vision from birth, nystagmus and photophobia and is consequent upon mutations in *CNGA3* or *CNGB3* [62]. Patients usually attain acuities of about 6/60 and have absent colour vision. Most patients are hyperopic. The fundus is usually normal, although some granularity of the central macula may develop with time. The ERG reveals an absent or severely reduced 30-Hz flicker response, but good rod ERGs following even a limited period of dark adaptation (Fig. 9.2C). Minor reduction in maximum ERG a-wave may reflect the absence of the cone contribution from this mixed response.

S-cone monochromatism is usually an X-linked disorder in which there is absent L- and M- cone function. The presentation in infancy is similar to rod monochromatism but the visual acuity is better (typically between 6/24 and 6/60) and the refractive error is usually myopic. Spectral sensitivity measurement can distinguish S-cone monochromatism from rod monochromatism, as can specialised colour vision testing [10], but these tests are not possible in infancy. ERG abnormalities are similar to those observed in the rod monochromat (Fig. 9.5C) except that the S-cone-specific ERG, a response to a short-wavelength stimulus recorded in the presence of longer wavelength adaptation, is preserved. A similar electrophysiological phenotype may be seen in achromatopsia associated with recessively inherited mutation in *GNAT2* [61].

9.4.4 Albinism

Albinism describes a group of inherited conditions characterised by disorders of melanin synthesis affecting the eyes (ocular albinism) or the eyes, skin and hair (oculocutaneous albinism). Children with albinism usually present with nystagmus and poor visual acuity in early infancy. Classical signs include iris transillumination, fundus hypopigmentation and foveal hypoplasia. There is a high incidence of strabismus and significant refractive error. In both oculocutaneous and ocular albinism, there is an abnormally high percentage of decussating temporal optic nerve fibres from each eye that project to the contralateral hemisphere. This intracranial misrouting is demonstrated by the presence of contralateral VEP predominance (Fig. 9.6), being of higher amplitude and/or shorter latency over the contralateral hemisphere [20, 67]. Flash VEPs are most sensitive to misrouting in infants and young children and pattern onset-offset VEPs are most sensitive in adolescents; between the ages of 5 and 14 years, the use of both techniques optimises sensitivity [67]. Pattern reversal stimulation is not appropriate; firstly, most patients have nystagmus and secondly, reversal VEPs are subject to the phe-

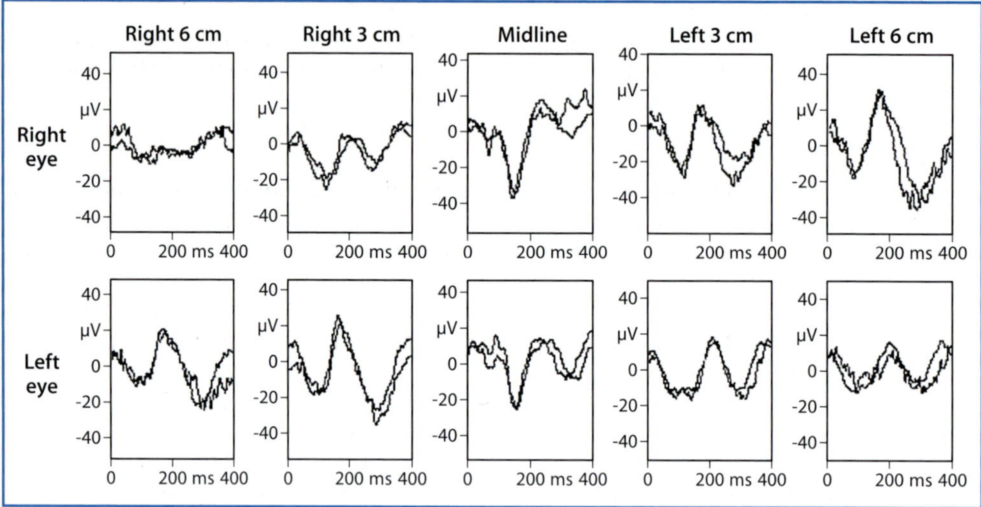

Fig. 9.6. Monocular flash VEPs in a 1-year-old patient recorded using five posteriorly situated electrodes; each referred to a mid frontal reference (Fz). Flash VEPs are of shorter latency and higher amplitude over the contralateral compared with the ipsilateral hemisphere, in keeping with the optic nerve misrouting associated with albinism

nomenon of paradoxical lateralisation [4]. Both of these factors confound accurate interpretation of pattern reversal VEPs but do not apply to VEPs elicited using brief pattern onset stimulation.

9.4.5 Optic Nerve Hypoplasia

Infants with severe bilateral optic nerve hypoplasia (ONH) usually present with nystagmus and poor vision. Although these patients have small pale optic discs, the optic nerve abnormality may easily be missed when examining a small infant with nystagmus. Electrophysiological testing is extremely useful in detecting visual pathway abnormalities and may prompt review of the optic disc appearance. It is important to make a specific diagnosis, as ONH may be associated with endocrine abnormalities, particularly growth hormone deficiency, which need treatment. Pattern and Flash VEPs show varying degrees of attenuation and delay [2, 49] and may be undetectable in severe cases. ERGs are normal and may be of high amplitude [13, 48].

Summary for the Clinician

Cone or cone-rod dystrophy

- **Patients with cone or cone-rod dystrophy typically present with progressive loss in visual acuity, abnormal colour vision, photophobia and often nystagmus**
- **The fundus may initially appear normal, but abnormalities can include peripheral hypopigmentation and/or pigment clumping, disc pallor, bull's eye maculopathy or macular atrophy**
- **Cone system photopic ERG's are reduced and usually delayed in cone dystrophy with additional involvement of rod-dominated scotopic ERGs in cone-rod dystrophy**
- **Pattern ERGs are usually markedly reduced or undetectable**

Leber congenital amaurosis

- **Severe visual impairment and roving eye movements or nystagmus from birth or early infancy**
- **Fundi are typically normal at presentation, but disc pallor, vessel attenuation and pigmentary changes may follow**

- **The ERG is severely reduced or undetectable from early infancy, indicating severe photoreceptor dysfunction**

Rod or S-cone monochromatism

- **Poor vision, nystagmus, photophobia and abnormal colour vision from birth**
- **Fundi are usually normal but maculae may appear granular**
- **Full-field ERGs reveal an absent or severely reduced photopic 30 Hz flicker response, but good rod ERGs following even a limited period of dark adaptation**

Albinism

- **Classical signs include foveal hypoplasia, iris transillumination and fundal hypopigmentation in addition to nystagmus**
- **VEPs are of higher amplitude and/or shorter latency over the contralateral hemisphere in keeping with an abnormally high percentage of decussating temporal fibres from each eye that project to the contralateral hemisphere**

9.5 Visual Impairment in Multisystem Disorders

The neuronal ceroid lipofuscinoses (NCLs) are a group of recessively inherited neurodegenerative storage disorders associated with progressive neurological failure and retinal degeneration. The juvenile onset form (Batten disease), relating to mutation in *CLN3*, is of particular interest as patients often present with visual acuity reduction prior to the development of neurological symptoms. At this stage, there may be a bull's eye maculopathy or the fundus may be normal. In the latter case, nonorganic visual loss may be suspected. Abnormal pattern ERGs indicate macular dysfunction [58]. The maximal ERG response is electronegative, but some patients will also show some a-wave reduction consistent with loss of photoreceptor outer segments [55, 84]. Photopic ERGs may also show a markedly reduced b:a ratio, a relatively unusual finding that may serve to alert to the diagnosis (Fig. 9.5 E); the flicker ERG is profoundly delayed. With time, the ERG becomes undetectable.

Peroxisomal disorders result from dysfunction or absence of peroxisomes and may be associated with pigmentary retinopathy resulting in severe ERG abnormalities [36]. Zellweger syndrome is characterised by infantile retinal degeneration that is associated with facial dysmorphia, hypotonia, psychomotor retardation, seizures, renal and hepatic abnormalities. Patients with neonatal adrenal leukodystrophy may present in infancy, but they generally survive until age 7–10 years. Flash ERGs have been documented as undetectable [27]. Less severe findings are present in infantile Refsum disease, so-called because of elevated serum phytanic acid.

Cortical visual impairment (CVI) is a condition resulting in bilateral visual impairment caused by nonocular damage to the visual pathways or cortex. The most common cause of CVI is hypoxic birth injury, although other causes include trauma, shunt failure leading to occipital lobe infarction, meningitis, encephalitis, congenital toxoplasmosis, neonatal herpes simplex, cardiac failure and infantile spasms. Flash ERGs may be useful in excluding a retinal cause of visual failure. Flash visual evoked potentials may confirm CVI and may be of prognostic value [17].

9.6 Investigation of Children Who Present with Unexplained Visual Acuity Loss

Visual loss in childhood may be due to macular disease, optic neuropathy or nonorganic visual loss, and electrophysiology not only allows these to be distinguished but may also indicate a specific diagnosis.

9.6.1 Macular Dystrophies

Inherited macular dysfunction can occur either in association with generalised retinal dysfunction or as disturbance of function confined to the macula (a macular dystrophy). Full-field ERG allows assessment of generalised retinal function and the pattern ERG P50 component allows assessment of macular function.

9.6.1.1 Stargardt Macular Dystrophy–Fundus Flavimaculatus

Stargardt macular dystrophy–fundus flavimaculatus (S-FFM) is an autosomal recessive disorder consequent upon mutation in *ABCA4* [1]. Patients often present in adolescence with progressive visual acuity reduction. On examination, there is usually macular atrophy and associated white flecks at the level of the retinal pigment epithelium. In children with S-FFM, there may be significant visual loss before there is significant fundus change, and it is in these cases where electrophysiological testing is most useful. Most patients with S-FFM have severe macular dysfunction and show severe PERG P50 reduction, even though visual acuity may be relatively well preserved. In some patients, dysfunction is confined to the macula (group 1) but in others there may be generalised involvement of the cone system (group 2) or rod and cone systems (group 3). The presence of a normal ERG at any stage during the course of the disorder appears to be associated with a good prognosis for retention of peripheral retinal function [53, 54]. Despite inter-sibling variation in clinical phenotypic features, such as fundus appearance and visual acuity, the electrophysiological grouping is concordant across sibling pairs [53], unlike patients with bulls' eye maculopathy [50, 43]. Typical findings in a young patient with S-FFM (group 1) are shown in Fig. 9.5D.

9.6.1.2 Best Vitelliform Macular Dystrophy

Best vitelliform macular dystrophy is an autosomal dominant disorder caused by mutations in *VMD2*, which encodes bestrophin [70]. Best disease usually has a childhood or teenage onset and in the early stages is typically characterised by a well-circumscribed vitelliform macular lesion, resulting from accumulation of lipofuscin at the level of the RPE. Visual acuity is usually normal until the subsequent vitelliruptive stage, resulting in disruption of overlying photoreceptors and eventual macular atrophy. The electrophysiology in Best disease is characteristic. Full-field ERGs are normal but the electro-oculogram (EOG) light rise is severely reduced or undetectable, in keeping with severe generalised dysfunction affecting the RPE–photoreceptor interface. The EOG is abnormal during the asymptomatic previtelliform stage. Pattern ERGs are typically normal until the vitelliruptive stage, when there is visual acuity loss and, at that stage, PERG reduction. Patients younger than about 6 years are unlikely to be able to comply with EOG testing, but as the disorder is dominantly inherited it is appropriate to test the parents.

9.6.1.3 X-Linked Juvenile Retinoschisis

Although, strictly, full-field ERG abnormalities imply generalised retinal dysfunction, X-linked retinoschisis (XLRS) may be referred to as a macular dystrophy. Patients typically present in the 1st or 2nd decade with reduced visual acuity, and macular abnormalities are present in most cases. Classically, these have a "spoke wheel" appearance due to the presence of foveal microcysts. The retinal cleavage may be revealed by optical coherence tomography [80]. With time, these radial cystic changes may give way to nonspecific macular atrophy. Peripheral schisis lesions are only present in 50 % of patients, mostly in the infero-temporal quadrant. In older patients with nonspecific macular atrophy, but no peripheral schisis, the diagnosis may not be obvious and electrophysiology may be instrumental in making the diagnosis or suggesting a candidate gene. An electronegative maximal ERG is typically present (Fig. 9.2D), although the degree of abnormality can vary and in rare cases b-wave amplitudes have been reported as normal [11]. Rod-specific ERGs are usually undetectable or markedly reduced in keeping with the intraretinal cleavage [80] and typical maximal response ERG b-wave abnormality. Photopic and 30-Hz flicker ERGs are usually subnormal and delayed. The ON- b-wave may be reduced with preservation of the OFF- d-wave in some patients [89], but in others the OFF- d-wave may also be affected. Pattern ERGs are usually markedly reduced in keeping with macular dysfunction [18, 80]. The presence of an electronegative ERG in a patient with a macular lesion, even if atypical, may suggest *XLRS1* as a suitable candidate gene for analysis. Severe cases of XLRS may also have an abnormal a-wave reflecting some photoreceptor loss, possibly consequent upon haemorrhage or full-thickness detachment early in life.

Summary for the Clinician

Stargardt–fundus flavimaculatus (S-FFM)

- Fleck lesions in the posterior pole extending to the mid-periphery, usually with central atrophy
- PERG usually undetectable – severe macular dysfunction
- Some patients have generalised ERG abnormalities that may be of prognostic value

Best disease

- Typically characterised in the early stages by a well-circumscribed vitelliform macular lesion
- Characterised by normal full-field ERGs but an absent or severely reduced EOG light rise
- Pattern ERGs are typically normal until the vitelliruptive stage, when there is visual acuity loss and PERG reduction

X-linked retinoschisis

- Classically, a "spoke wheel" appearance at the fovea that is replaced by nonspecific macular atrophy with age
- Electronegative ERG appearance indicating dysfunction post-phototransduction or inner retinal
- Pattern ERGs are usually markedly reduced

9.6.2 Optic Nerve Dysfunction

9.6.2.1 Familial Optic Atrophy

The commonest cause of familial optic nerve dysfunction is dominant optic atrophy (DOA), related to mutation in *OPA1*. Patients typically present with painless, progressive visual acuity loss that may be asymmetrical. Other clinical features include centrocaecal scotoma, dyschromatopsia, pallor of the optic disc and loss of the papillomacular bundle [16, 82]. Histopathological studies suggest that the fundamental pathology is degeneration of the retinal ganglion cells [44]. The PERG shows N95 loss that can occur before a VEP abnormality. The PVEP is often markedly delayed and can vary in amplitude from subnormal to undetectable in end-stage disease. In severe long-standing disease, significant PERG P50 component amplitude reduction may occur, often accompanied by a shortening of implicit time, in keeping with the loss of ganglion cell contribution to both the N95 and P50 components [42, 81]. Typical findings are shown in Fig. 9.7.

Most patients with Leber hereditary optic neuropathy (LHON) present with acute painless sequential bilateral disc swelling and visual loss between 11 and 30 years of age, but there are reports of much earlier and much later age of onset [8, 41]. There are few reports of the PERG in LHON, but N95 reduction may occur [8, 39]. This is accompanied by a normal PERG P50 component and normal full-field ERGs. One case report [59] describes recordings taken 3 days after the acute onset of visual loss in the second eye of a young male patient (11778 mutation). There had been sudden reduction in vision in the first eye 3 weeks earlier. Both eyes showed prominent N95 reduction in the PERG, but P50 was normal and there was no interocular asymmetry. The N95 loss in the more recently affected eye was attributed to primary ganglion cell dysfunction; more time would be required for retrograde degeneration to have occurred.

9.6.2.2 Compressive Lesions

Optic nerve glioma in children may be associated with painless visual loss, proptosis or squint, although patients are often asymptomatic, especially when associated with neurofibromatosis. Optic disc swelling and atrophy may occur. There may be chiasmal involvement and presentation will depend upon the location of the tumour and the age of the patient. Pattern VEPs often show marked attenuation, broaden-

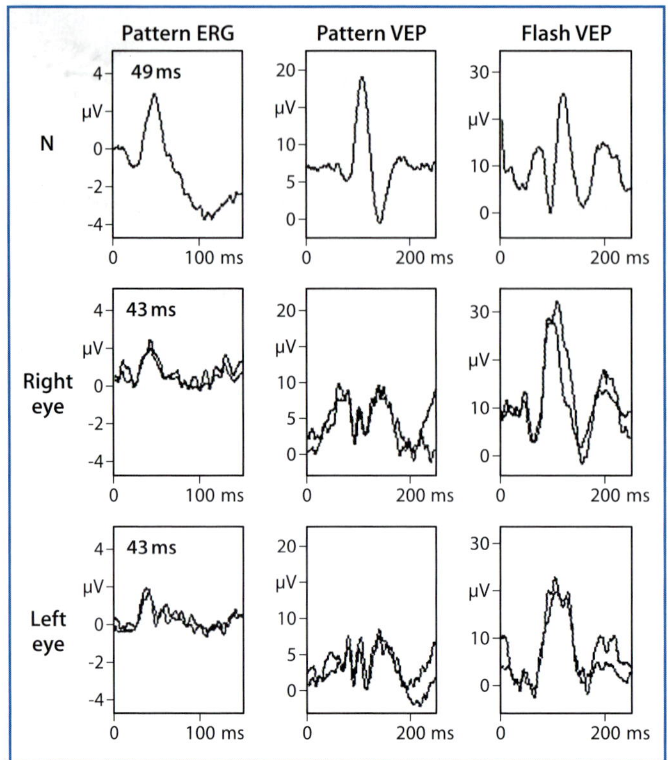

Fig. 9.7. Pattern and flash VEPs and pattern ERGs from a normal subject (*N*) and from right and left eyes of a 9-year-old patient with dominant optic atrophy. Pattern VEPs are abnormal, PERG N95:P50 amplitude ratio is reduced and P50 is of shortened implicit time, consistent with ganglion cell disease (see text for details)

ing and delay. Flash VEPs may be less severely affected. With chiasmal involvement, the occipital distribution of VEPs from the fellow eye may additionally demonstrate a degree of interhemispheric asymmetry.

The signs and symptoms in craniopharyngioma vary greatly depending on the neural structures affected but commonly involve headache, vomiting and visual disturbance [19]. Nystagmus has been reported in some cases. Anterior extension to the optic chiasm can result in bitemporal hemianopia, unilateral temporal hemianopia, papilledema, or unilateral/bilateral decrease in visual acuity. Children are often inattentive to visual loss and formal testing may be required. Monocular pattern VEPs frequently reveal a crossed asymmetry where there is an abnormal distribution over the two hemispheres which reverses on monocular stimulation of the other eye and which is opposite in nature to that seen in the misrouting of albinism. Stimulus parameters are of crucial importance to accurate localisation. In general, use of a large field, large check stimulus gives paradoxical lateralisation [4, 34], whereas a small field, small check stimulus gives anatomical lateralisation. Uncrossed asymmetries have also been reported to reflect unilateral post-chiasmal compression [49].

Summary for the Clinician

Familial optic atrophy

- **The PERG shows N95 loss that can occur before a VEP abnormality in DOA. PERG P50 component amplitude reduction may occur in severe long-standing disease significant, usually accompanied by a shortening of implicit time**
- **The PVEP may be markedly delayed and can vary in amplitude from subnormal to undetectable in end-stage disease**

9.7 Unexplained Visual Loss in the Normal Child

In most children that present with acquired visual loss, the cause of the impairment is revealed by careful ophthalmological examination. However, some children with retinal dystrophies may have a normal fundus or very subtle changes in the early stages and electrophysiological testing is fundamental to making the correct diagnosis. Equally, there is a higher incidence of nonorganic visual loss in a paediatric population. Any acuity reduction in a child should probably be regarded as organic until proven otherwise. The objective data provided by electrophysiology is extremely helpful in the diagnosis of nonorganic visual loss.

Children with high ametropia have a significantly higher rate of retinal electrophysiological abnormalities compared with lower refractive errors or emmetropia [26]. Electrophysiological testing, to rule out associated retinal pathology, should be considered in cases of high ametropia in childhood when correction of the refractive error does not result in normal acuity.

9.7.1 Amblyopia

Children suspected of being amblyopic are generally referred for electrodiagnostic testing in order to exclude other pathologies, e.g., when visual acuity has not improved with patching and the fundi are normal or when visual acuity is reduced bilaterally. In amblyopic eyes, pattern visual evoked potentials often show amplitude reduction and/or mild to moderate delay [75, 79] that is not due to optical factors [52]. Generally, latency abnormalities in the major positive (P100) component tend to be milder in anisometropic than with strabismic amblyopia. Pattern VEPs may also play a useful role in monitoring the effects of patching therapy in amblyopic and fellow eyes [83, 87].

9.7.2 Nonorganic Visual Loss

The VEP, combined with other electrophysiological tests, is crucial to the diagnosis of nonorganic visual loss. Electrophysiological testing may demonstrate normal function in the presence of symptoms that suggest otherwise or may quantify the level of genuine dysfunction in the presence of functional overlay. Flash VEPs in nonorganic visual loss are normal [33, 51]. A well-formed pattern reversal VEP is incompatible with a visual acuity of approximately 6/36 or worse [32]. The pattern onset or appearance VEP (PaVEP) is more susceptible to blur than the pattern reversal VEP and it is the authors' experience that the PaVEP enables a more direct relationship to be established between visual acuity and the presence or absence of a response to small check sizes of varying contrast. Constant encouragement and direct monitoring of fixation and compliance are essential in all patients suspected of hysteria or malingering and will often result in improved patient cooperation. Careful observation of the background electroencephalographic (EEG) input and the developing averaged VEP is advisable; children may find the alternating checkerboard hypnotic and the appearance of an alpha rhythm in the ongoing EEG may indicate drowsiness or loss of concentration. Equally, a tendency for the P100 component to broaden or increase in latency in the acquired average suggests that accommodation or fixation is unsatisfactory. It may be necessary to stop averaging after fewer sweeps than usual to prevent waveform deterioration. Simultaneous PERG recording may be beneficial. The PERG P50 component is very susceptible to deterioration with poor compliance, and a normal PERG can only be obtained with satisfactory fixation and accommodation. Routine ERG should also be performed; ERGs can be markedly abnormal in retinal dysfunction with no or minimal fundus abnormality but constricted visual fields, and field loss is often a feature of nonorganic visual loss. PERG and PVEP findings may be normal in such conditions if the maculae are spared.

Normal electrophysiology does not preclude the presence of some underlying organic disease [31, 38], but the demonstration of normal electrophysiology can be reassuring, both for the clinician and for concerned parents. Particular caution must be exercised if there is a possibility of cortical dysfunction. Electrophysiological examination is always advisable if there is any doubt.

Summary for the Clinician

- **Visual acuity loss in a child should probably be regarded as organic until proven otherwise**
- **Electrophysiology in a child with functional visual loss will either reveal normal function, or may suggest a degree of functional overlay superimposed upon genuine underlying dysfunction**

9.8 Conclusions

The objective data provided by electrophysiological testing are fundamental to the management of the child with suspected visual pathway dysfunction. A flexible approach to testing children is advocated, without the routine use of sedation, performing more demanding testing protocols in children who are able to cooperate and limiting recordings in the younger patients to address the most salient diagnostic questions. The wide diversity of disorders is reflected in the range of ERG, PERG and VEP abnormalities.

Electrophysiological phenotyping is of great importance not only in terms of diagnostic accuracy and the characterisation of the disorder, but also in prognosis by distinguishing between severe and relatively benign disease, both of which may initially present similar clinical features, or by distinguishing between progressive and stationary disorders that may present with similar symptoms. The importance of phenotype-genotype correlations is likely to increase with time and, if treatment intervention for the inherited disorders becomes available, it is likely that electrophysiological examination will facilitate suitable patient identification and will be the likely outcome measure in the evaluation of treatment efficacy.

References

1. Allikmets R, Singh N, Sun H, Shroyer NF, Hutchinson A, Chidambaram A, Gerrard B, Baird L, Stauffer D, Peiffer A, Rattner A, Smallwood P, Li Y, Anderson KL, Lewis RA, Nathans J, Leppert M, Dean M, Lupski JR (1997) A photoreceptor cell-specific ATP-binding transporter gene (ABCR) is mutated in recessive Stargardt macular dystrophy. Nat Genet 15:236–246
2. Apkarian P Spekreijse H (1990) The use of the electroretinogram and visual evoked potentials in ophthalmogenetics. In: Desmedt JE (ed) Visual evoked potentials. Elsevier, Amsterdam, pp 169–228
3. Arden GB, Carter RM, Hogg CR, Powell DJ, Ernst WJ, Clover GM, Lyness AL, Quinlan MP (1983) A modified ERG technique and the results obtained in X-linked retinitis pigmentosa. Br J Ophthalmol 67:419–430
4. Barrett G, Blumhardt L, Halliday AM, Halliday E, Kriss A (1976) Paradoxical reversal of lateralization of the half-field pattern-evoked response with monopolar and bipolar electrode montages. J Physiol 258:63P–64P
5. Bech-Hansen NT, Naylor MJ, Maybaum TA, Pearce WG, Koop B, Fishman GA, Mets M, Musarella MA, Boycott KM (1998) Loss-of-function mutations in a calcium-channel alpha1-subunit gene in Xp11.23 cause incomplete X-linked congenital stationary night blindness. Nat Genet 19:264–267
6. Bech-Hansen NT, Naylor MJ, Maybaum TA, Sparkes RL, Koop B, Birch DG, Bergen AA, Prinsen CF, Polomeno RC, Gal A, Drack AV, Musarella MA, Jacobson SG, Young RS, Weleber RG (2000) Mutations in NYX, encoding the leucine-rich proteoglycan nyctalopin, cause X-linked complete congenital stationary night blindness. Nat Genet 26:319–323
7. Berninger TA, Arden GB (1988) The pattern electroretinogram. Eye [Suppl 2]:S257–S283
8. Berninger TA, Bird AC, Arden GB (1989) Leber's hereditary optic atrophy. Ophthalmic Paediatr Genet 10:211–227
9. Berson EL, Rosen JB, Simonoff EA (1979) Electroretinographic testing as an aid in detection of carriers of X-chromosome-linked retinitis pigmentosa. Am J Ophthalmol 87:460–468
10. Berson EL, Sandberg MA, Rosner B, Sullivan PL (1983) Color plates to help identify patients with blue cone monochromatism. Am J Ophthalmol 95:741–747
11. Bradshaw K, George N, Moore A, Trump D (1999) Mutations of the XLRS1 gene cause abnormalities of photoreceptor as well as inner retinal responses of the ERG. Doc Ophthalmol 98:153–173

12. Brecelj J (2003) From immature to mature pattern ERG and VEP. Doc Ophthalmol 107:215–224
13. Brecelj J, Stirn-Kranjc B (2004) Visual electrophysiological screening in diagnosing infants with congenital nystagmus. Clin Neurophysiol 115:461–470
14. Brecelj J, Strucl M, Zidar I, Tekavcic-Pompe (2002) Pattern ERG and VEP maturation in children. Clin Neurophysiol 113:1764–1770
15. Bush RA, Sieving PA (1994) A proximal retinal component in the primate photopic ERG a-wave. Invest Ophthalmol Vis Sci 35:635–45
16. Caldwell JBH, Howard RO, Riggs LA (1971) Dominant juvenile optic atrophy: a study of two families and review of the hereditary disease in childhood. Arch Ophthalmol 85:133–147
17. Clarke MP, Mitchell KW, Gibson M (1997) The prognostic value of flash visual evoked potentials in the assessment of non-ocular visual impairment in infancy. Eye 11:398–402
18. Clarke MP, Mitchell KW, McDonnell S (1997) Electroretinographic findings in macular dystrophy. Doc Ophthalmol 92:325–339
19. De Vries L, Lazar L, Phillip M (2003) Craniopharyngioma: presentation and endocrine sequelae in 36 children. J Pediatr Endocrinol Metab 16:703–710
20. Dorey SE, Neveu MM, Burton LC, Sloper JJ, Holder GE (2003) The clinical features of albinism and their correlation with visual evoked potentials. Br J Ophthalmol 87:767–772
21. Downes SM, Holder GE, Fitzke FW, Payne AM, Warren MJ, Bhattacharya SS, Bird AC (2001) Autosomal dominant cone and cone-rod dystrophy with mutations in the guanylate cyclase activator 1A gene-encoding guanylate cyclase activating protein-1. Arch Ophthalmol 119:96–105
22. Downes SM, Payne AM, Kelsell RE, Fitzke FW, Holder GE, Hunt DM, Moore AT, Bird AC (2001) Autosomal dominant cone-rod dystrophy with mutations in the guanylate cyclase 2D gene encoding retinal guanylate cyclase-1. Arch Ophthalmol 119:1667–1673
23. Dryja TP (2000) Molecular genetics of Oguchi disease, fundus albipunctatus, and other forms of stationary night blindness: LVII Edward Jackson Memorial Lecture. Am J Ophthalmol:130 547–563
24. Fishman GA, Kumar A, Joseph ME, Torok N, Anderson RJ (1983) Usher's syndrome, ophthalmic and neuro-otologic findings suggesting genetic heterogeneity. Arch Ophthalmol 101: 1367–1374
25. Fishman GA, Birch DG, Holder GE, Brigell MG (2001) Electrophysiologic testing in disorders of the retina, optic nerve and visual pathway. Ophthalmology monographs No. 2. The Foundation of the American Academy of Ophthalmology, San Francisco
26. Flitcroft DI, Adams GG, Robson AG, Holder GE (2004) Retinal dysfunction and refractive errors. An electrophysiological study of children. Br J Ophthalmol 89:484–488
27. Folz SJ, Trobe JD (1991) The peroxisome and the eye. Surv Ophthalmol 35:353–368
28. Fulton AB, Hansen RM, Westall CA (2003) Development of ERG responses: the ISCEV rod, maximal and cone responses in normal subjects. Doc Ophthalmol 107:235–241
29. Gelbart SS, Hoyt CS (1988) Congenital nystagmus: a clinical perspective in infancy. Graefes Arch Clin Exp Ophthalmol 226:178–180
30. Haider NB, Jacobson SG, Cideciyan AV, Swiderski R, Streb LM, Searby C, Beck G, Hockey R, Hanna DB, Gorman S, Duhl D, Carmi R, Bennett J, Weleber RG, Fishman GA, Wright AF, Stone EM, Sheffield VC (2000) Mutation of a nuclear receptor gene, NR2E3, causes enhanced S cone syndrome, a disorder of retinal cell fate. Nature Genet 24:127–131
31. Halliday AM (1973) Evoked responses in organic and functional sensory loss. In: Fessard A, LeLord (eds) Activités Évoquées et Leur Conditionnement Chez l'Homme Normal et en Pathologie Mentale. Institut National de la Sante et de la Recherche Medicale, Paris, pp 189–212
32. Halliday AM, Macdonald WI (1981) Visual evoked potentials. In: Stalberg E, Young RR (eds) Neurology 1. Clinical neurophysiology. Butterworths, London, pp 228–258
33. Harding GFA (1974) The visual evoked response. Adv Ophthalmol 28:2–28
34. Harding GFA, Smith GF, Smith PA (1980) The effect of various parameters on the lateralization of the VEP. In: Barber C (ed) Evoked potentials. MTP Press, pp 213–218
35. Heckenlively JR (1988) Retinitis pigmentosa. JB Lippincott, Philadelphia
36. Hittner HM, Kretzer FL, Mehta RS (1981) Zellweger syndrome. Lenticular opacities indicating carrier status and lens abnormalities characteristic of homozygotes. Arch Ophthalmol 99:1977–1982
37. Holder GE (1987) Significance of abnormal pattern electroretinography in anterior visual pathway dysfunction. Br J Ophthalmol:71:166–171
38. Holder GE (1991) Electrodiagnostic testing in malingering and hysteria. In: Heckenlively JR, Arden GB (eds) Principles and practice of clinical neurophysiology of vision. Mosby Year Book, St Louis, pp 549–556
39. Holder GE (1997) The pattern electroretinogram in anterior visual pathway dysfunction and its relationship to the pattern visual evoked potential: A personal clinical review of 743 eyes. Eye 11: 924–934

40. Holder GE (2001) Pattern ERG and an integrated approach to visual pathway diagnosis. Prog Retin Eye Res 20:531–561
41. Holder GE (2004) Electrophysiological assessment of optic nerve disease. Eye 18:1133–1143
42. Holder GE, Votruba M, Carter AC, Bhattacharya SS, Fitzke FW, Moore AT (1999) Electrophysiological findings in dominant optic atrophy (DOA) linking to the OPA1 locus on chromosome 3q 28-qter. Doc Ophthalmol 95:217–228
43. Holder GE, Robson AG, Hogg CR, Kurz-Levin M, Lois N, Bird A (2003) Pattern ERG: clinical overview, and some observations on associated fundus autofluorescence. Doc Ophthalmol 106:17–23
44. Johnston PB, Gaster RN, Smith VC, Tripathi RC (1979) A clinicopathological study of autosomal dominant optic atrophy. Am J Ophthalmol 88: 868–875
45. Kabanarou SA, Holder GE, Fitzke FW, Bird AC, Webster AR (2004) Congenital stationary night blindness and a "Schubert-Bornschein" type electrophysiology in a family with dominant inheritance. Br J Ophthalmol 88:1018–1022
46. Koh AH, Hogg CR, Holder GE (2001) The incidence of negative ERG in clinical practice. Doc Ophthalmol:102:19–30
47. Kriss A (1994) Skin ERGs: their effectiveness when recording from young children and comparison with ERGs recorded using various types of electrode. Int J Psychophysiol 16:137–146
48. Kriss A, Russell-Eggitt I (1992) Electrophysiological assessment of visual pathway function in infants. Eye 6:145–153
49. Kriss T, Thompson D (1997) Visual electrophysiology. In: Taylor D (ed) Paediatric ophthalmology. Blackwell, Oxford, pp 93–121
50. Kurz-Levin MM, Halfyard AS, Bunce C, Bird AC, Holder GE (2002) Clinical variations in assessment of bull's-eye maculopathy. Arch Ophthalmol 120:567–575
51. Lazarus GM (1974) A clinical application of the visual evoked potential in the diagnosis of ophthalmic and neuroophthalmic pathology-organic and functional lesions. Am Optom Assoc 45:1056–1063
52. Levi DM, Harwerth RS (1978) Contrast evoked potentials in strabismic and anisometropic amblyopia. Invest Ophthalmol Vis Sci 17:571–575
53. Lois N, Holder GE, Fitzke FW, Plant C, Bird AC (1999) Intrafamilial variation of phenotype in Stargardt macular dystrophy-Fundus flavimaculatus. Invest Ophthalmol Vis Sci 40:2668–2675
54. Lois N, Holder GE, Bunce C, Fitzke FW, Bird AC (2001) Phenotypic subtypes of Stargardt macular dystrophy-fundus flavimaculatus. Arch Ophthalmol 119:359–369
55. Mantel I, Brantley M, Bellmann C, Robson AG, Holder GE, Taylor A, Anderson G, Moore AT (2004) Juvenile neuronal ceroid lipofuscinosis (Batten Disease) CLN3 Mutation (Chrom 16p11.2) with different phenotypes in a sibling pair and low intensity in vivo autofluorescence. Klin Monatsbl Augenheilkd 221:27–30
56. Marmor MF, Zrenner E (1993) Standard for clinical electro-oculography. Doc Ophthalmol 85:115–124
57. Marmor MF, Holder GE, Seeliger MW, Yamamoto S (2004) Standard for clinical electroretinography (2004 update) Doc Ophthalmol 108:107–114
58. Marshman WE, Lee JP, Jones B, Schalit G, Holder GE (1998) Duane's retraction syndrome and juvenile Batten's disease: a new association? Aust N Z J Ophthalmol 26:251–254
59. Mauguiere F, Holder GE, Luxon LM, Pottinger R (1995) Evoked potentials: abnormal waveforms and diagnostic yield of evoked potentials. In: Osselton J, Binnie C, Cooper R, Fowler C, Mauguiere F, Prior P (eds) A manual of clinical neurophysiology. Butterworth-Heinemann, Oxford, pp 431–481
60. Meredith SP, Reddy MA, Allen LE, Moore AT, Bradshaw K (2004) Full-field ERG responses recorded with skin electrodes in paediatric patients with retinal dystrophy. Doc Ophthalmol 109:57–66
61. Michaelides M, Aligianis IA, Holder GE, Simunovic M, Mollon JD, Maher ER, Hunt DM, Moore AT (2003) Cone dystrophy phenotype associated with a frameshift mutation (M280fsX291) in the alpha-subunit of cone specific transducin (GNAT2) Br J Ophthalmol 87:1317–1320. Erratum in: Br J Ophthalmol 88:314
62. Michaelides M, Hunt DM, Moore AT (2004) The cone dysfunction syndromes. Br J Ophthalmol 88:291–297
63. Milam AH, Rose L, Cideciyan AV, Barakat MR, Tang WX, Gupta N, Aleman TS, Wright AF, Stone EM, Sheffield VC, Jacobson SG (2002) The nuclear receptor NR2E3 plays a role in human retinal photoreceptor differentiation and degeneration. Proc Natl Acad Sci USA 99:473–478
64. Miyake Y, Yagasaki K, Horiguchi M, Kawase Y, Kanda T (1986) Congenital stationary night blindness with negative electroretinogram. A new classification. Arch Ophthalmol 104:1013–1020
65. Miyake Y, Yagasaki K, Horiguchi M, Kawase Y (1987) On- and off-responses in photopic electroretinogram in complete and incomplete types of congenital stationary night blindness. Jpn J Ophthalmol 31:81–87; Ophthalmol 109:44–48

66. Miyake Y, Shiroyama N, Sugita S, Horiguchi M, Yagasaki K (1992) Fundus albipunctatus associated with cone dystrophy. Br J Ophthalmol 76:375–379
67. Neveu MM, Jeffery G, Burton LC, Sloper JJ, Holder GE (2003) Age-related changes in the dynamics of human albino visual pathways. Eur J Neurosci 18:1939–1949
68. Newman NJ (1993) Optic disc pallor: a false localizing sign. Surv Ophthalmol 37:273–282
69. Noble KG, Carr RE, Siegel IM (1990) Autosomal dominant congenital stationary night blindness and normal fundus with an electronegative electroretinogram. Am J
70. Petrukhin K, Koisti MJ, Bakall B, Li W, Xie G, Marknell T, Sandgren O, Forsman K, Holmgren G, Andreasson S, Vujic M, Bergen AA, McGarty-Dugan V, Figueroa D, Austin CP, Metzker ML, Caskey CT, Wadelius C (1998) Identification of the gene responsible for Best macular dystrophy. Nat Genet 19:241–247
71. Regan, D (1989) Human brain electrophysiology. Elsevier, New York
72. Robson AG, El-Amir A, Bailey C, Egan CA, Fitzke FW, Webster AR, Bird AC, Holder GE (2003) Pattern ERG correlates of fundus autofluorescence abnormalities in patients with retinitis pigmentosa and normal visual acuity. Invest Ophthalmol Vis Sci 44:3544–3550
73. Robson AG, Egan CA, Luong VA, Bird AC, Holder GE, Fitzke FW (2004) Comparison of fundus autofluorescence with photopic and scotopic fine matrix mapping in patients with retinitis pigmentosa and normal visual acuity. Invest Ophthalmol Vis Sci 45:4119–4125
74. Sadun AA (1990) Distinguishing between clinical impairments due to optic nerve or macular disease. Metab Pediatr Syst Ophthalmol 13:79–84
75. Shawkat FS, Kriss A, Timms C, Taylor DS (1998) Comparison of pattern-onset, -reversal and -offset VEPs in treated amblyopia. Eye 12:863–869
76. Shiells RA, Falk G (1999) Contribution of rod, on-bipolar, and horizontal cell light responses to the ERG of dogfish retina. Vis Neurosci 16:503–511
77. Sieving PA (1993) Photopic ON and OFF-pathway abnormalities in retinal dystrophies. Trans Am Ophthalmol Soc 91:701–773
78. Simunovic MP, Moore AT (1998) The cone dystrophies. Eye 12:553–565
79. Sokol S (1983) Abnormal evoked potential latencies in amblyopia. Br J Ophthalmol 67:310–314
80. Stanga PE, Chong NH, Reck AC, Hardcastle AJ, Holder GE (2001) Optical coherence tomography and electrophysiology in X-linked juvenile retinoschisis associated with a novel mutation in the XLRS1 gene. Retina 21:78–80
81. Viswanathan S, Frishman LJ, Robson JG (2000) The uniform field and pattern ERG in macaques with experimental glaucoma: removal of spiking activity. Invest Ophthalmol Vis Sci 41:2797–2810
82. Votruba M, Fitzke FW, Holder GE, Carter A, Bhattacharya SS, Moore AT (1998) Clinical features in affected individuals from 21 pedigrees with dominant optic atrophy. Arch Ophthalmol 116:351–358
83. Watts PO, Neveu MM, Holder GE, Sloper JJ (2002) Visual evoked potentials in successfully treated strabismic amblyopes and normal subjects. J AAPOS 6:389–392
84. Weleber RG (1998) The dystrophic retina in multisystem disorders: the electroretinogram in neuronal ceroid lipofuscinosis. Eye 12:580–590
85. Weleber RG (2002) Infantile and childhood retinal blindness: a molecular perspective (The Franceschetti Lecture) Ophthalmic Genet 23:71–97
86. Westall CA, Panton CM, Levin AV (1998) Time courses for maturation of electroretinogram responses from infancy to adulthood. Doc Ophthalmol 96:355–379
87. Wilcox LM Jr, Sokol S (1980) Changes in the binocular fixation patterns and the visually evoked potential in the treatment of esotropia with amblyopia. Ophthalmology 87:1273–1281
88. Woodruff SA, Fraser S, Burton LC, Holder GE, Sloper JJ (2004) Evaluation of the electrodiagnostic investigation of children using the Greenwich Grading System. Eye 18:15–19
89. Yamamoto S, Hayashi M, Tsuruoka M, Ogata K, Tsukahara I, Yamamoto T, Takeuchi S (2002) Selective reduction of S-cone response and on-response in the cone electroretinograms of patients with X-linked retinoschisis. Graefes Arch Clin Exp Ophthalmol 240:457–460

Clinical and Molecular Genetic Aspects of Leber's Congenital Amaurosis

10

Robert Henderson, Birgit Lorenz, Anthony T. Moore

Core Messages

- Leber's congenital amaurosis (LCA) is a severe generalized retinal dystrophy which presents at birth or soon after with nystagmus and poor vision and is accompanied by a nonrecordable or severely attenuated ERG
- As some forms are associated with better vision during childhood and nystagmus may be absent, a wider definition is early onset severe retinal dystrophy (EOSRD) with LCA being the most severe form
- It is nearly always a recessive condition but there is considerable genetic heterogeneity
- There are eight known causative genes and three further loci that have been implicated in LCA/EOSRD
- The phenotype varies with the genes involved; not all are progressive. At present, a distinct phenotype has been elaborated for patients with mutations in *RPE65*
- Although LCA is currently not amenable to treatment, gene therapy appears to be a promising therapeutic option, especially for those children with mutations in *RPE65*

10.1 Introduction

Leber's congenital amaurosis, an infantile onset form of rod-cone dystrophy, is usually inherited as an autosomal recessive trait. First described by Theodor Leber in 1869 and 1871 [71], it accounts for 3–5% of childhood blindness in the developed world [108] and has an incidence of about 2–3 per 100,000 live births [119, 50]. It occurs more frequently in communities where consanguineous marriages are common [128].

10.1.1 Clinical Findings

LCA is characterized clinically by severe visual impairment and nystagmus from early infancy associated with a nonrecordable or substantially abnormal rod and cone electroretinogram (ERG) [32, 31, 118]. The pupils react sluggishly and, although the fundus appearance is often normal in the early stages, a variety of abnormal retinal changes may be seen. These include peripheral white dots at the level of the retinal pigment epithelium, and the typical bone-spicule pigmentation seen in retinitis pigmentosa.

Other associated findings include the oculodigital sign, microphthalmos, enophthalmos, ptosis, strabismus, keratoconus [28], high refractive error [143], cataract, macular coloboma, optic disc swelling, and attenuated retinal vasculature.

10.1.2 Differential Diagnosis

It is now recognised that LCA represents the most severe end of the spectrum of infantile onset retinal dystrophies. Some genes originally described as causing LCA have since been shown to have a less severe clinical phenotype–with less nystagmus, normal pupil reactions, and better vision despite an absent ERG

Table 10.1. Systemic disorders with associated LCA findings

Disorder	MIM No.	Systemic features
Senior-Loken syndrome	MIM 266900	Kidney disease (nephronophthisis)
Mainzer-Saldino syndrome	MIM 266920	Skeletal anomalies including osteopetrosis giving cone shaped epiphyses of the hand bones and ataxia
Lhermitte-Duclos syndrome	MIM 158350	Cerebellar hyperplasia, macrocephaly and seizures
Joubert syndrome	MIM 213300	Cerebellar hypoplasia, oculomotor difficulties and respiratory problems
Alstrom syndrome	MIM 203800	Cardiomyopathy, deafness, obesity and diabetes
Bardet-Biedl syndrome	MIM 209900	Mental retardation, polydactyly, obesity and hypogonadism, abnormality in renal structure, function, or both
Infantile Refsum disease	MIM 266510	Abnormal accumulation of phytanic acid leading to peripheral neuropathy, ataxia impaired hearing, and bone and skin changes
Zellweger disease	MIM 214100	Cerebrohepatorenal syndrome
Neonatal adrenoleucodystrophy	MIM 202370	Similar in biochemical terms to Zellweger syndrome; it has characteristic facies, adrenal atrophy, and degenerative white matter changes
Infantile Batten disease	MIM 256730	Histopathologically: total derangement of cortical cytoarchitecture with severe degeneration of white matter. Clinically: rapid psychomotor deterioration, ataxia, and muscular hypotonia; microcephaly and myoclonic jerks are also features

[99]. This has led some to use the term early onset severe retinal dystrophy (EOSRD) to describe severe rod-cone dystrophies of infantile onset.

The main differential diagnosis is from other causes of infantile nystagmus [14, 76] particularly early onset static retinal conditions such as congenital stationary night blindness [5] and the various forms of achromatopsia [90]. The clinical features, and in particular the ERG findings, allow these disorders to be distinguished from LCA. Although most children with LCA have disease confined to the eye; there are a number of recessively inherited systemic disorders such as Joubert syndrome, and the peroxisomal disorders in which an early onset retinal dystrophy similar to LCA may form part of the syndrome (Table 10.1). Usually the other systemic findings allow these disorders to be distinguished from LCA but in some disorders, for example Alstrom syndrome [117] and juvenile nephronothisis [7, 30, 132] the systemic features may not become apparent until later childhood.

10.2 Molecular Genetics

LCA is usually inherited as an autosomal recessive disorder, although there are a few reports of autosomal dominant inheritance [33, 102, 135]. Although it had been recognised as early as 1963 that there was more than one causative gene [142], it is only recently that the true extent of the genetic heterogeneity has been identified. To date, eight genes (*GUCY2D* [103], *AIPL1* [123], *RPE65* [84, 44], *RPGRIP1* [27, 40], *CRX* [35, 56], *TULP1* [9, 43, 46], *CRB1* [79], *RDH12* [58, 101]) and a three further loci (LCA3 [126], LCA5 [93] and LCA9 [62]) have been reported in LCA/EOSRD. Furthermore, mutations in two other genes (*LRAT* [131] and *MERTK* [87]) are associated with a very early onset form of RP that could also be classified as EOSRD. All together these genes account for between 20% and 50% of cases of LCA cases and it is evident that more genes remain to be discovered [48, 18] (Figs. 10.1, 10.2).

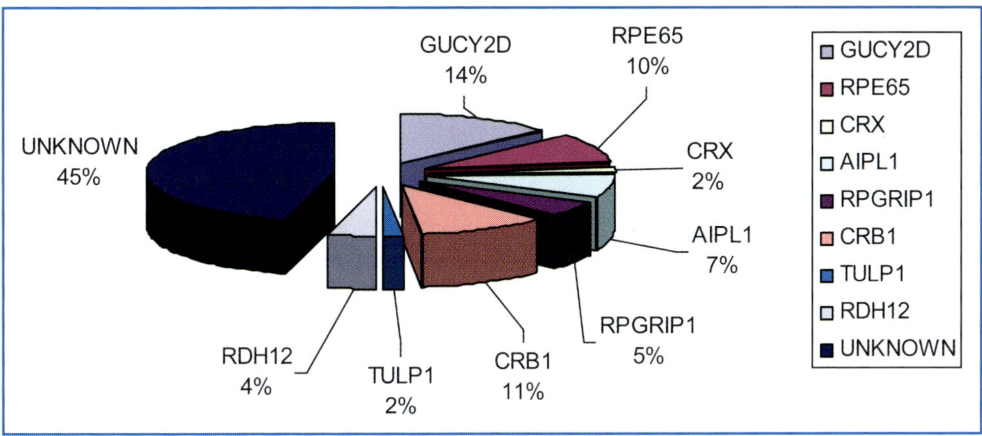

Fig. 10.1. Median frequency of disease genes in LCA/EOSRD

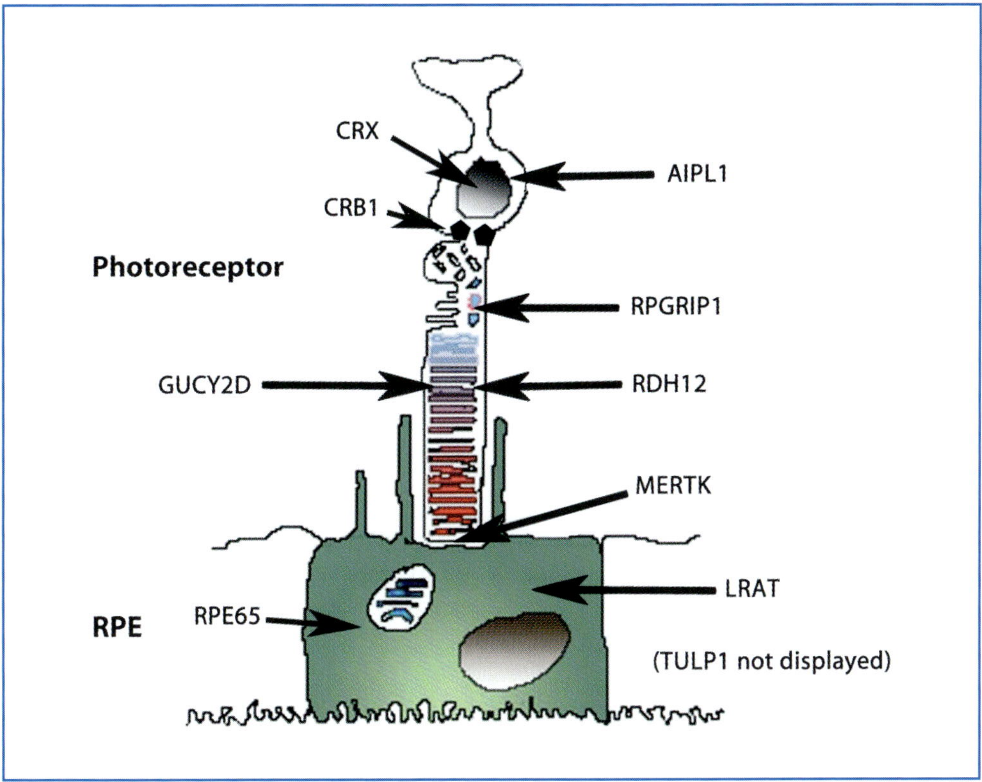

Fig. 10.2. Putative sites of gene expression for LCA/EOSRD

10.2.1 GUCY-2D (LCA1 Locus)

GUCY-2D (17p13.1) was the first gene identified as causative in LCA [103]. The prevalence of mutations of *GUCY-2D* in LCA is much higher (70 %) in cases from Mediterranean countries [49]. *GUCY-2D* encodes a human photoreceptor specific guanylate cyclase which plays a key role in phototransduction. Guanylyl cyclase catalyzes the conversion of guanosine triphosphate (GTP) to cyclic guanosine monophosphate (cGMP). Guanylate cyclase function is important in restoring levels of cGMP levels, which keeps open the gated cation channels allowing recovery of the dark state after phototransduction. Mutations in the gene would lead to permanent closure of the c-GMP gated cation channels with resultant hyperpolarisation of the plasma membrane.

Recessive mutations in *GUCY-2D* are associated with LCA and the causative mutations have been reported in the extracellular, kinase-like, dimerisation, and catalytic domains [104, 116]. Heterozygous mutations in the same gene have been reported to cause an autosomal dominant cone rod dystrophy [26, 105, 134] (http://www.retina-international.org/sci-news/gcmut.htm).

Histological examination of the eyes from an 11-year-old LCA donor with a known *GUCY-2D* mutation, who had light perception vision and a nondetectable ERG at the time of death, showed regional loss of photoreceptors. There were no identifiable photoreceptors in the mid-peripheral retina, but rods and cones lacking outer segments were present in the macula and peripheral retina, although in reduced numbers. The inner nuclear layer was found to be of normal thickness but horizontal cell, amacrine and ganglion cell numbers were decreased [91]. The fact that there were significant numbers of residual photoreceptors and inner retinal neurons despite a visual acuity of light perception gives rise to some optimism that any future therapy may lead to improved retinal function. However, visual improvement following successful therapy may be limited by sensory deprivation amblyopia unless treatment was given in early infancy.

10.2.1.1 Genotype–Phenotype Correlations

The findings of high hyperopia (>+7 DS), severe photophobia, poor vision of count fingers (CF) or light perception (LP) in addition to the presence of early peripheral and macular degeneration with bone spicule pigments in the periphery, disc pallor and vessel attenuation has been suggested by Perrault et al. to be pathognomonic of the *GUCY-2D* mutation [103]. Other groups have, however, reported LCA patients with *GUCY-2D* mutations who have no significant photophobia, better visual acuity (20/200), and mild to moderate hyperopia [25].

10.2.2 RPE65 (LCA2)

Mutations in *RPE65* are associated with a number of different retinal degenerations, including LCA [44, 84, 95, 121], autosomal recessive RP [93], and an early onset severe rod-cone dystrophy [77] (http://www.retina-international.org/sci-news/rpe65mut.htm). Mutations in *RPE65* account for 3–16 % of cases of LCA/EOSRD in various series [25, 40, 48, 80, 95, 130]. The *RPE65* gene localizes to 1p31.2 and consists of 14 exons. It encodes two distinct forms of a 65-kD protein specific to the smooth endoplasmic reticulum (ER) of the retinal pigment epithelium: a retinal pigment epithelium (RPE) membrane-associated form (mRPE65) and a lower molecular weight soluble form (sRPE65)[83]. RPE65 plays a key role in the metabolism of vitamin A within the retina. RPE65 serves as a binding protein for all-*trans*-retinyl esters [41, 57] Analysis of *RPE65* knockout mice shows that it is involved in the isomerisation of all-*trans*-retinol to 11-*cis*-retinol within the RPE [107]. Xue et al. [148] demonstrated that the membrane associated form is triply palmitoylated and is a chaperone for all-*trans* retinyl esters, allowing their entry into the visual cycle for processing into 11-cis retinal. The soluble form of RPE65 is not palmitoylated and is a chaperone for vitamin A. The two chaperones are interconverted by lecithin acyl transferase (LRAT) acting as a palmitoyl transferase catalyzing the mRPE65 to sRPE65 conversion, like a molecular switch controlling the quantity of chromophore required by the visual cycle [148]. Recent evidence suggests RPE65, when coexpressed with LRAT in QBI-293A or COS-1 cells, efficiently generates 11-*cis* retinol from *all-trans* retinyl ester, suggesting that it is an enzyme responsible for the isomerohydrolase activity [150].

Knockout mice show oil-like droplets in the RPE composed of accumulations of these all-trans retinyl esters [109]. However, it is unlikely that the accumulation of these esters is responsible for the photoreceptor degeneration. Further experiments in *RPE65*$^{-/-}$ mice have demonstrated a high concentration of the apoprotein opsin, mostly unphosphorylated and unbound to arrestin [109, 115]. Spontaneous opsin activity has been subsequently shown to lead to retinal degeneration through a mechanism as yet poorly understood [147], and this may be a key factor in photoreceptor cell death in early onset retinal dystrophy associated with mutations of *RPE65*.

Histological examination of 33-week embryonic human retina with a known *RPE65* mutation showed extensive structural degeneration with RPE, neural retina, choriocapillaris and Bruch's membrane, all showing severe changes compared to age-matched controls [107]. This suggests that some of the retinal degeneration in this form of LCA may occur before birth. It has been argued that the extensive retinal degeneration seen in this foetus may not be char-

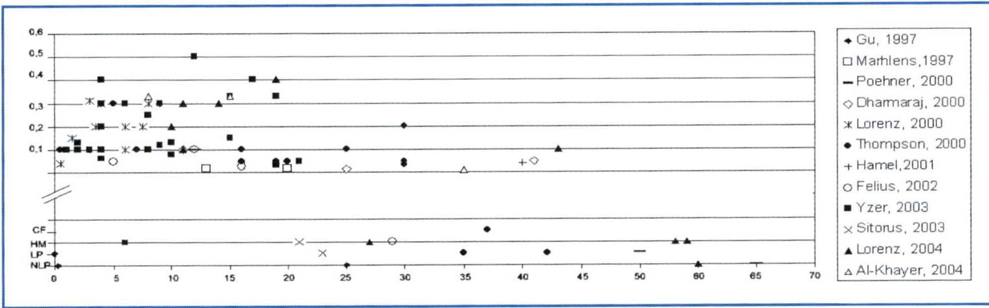

Fig. 10.3. Scatterplot of VA data of patients with known mutations in RPE65. VA in dependence on age (51 patients, 114 VA data). Most patients had measurable visual acuities at least during the first decade, with a clustering between 0.1 and 0.3 From [99]. With permission from *Graefe's Archive*

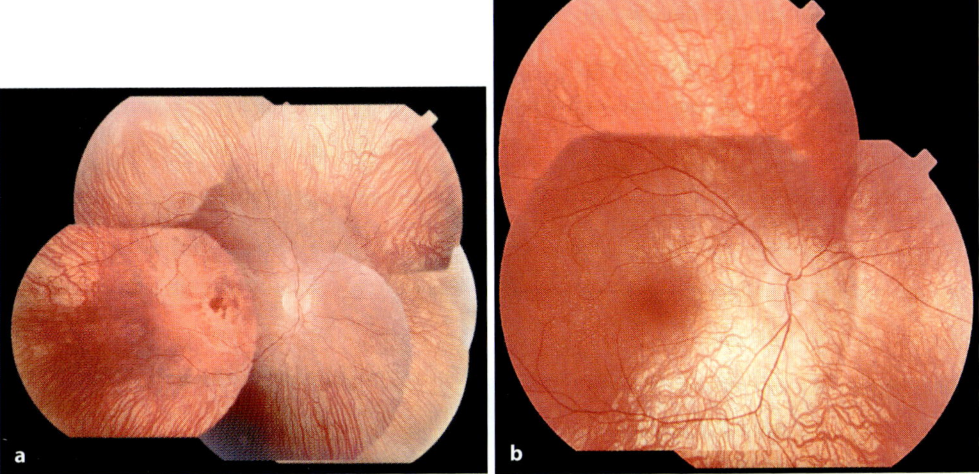

Fig. 10.4 a, b. Fundus of two patients with RPE65 mutations. **a** HJ at 6 years. IVS1 + 5G-A/144insT. For details see [77]. **b** BR at 7 years. IVS1 + 5G-A/114delA +T457N. For details see [77]

acteristic, as clinically infants with *RPE65* mutations have a normal fundus and reasonable visual acuity and fields [99].

10.2.2.1 Genotype–Phenotype Correlations

Infants with *RPE65* mutations perform visual tasks best in bright light [77, 106] and often show light-staring behaviour. The infants have poor but useful vision in early life (6/18–6/60), which may show initial improvement [106] (though this may represent a form of delayed visual maturation) but then declines through school age years. A number of patients retain residual islands of peripheral vision into the third decade of life [130] and later [99]. Progressive visual field loss and vision reduced to LP in the fifth and sixth decades is usual [3]. Refractive errors are variable with high or mild hyperopia, emmetropia or myopia being reported [25, 99] (Fig. 10.3).

Fundus autofluorescence (FAF) imaging has shown to be absent in children with early onset severe retinal dystrophy who have compound heterozygous or homozygous *RPE65* mutations. They have a near normal fundus appearance on ophthalmoscopy and preserved RPE and photoreceptors on OCT (Fig. 10.4). Absence of fundus autofluorescence in *RPE65*$^{-/-}$ mice has been shown to be secondary to failure of lipofuscin fluorophore manufacture, which depends upon normal function of the visual cycle [60, 78]. Similar lack of fundus autofluorescence is also seen in human subjects (Fig. 10.5). FAF imaging is therefore an extremely useful tool for screening patients with retinal dystrophies that may be due to *RPE65* mutations; the restoration of normal autofluorescence may be an early sign of successful therapeutic effect in future treatment trials [78].

10.2.3 CRX

The third gene found to be responsible for LCA was *CRX* [35, 55, 125], a photoreceptor homeobox gene localizing to 19q13.3 [16]. CRX mutations have been reported in a number of differing retinal phenotypes, including early onset autosomal dominant cone-rod dystrophy [34], autosomal dominant RP [125], autosomal dominant LCA [35, 102] and recessive LCA [127]. *CRX* has been found to account for between 0.6 % and 6 % of mutations in LCA patients [25, 34, 48, 80, 112].

CRX encoding a 299-aminoacid protein which belongs to the paired class of homeodomain proteins with three highly conserved motifs: the homeodomain, a WSP domain and an OTX tail. It functions as a transcription factor and in vitro, the protein recognises a specific sequence that is found in the promoters of many photoreceptor-specific genes, including rhodopsin, arrestin, the β-subunit of rod cGMP-phosphodiesterase, and interphotoreceptor retinoid-binding protein (IRBP) [16, 36]. In vivo, many of these genes seem to require *CRX* for normal expression [37]. *CRX* knockout mice have reduced levels of expression of many photoreceptor-specific genes, leading to subsequent retinal degeneration [75]. The *CRX* protein forms a complex with another transcription factor – *NRL* – and works synergistically to activate the rhodopsin promoter [16] to much greater effect than either alone.

Mutations in *CRX* have been implicated in both dominant ad recessive forms of LCA. Reported mutations include: a homozygous *CRX* mutation [127]; a heterozygous *CRX* mutation resulting in a four amino acid deletion [125]; a heterozygous null mutation [102, 120]; and a heterozygous frameshift mutation identified in a mother and son with LCA [64] (http://www.retina-international.org/scinews/crxmut.htm). There are a number of possible explanations for the finding of heterozygous mutations in some patients including the presence of an unidentified mutation on the other *CRX* allele; an additional mutation in another gene (digenic inheritance) or the possibility that some *CRX* mutants work in a dominant-negative manner to interfere with wild-type *CRX* function [111].

10.2.3.1 Genotype–Phenotype Correlations

CRX mutations have been identified in association with LCA, retinitis pigmentosa and cone rod dystrophy. Although this phenotypic vari-

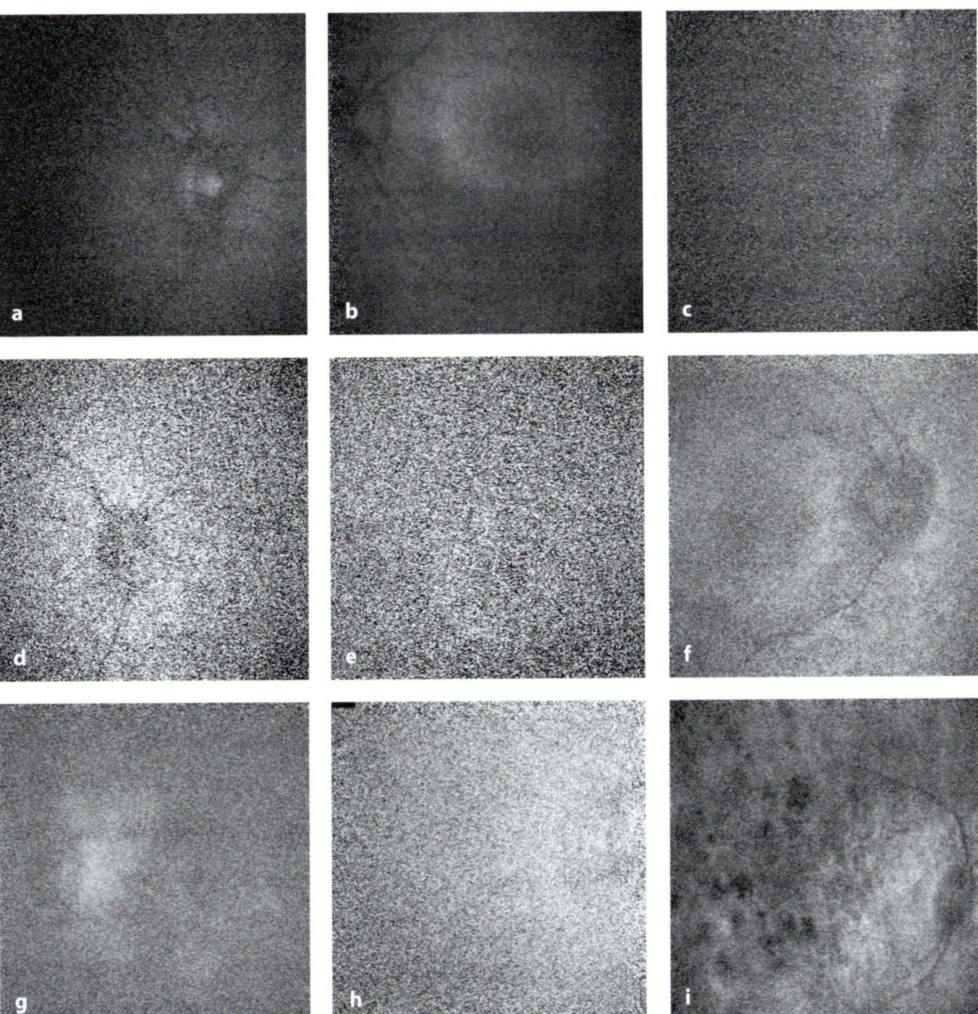

Fig. 10.5 a–i. Fundus autofluorescence (Heidelberg Retina Angiograph, HRA, Heidelberg Engineering) in patients with early onset severe retinal dystrophy (EOSRD) associated with mutations in RPE65. Overall image brightness does not reflect the absolute amount of fundus autofluorescence (AF). Please note very similar brightness at optic disc and retina in all images displayed. This results from lack of AF. **a** Patient LJ at 10 years of age. Nearly absent AF in both eyes. Shown is the right eye. **b** Patient LH at 14 years of age. Very low AF in both eyes, perimacular slightly brighter circle. Left eye is shown. LJ and LH are siblings. **c** Patient HJ at 11 years. Nearly absent AF in both eyes. Right eye is shown. **d** Patient BR, aged 11 years. No detectable AF in both eyes. Right eye is shown. **e** Patient CG at 19 years of age. No detectable AF in both eyes. Right eye is shown. **f** Patient CY aged 27 years. Very low AF in both eyes, peripapillary image is a little brighter. Right eye is shown. CG and CY are siblings. **g** Patient KM at 54 years. Nearly absent AF in both eyes. Shown is the left eye. **h** Patient KG at 43 years. Nearly absent AF in both eyes. Right eye is shown. KM and KG are siblings. **i** Patient FT at 55 years of age. Very low AF in both eyes, oval areas of nondetectable AF at the posterior pole corresponding clinically to atrophic areas, temporal of the optic disc, some AF visible. The signal may come from the sclera. Right eye is shown. With permission from Ophthalmology. For detailed explanation see [78]

ability may in the main be due to allelic heterogeneity, other modifying genes or environmental factors are likely to play a role, as the same *CRX* mutation may produce clinically highly disparate phenotypes. For example, some patients with c.436del12 bp were diagnosed with LCA, while one retained vision of 20/80 at age 27 years [125].

The fundal appearances associated with *CRX* mutations include attenuated retinal vessels, intraretinal pigment deposits, and areas of retinal atrophy, including macular atrophy (coloboma). Some patients are reported as having normal fundi in infancy [25]. Moderate hyperopia is often found [25, 801, 111], though Rivolta et al. [111] showed that when the average refractive error of published cases of all *CRX* mutations was calculated, the outcome was slightly myopic. This, they argued, indicates that hyperopia is associated with poor vision in early life rather than with the *CRX* mutations per se.

10.2.4 AIPL1 (LCA4)

AIPL1 (aryl-hydrocarbon interacting protein-like 1), described by Sohocki et al. [123], was the fourth of the LCA genes to be identified and accounts for 3.4–11% [24, 48, 66, 124] of cases. It has also been identified as putatively causative in autosomal dominant cone-rod dystrophy and retinitis pigmentosa (RP) [124] (http://www.retina-international.org/sci-news/aipl1mut.htm), though Cremers [18] has expressed some doubt about this.

The *AIPL1* gene (located on 17p13.2) encodes a 384-aminoacid protein that contains three tetratricopeptide (TPR) motifs. TPR domains are sites of protein–protein interaction, and it is thought that the *AIPL1* protein, through this motif, interacts and aids in the processing of farnesylated proteins [151] which are responsible for attachment to cell membranes, in other words, maintaining photoreceptor architecture.

AIPL1 has also been shown to interact with NEDD8 ultimate buster-1 (*NUB1*), which is an interferon inducible protein; both *NUB1* and *AIPL1* are expressed within the developing cone and rod photoreceptors but co-localise solely within the rods of the mature retina [2, 123, 139]. This suggests that *AIPL1* is essential for the normal development of photoreceptor cells. *NUB1* is located predominantly within the nuclear component of cells as compared to *AIPL1*, which is largely cytoplasmic [137, 139]. It has now been shown that *AIPL1* can modulate protein translocation through enhanced farnesylation, and acts in a chaperone-like manner escorting prenylated proteins to their target membranes, suggesting that *AIPL1* is an important modulator of *NUB1* cellular function [138]. *AIPL1* mutations implicated in LCA have been shown in vitro not to interact with *NUB1* suggesting that this lack of interaction may be a key factor in the abnormal retinal function seen in the LCA retina [59].

10.2.4.1 Genotype–Phenotype Correlations

Much of the phenotypic description given below is from the study of 26 probands with the *AIPL1* mutation described by Dharmaraj et al. [24]. Affected individuals had a severe phenotype with poor vision, maculopathy, significant pigmentary changes, disc pallor, with the later development of keratoconus and cataract in up to one-third of cases.

Nyctalopia was found in half, and photoaversion and photoattraction were described but were uncommon. Levels of visual acuity were generally very poor with most patients having HMs or light perception. No patient had better vision than 20/400. The most common refractive error was moderate hyperopia, though mild myopia was occasionally found.

Maculopathy was present in 80% (16/20) in this study and in the remaining four probands, who were all aged 2–6 years, an abnormal indistinct foveal reflex was noted. All patients had some form of pigmentary retinopathy from mild mid-peripheral salt and pepper appearance to a severe chorioretinopathy. In addition, varying degrees of optic nerve pallor were seen in all patients after the age of 6 (Fig. 10.6).

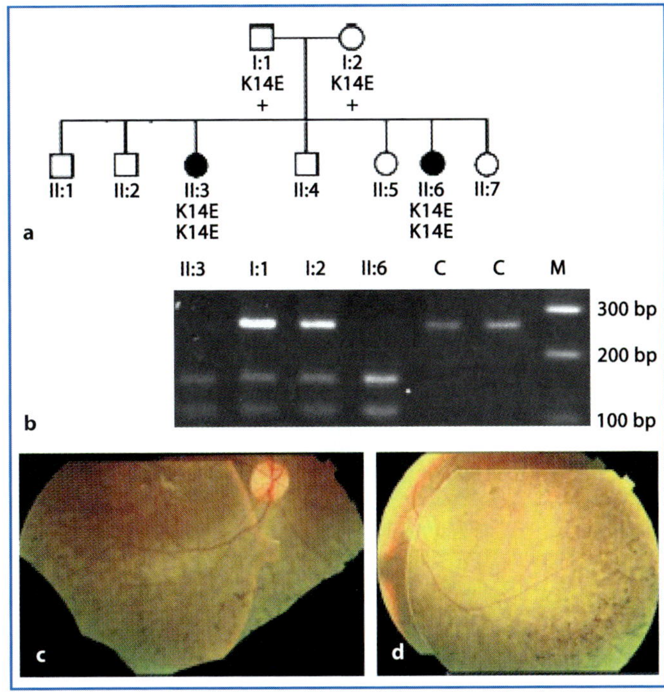

Fig. 10.6. a Pedigree of family with AIPL1 mutation K14E. **b** *Xmn*I restriction digest for the homozygous K14E mutation. The mutation creates a novel restriction site, as shown by the restriction fragments of 152 and 103 bp from the 255-bp amplimer (C control, M marker). Fundus photograph of case 3 (II:3) at age 22 years: **c** right eye, **d** left eye

10.2.5 RPGRIP1 (LCA6)

RPGRIP1 (14q11.2) is the fifth (and largest with 25 exons) of the genes responsible for the LCA phenotype [27]. It accounts for between 4.5% and 6% of LCA cases [6, 27, 40, 48] (http://www.retina-international.org/sci-news/rpgripmu.htm).

The X-linked RP3 locus encodes several spliced isoforms of the retinitis pigmentosa GTPase regulator (RPGR) [63, 89, 113, 141]. The RPGR interacting protein (RPGRIP) is a structural component of the ciliary axoneme and is known to localize in the photoreceptor connecting cilium [51] and the amacrine cells of bovine retina [13, 85]. RPGR interacts directly in vivo and in vitro with the RPGR interacting domain (RID) at the C-terminus of *RPGRIP1*, and both proteins co-localise to the outer segment of photoreceptors in the bovine and human retina [114].

Several *RPGRIP1* isoforms have also been found and are expressed at a number of different subcellular locations across species, including at the nuclear rims and axonal processes in a subset of amacrine cells located at the proximal edge of the inner nuclear layer (INL) [13]. These *RPGRIP1* isoforms have also been shown to co-localise with RanBP2, a component of the nuclear pore complex which has been implicated in the rate-limiting steps of nuclear-cytoplasmic trafficking processes.

RPGRIP knockout mice initially develop a full complement of photoreceptors, but the outer segments rapidly become disorganized with pyknotic nuclei indicating cell death, and there is almost complete loss of photoreceptors by 3 months of age. The photoreceptor degeneration is more severe than that seen in the $RPGR^{-/-}$ mice [149]. It has also been established in the murine knockout model that *RPGRIP* is not essential for transporting or restricting proteins across the connecting cilium (CC); nor is it thought to be essential for development or maintenance of the core CC structure. However, the outer segment arrangement of disks is grossly altered in a manner not seen in the $RPGR^{-/-}$ mice. The mechanism of photoreceptor cell death associated with *RPGRIP1* mutations is currently poorly understood.

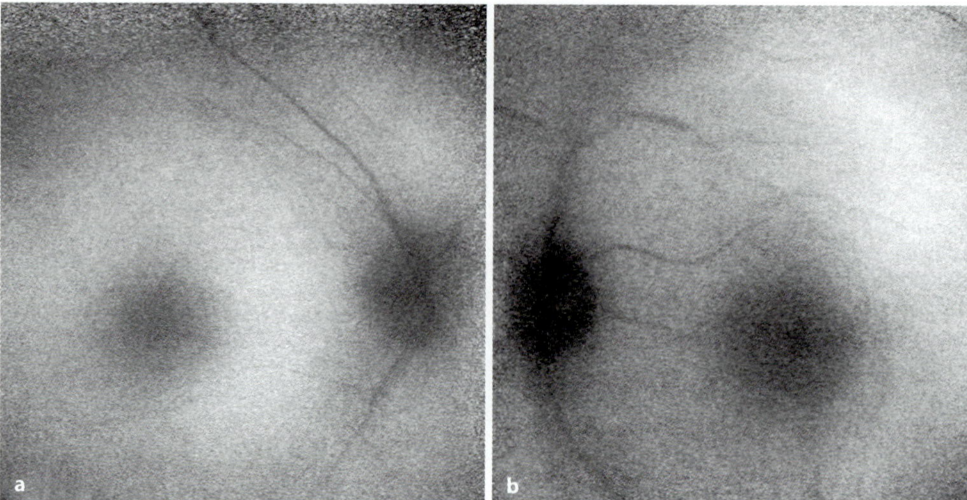

Fig. 10.7 a, b. Fundus autofluorescence (Heidelberg Retina Angiograph, HRA, Heidelberg Engineering) in patients with early onset severe retinal dystrophy (EOSRD) not associated with RPE65 or LRAT mutations. **a** Patient HaA at 7 years of age. Limited cooperation and photophobia affect image quality. Fundus autofluorescence AF is clearly present in both eyes. Right eye is shown. **b** Patient MT at 10 years of age. Limited cooperation due to photophobia and nystagmus influence image quality. AF is clearly present in both eyes. Left eye is shown. From [78], with permission

10.2.5.1 Genotype–Phenotype Correlations

The phenotype of the *RPGRIP1* LCA patients is relatively severe, with nystagmus and severely reduced visual acuities from a young age. Dryja's original paper [27] reports a 26-year-old with LP vision, moderate vascular attenuation, and no intraretinal pigmentation; another 15-year-old had LP vision, low hyperopia and mid-peripheral pigmentation. Hanein et al. [48] report early photophobia as an early sign in patients with *RPGRIP1* mutations (Fig. 10.7).

10.2.6 TULP1

The gene (*TULP1*) encoding the Tubby like protein 1 on 6p21.3 is part of a family of tubby genes (tub, tubby 1–3). *TULP1* was identified as a cause of an autosomal recessive retinal degeneration in several isolated families [43, 46] and large pedigrees living in the Dominican Republic [9]. Several mutations in the *TULP1* gene are associated with early onset, severe retinal degeneration consistent with LCA (http://www.retina-international.org/sci-news/tulpmut.htm). *TULP1* mutations accounts for a minority of Leber's cases (1.7% [48]).

The TULP genes are characterized by the tubby domain, a highly conserved region of about 260 amino acids, located at the carboxyl terminus of all TULP-family proteins. The four members of the family are localised primarily to nervous tissue [12] and all are expressed in the retina [92]. Tubby mice display a three-part phenotype of blindness, deafness, and maturity onset obesity. The exact role of the Tubby-like proteins remains to be fully elucidated.

TULP1 is found expressed by human retinal neuroblasts at 8.4 foetal weeks, suggesting a fundamental role in retinal differentiation; it is not expressed in mature rod or cone outer segments in either human or mouse [52], nor indeed is it seen in the nuclei of adult mouse photoreceptors [46]. Some evidence suggests that *TULP1* is a transcription factor involved in control of other photoreceptors genes [11].

TULP1 knockout mice show a retinal degeneration, but not the other characteristic phenotypes – obesity or deafness – seen in mice with $TUB^{-/-}$ mutations [53]. Histological analysis in the mouse model shows there to be a marked degeneration of the photoreceptor layer.

10.2.6.1 Genotype–Phenotype Correlations: TULP1

Initially, patients found to have *TULP1* mutations by candidate gene screening were from populations with the clinical diagnosis of RP [43, 46]; however, the retinal degeneration resulting from the IVS14+1, GA *TULP1* mutation [9, 74] is an atypical form of RP and fits a clinical category that is better described as LCA. Subsequent analysis of a large LCA group (n=179) found *TULP1* involvement in 1.7% [48]. Clinical features include nystagmus, poor vision from an early age ranging from 20/200, LP, nyctalopia and early immeasurable rod function, and impaired or absent cone function on electroretinography [46]. Older patients may show macular abnormalities (yellow macular deposits or a bull's eye maculopathy) and optic disc pallor. Myopic refractive errors have also been described. However, in contrast to tubby mice, *Tulp1* (–/–) mice exhibited normal hearing ability and, surprisingly, normal body weight despite the fact that both TUB and TULP1 are expressed in the same neurons within the hypothalamus in areas known to be involved in feeding behaviour and energy homeostasis.

10.2.7 CRB1

The Crumbs homologue 1 gene (*CRB1*) maps to 1q31.3 and consists of 11 exons; it is expressed specifically in the brain and retina [22], though the truncated secreted protein CRB1s is also expressed during skin development [144]. It was first described as responsible for a distinctive form of autosomal recessive RP, referred to as RP12, which exhibited preservation of the para-arteriolar RPE. Subsequently, several cohorts of LCA probands were analysed and *CRB1* variants were found in 9–13% [23, 48, 79], though in one study no *CRB1* mutations were identified. [21] (http://www.retina-international.org/sci-news/crb1mut.htm).

CRB1 is analogous to the Drosophila Melanogaster Crumbs protein ; it contains 19 epidermal growth factor (EGF) -like domains, a transmembrane domain, three laminin A globular-like domains, and a 37-amino acid cytoplasmic tail [23]. The Crumbs protein localises to the apical membrane in Drosophila and acts as a regulator of epithelial polarity [129, 145]. Antibodies raised against the cytoplasmic domain of *CRB1* reveal its distribution at the apical membrane of all retinal epithelial cells, the rod and cone photoreceptors and Muller cells in the adult mouse retina. In rod and cone photoreceptors, *CRB1* is confined to the inner segments, where it is specifically located at the zonula adherens (ZA). CRB has a role in the maintenance of the ZA integrity and stalk membrane formation during photoreceptor cell (PRC) development in Drosophila [100].

The defects in CRB rd8 mutant mice show similarities to those in the fly model: the external limiting, membrane and zonula adherens are fragmented and shortened photoreceptor inner and outer segments are observed as early as 2 weeks after birth, suggesting that there is a developmental defect rather than a degenerative process [88]. Studies in the *CRB1*$^{-/-}$ mice suggest that CRB1 has a key role in formation of the adherens junctions that make up the outer limiting membrane. It is required for the maintenance of a single, organized layer of PRCs. In the absence of the normal gene product, the adhesion between PRCs and Muller cells is temporarily lost, following light exposure, resulting in dramatic structural and functional changes. These changes were exacerbated by prolonged exposure to light [136].

10.2.7.1 Genotype-Phenotype Correlations

In humans with CRB1 mutations, retinal thickness as measured by OCT is significantly increased (1.5 times thicker), with a coarse lamination pattern [54]. (Fig. 10.8). In the original description [79], two fairly consistent phenotypic features were described: the presence of

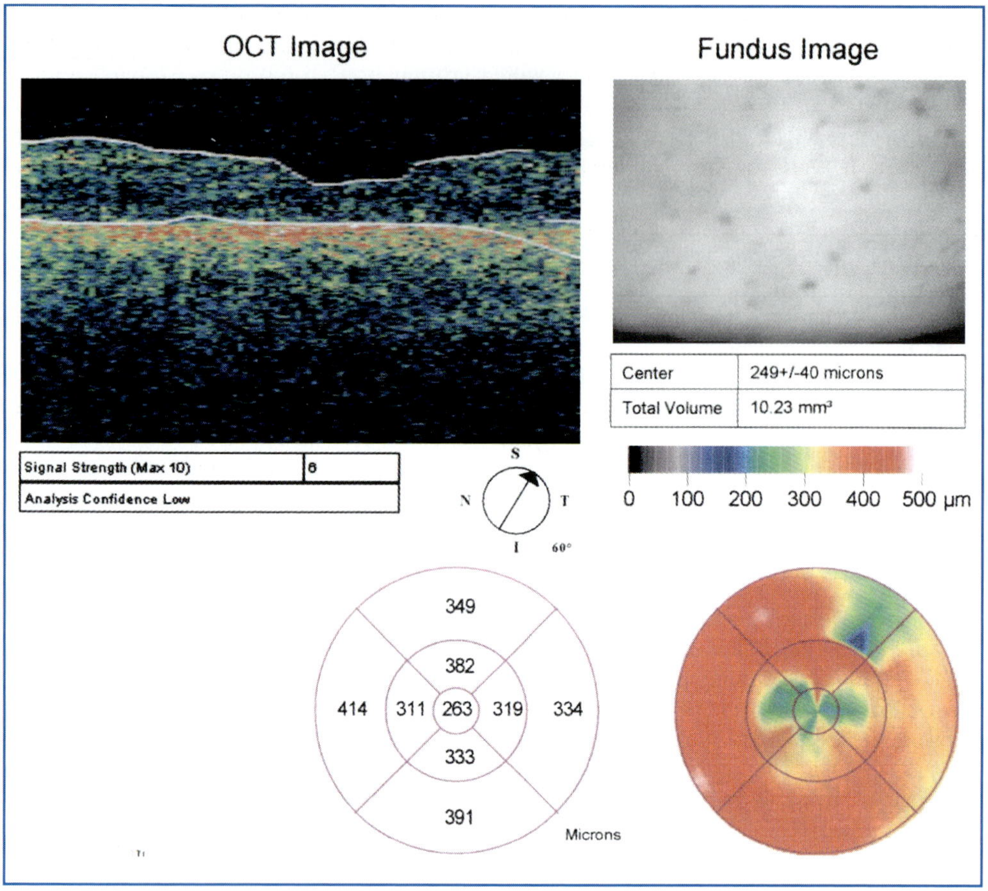

OCT Image

Fundus Image

Center	249+/-40 microns
Total Volume	10.23 mm³

0 100 200 300 400 500 µm

Signal Strength (Max 10)	6
Analysis Confidence Low	

S N T I 60°

349 382 414 311 263 319 334 333 391

Microns

Fig. 10.8. Optical coherence tomography scan Zeiss OCT-3 (Zeiss Humphrey, Dublin, CA), 15-year-old Caucasian male with homozygous C948Y mutation in CRB1 showing thickened retinal appearance

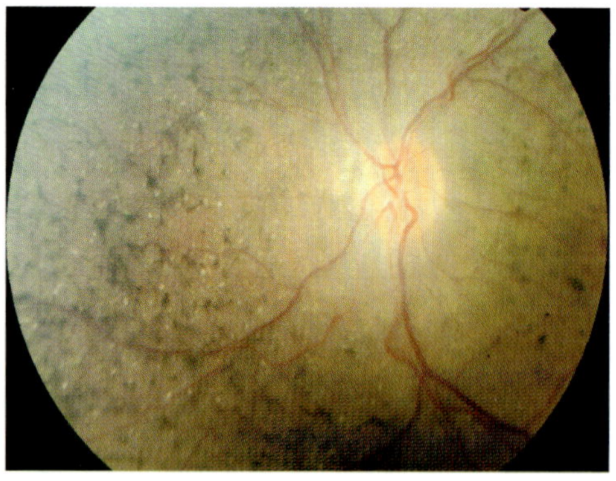

Fig. 10.9. Six-year-old male with heterozygous G850S mutation in CRB1 showing white dots and pigment at level of the RPE

moderate to high hyperopia; and the relatively early appearance of white spots at the level of the RPE and pigment clumping (Fig. 10.9). The preservation of the peri-arteriolar retinal pigment epithelium (characteristic of RP12) is seen occasionally [79]. Hanein et al. report early macular reorganisation in the first decade of life as being characteristic of CRB1 mutations [48].

10.2.8 RDH12

RDH12 mutations were first reported simultaneously in several west Austrian families [58], possibly as a founder mutation, and in a significant subset (4.1%) of unrelated LCA patients in France [101] (http://www.retina-international.org/sci-news/rdh12mut.htm). *RDH12* maps close to the LCA3 locus [126] on 14q24.1, though whilst the linkage analysis performed gave a significant lod score at this locus (3.24–3.87) a maximum lod score of 13.29 was obtained 10 Mb distally. It remains to be seen whether the families mapped to the LCA3 locus have RDH12 mutations or whether there is another LCA gene in the same region.

RDH12 is a photoreceptor-specific gene involved in the production of 11-*cis* retinal from 11-*cis* retinol during regeneration of the cone visual pigments [45], though it has dual substrate specificity for both the -*cis* and -*trans* retinoids. Whether it is the decrease in 11-cis synthesis and/or accumulation of the all-trans retinal within the photoreceptors that causes the severe LCA phenotype is not yet known.

10.2.8.1 Genotype–Phenotype Correlations

Both of the original papers reporting *RDH12* mutations described a severe phenotype with onset of symptoms in early childhood with nystagmus, attenuation of the arterioles, bone spicule intraretinal pigmentation, mild to moderate hypermetropia and macular atrophy with severe visual loss before the end of the second decade [58, 101]. Early visual assessments during childhood differ between individuals mapping to the LCA3 locus [126] and those with *RDH12* mutations, with acuities ranging from 5/200-LP in LCA 3 but the clinical course in RDH12 being similar to that of RPE65 with initial slight improvement in vision (1/10–2/10) followed by later progressive deterioration [101].

10.2.9 Other Loci

There are several other loci reported for LCA. These include LCA3 on 14q24 [126], LCA5 on 6q11–16 [93]; and LCA9 on 1p36 [62]. In addition, early onset retinal dystrophies have been reported with mutations in LRAT located on 4q31 [131] and MERTK on 2q14.1 [87].

Linkage to the LCA5 locus at 6q11–16 was confirmed from 13 members of a large consanguineous family from Pakistan [93]. Best corrected visual acuities were PL and nystagmus was present in all affected members. A unilateral vitreous opacity was found in the three eldest members. Macular atrophy appearing more severe with age was noted, and progressive changes in the retinal periphery were observed with white dots at the level of the RPE in the youngest member, which changed to a grey-green pigmentary disturbance in the older members.

The LCA9 (1p36) locus was identified through homozygosity mapping in a large consanguineous family of Pakistani origin. The phenotype is one of severe visual impairment (PL) from birth, photophobia, nystagmus and posterior subcapsular lens opacities. Fundus examination showed optic disc pallor, retinal vascular attenuation, macular staphyloma and pigmentary disturbance, with white dots at the level of the RPE [62].

Lecithin retinol acyl transferase (LRAT-4q31.2) mutations have been associated with EOSRD [131]. LRAT is an enzyme present mainly in the RPE and the liver; it converts all-*trans*-retinol into all-*trans*-retinyl esters, and therefore plays a key role in the retinoid cycle, replenishing the 11-*cis*-retinal chromophore of rhodopsin and cone pigments. LRAT knockout mice revealed rod segments that are approximately 35% shorter than wild type and have severely attenuated ERGs [10]. The phenotype identified so far in humans is similar to that of RPE65, with night blindness and poor vision from early childhood. There is severe early loss of peripheral visual field, and fundus examination shows peripheral RPE atrophy with little pigment migration into the retina.

MERTK was identified as a rare cause of EOSRD [85] mutations in three patients with an early onset form of autosomal recessive RP [39]. It encodes a receptor tyrosine kinase found in RPE cells that is required for phagocytosis of shed photoreceptor outer segments. The absence of MERTK results in accumulation of outer segment debris, which subsequently leads to progressive loss of photoreceptor cells [19]. A naturally occurring animal model with a *MERTK* mutation, the RCS rat, has been extensively investigated [19].

The patients described with MERTK mutations are reported to have childhood onset nyctalopia, preserved visual fields, relatively mild RPE changes with a bull's eye lesion at the macular, absence of pigment migration to the RPE, and recordable autofluorescence [87, 133].

10.3 Heterozygous Carriers

Several groups have looked at the phenotypic characteristics of the heterozygous carriers in families with LCA [25, 38]. In one cohort, 22 of the 30 LCA carriers (73.3%) had a phenotype determined from detailed ERG measurements and/or retinal examination. None experienced significant subjective visual difficulty. Visual acuities were normal and there was no refractive error trend associated with a genotype. Fundus findings most commonly seen were white drusen-like deposits, present in RPE65 carriers (88%), a finding previously noted [77], CRB1 carriers (75%) and RPGRIP1 carriers (57%).

10.4 Future Therapeutic Avenues

There are three promising potential treatment strategies for LCA: (a) gene therapy, (b) retinal/RPE transplantation, and (c) pharmacological therapy. None have yet been the subject of a clinical trial in humans.

10.4.1 Gene Therapy

Gene therapy is by its very nature gene-specific and requires that the patient's individual mutations are known. For any gene therapy, trial patients will be selected on the basis of their genotype and this requires that patients with LCA/EOSRD are accurately genotyped, which, given the heterogeneity of the disorder, is a significant undertaking. Gene therapy appears to be a very promising approach and has been shown to be effective in some animal models. Both the Briard dog, a large animal model of EORD, which has a naturally occurring homozygous 4-bp deletion in the *RPE65* gene and the *RPE65*$^{-/-}$ mouse have been treated with gene therapy techniques using viral vectors. In utero gene therapy in the *RPE65*$^{-/-}$ mouse resulted in restoration of visual function and measurable rhodopsin in the outer retina [20]. Treatment also results in a decrease in retinyl ester droplets and an increase in shortwave cone opsin cells [67]. In the LCA dog model, animals treated with subretinal injections of adenoassociated virus (AAV) containing cDNA of canine *RPE65*, all electrophysiological parameters, pupillometry, and behavioural testing showed significant signs of improvement [1]. An unexpected finding was that on long-term follow-up, significant improvement in photopic ERG responses were found in the contralateral untreated eye [97]. This surprising finding is unexplained.

The main concern with this mode of treatment relates to the potential for a sight-threatening uveitic response to the novel protein. Lewis rats immunized with RPE65 developed acute and severe inflammatory eye disease that affected most ocular tissues [47]. Uveitis developed in 75% of transgene-treated eyes in the null mutation dogs but only one eye (8%) was refractory to treatment [96]. Human gene therapy trials are planned for LCA patients with *RPE65* mutations in the near future [4].

10.4.2 Retinal Transplantation and Stem Cell Therapy

Several experimental surgical approaches to retinal cell rescue, including cell transplantation and stem cell therapy have been pursued in the last few years. The advantages of these approaches are that they are not mutation-specific and in theory they could be performed late in the disease process. However, preventing tissue rejection and in the case of photoreceptor transplantation ensuring that the transplant integrates with host retinal tissue remain formidable challenges.

RPE transplantation holds out a greater prospect of success than photoreceptor transplantation, as functioning synapses do not need to be established. It has been investigated in a number of animal models. Transplantation of normal RPE into the subretinal space of *RPE65*$^{-/-}$ mice increases ERG amplitude and reduces anatomic deterioration without signs of inflammation [42]. These effects, however, do not seem to be maintained, suggesting that transplanted RPE cells have a limited life span.

Transplantation of either embryonic dissociated cells or retinal sheets in to the subretinal space of rodent models of retinal degeneration demonstrate that transplants survive and differentiate and that neuronal fibres originating from the transplant develop synapses with the host retina which are at least sufficient to mediate a simple light-dark preference [8, 67]. It is unclear whether the effects of the transplant are mediated via these putative synapses or by the production by the graft of trophic growth factors which preserve some host retinal function.

Another generic approach to the treatment of retinal dystrophies has been to provide an alternative RPE cell type to replace the physiological function of defective cells [82]. ARPE19 cells, when transplanted into the retina of young RCS rats, slows the progress of photoreceptor loss [17]. Similarly, the transplantation of Schwann cells rescues photoreceptors in both RCS rats and rho$^{-/-}$ mice [61, 69, 70, 86]; this is thought to be mediated though release of neuroprotective paracrine factors. It has also been demonstrated that normal rod photoreceptors release a cone survival factor (rod-derived cone viability factor –rdCVF [71]). Transplanting small amounts of rods can rescue cones in a murine model [72, 94].

Stem cell therapy holds out the prospect of retinal tissue replacement and repair, but research in this area is still in its infancy. Experimental transplantation of brain-derived stem cells [81, 146], bone marrow derived neural stem cells [98], and retinal progenitor cells [15] have had mixed results. Retinal progenitor cells have been isolated, expanded and grafted into the degenerating retina of mature rho$^{-/-}$ mice. A subset of the grafted cells developed into mature neurons and photoreceptors, with rescue of the outer nuclear layer and integration of donor cells into the inner retina. Engrafted mice showed improved light-mediated behaviour [64].

10.4.3 Pharmacological Therapies

In retinal dystrophies due to *RPE65* mutations, there is an inability to form 11-cis retinal and this has led to vitamin A supplements being given to *RPE65*$^{-/-}$ mice in the form of oral 9-cis retinal. Within 48 h, there was a significant improvement in rod function with formation of rod photopigment [140]. Whether these results can be translated in humans, once safety and efficacy issues are resolved, remains to be seen.

Other neuroprotective factors are being assessed in mice models of RP. Basic fibroblast growth factor increases the life of photoreceptors in the RCS rat [29], and recently systemic erythropoietin has been shown to have neuroprotective and neurotrophic actions in the central and peripheral nervous systems including the retina in rds/peripherin models of retinal degeneration [110].

Summary for the Clinician

- **LCA/EOSRD is a recessive condition leading to severely impaired vision from birth or infancy**
- **It is distinguished from other diagnoses on the basis of a nonrecordable ERG**

- **There are several known syndromic causes that must be excluded**
- **Genotype-phenotype correlations are being established though are still in an early stage of refinement and include:**
  - ***GUCY2D*: severe pigmentary dystrophy, high hyperopia, and photophobia**
  - ***RPE65*: better vision until late school years, extreme light dependence of visual performance in infancy and childhood, nyctalopia, absence of retinal autofluorescence even though the fundal appearance is still almost normal**
  - ***AIPL1*: pigmentary retinopathy, maculopathy and optic nerve pallor with keratoconus and cataract in up to one-third of cases**
  - ***CRB1*: early appearance of white spots and pigment clumping at the level of the RPE, and thickened retinal appearance as seen on OCT**
- **Several different therapeutic avenues are now being explored: Gene therapy appears to be the most promising approach and the first gene therapy trials for *RPE65* mutations are likely to start in the next 2–3 years**

References

1. Acland GM, Aguirre GD, Ray J et al (2001) Gene therapy restores vision in a canine model of childhood blindness. Nat Genet 28:92–95
2. Akey DT, Zhu X, Dyer M et al (2002) The inherited blindness associated protein AIPL1 interacts with the cell cycle regulator protein NUB1. Hum Mol Genet 11:2723–2733
3. Al-Khayer K, Hagstrom S, Pauer G et al (2004) Thirty-year follow-up of a patient with Leber congenital amaurosis and novel RPE65 mutations. Am J Ophthalmol 137:375–377
4. Ali R (2004) Prospects for gene therapy. Novartis Found Symp 255:165–172
5. Allen LE, Zito I, Bradshaw K et al (2003) Genotype-phenotype correlation in British families with X linked congenital stationary night blindness. Br J Ophthalmol 87:1413–1420
6. Allikmets R (2004) Leber congenital amaurosis: a genetic paradigm. Ophthalmic Genet 25:67–79
7. Alsing A, Christensen C (1988) Atypical macular coloboma (dysplasia) associated with familial juvenile nephronophthisis and skeletal abnormality. Ophthalmic Paediatr Genet 9:149–155
8. Aramant RB, Seiler MJ (1995) Fiber and synaptic connections between embryonic retinal transplants and host retina. Exp Neurol 133:244–255
9. Banerjee P, Kleyn PW, Knowles JA et al (1998) TULP1 mutation in two extended Dominican kindreds with autosomal recessive retinitis pigmentosa. Nat Genet 18:177–179
10. Batten ML, Imanishi Y, Maeda T et al (2004) Lecithin-retinol acyltransferase is essential for accumulation of all-trans-retinyl esters in the eye and in the liver. J Biol Chem 279:10422–10432
11. Boggon TJ, Shan WS, Santagata S et al (1999) Implication of tubby proteins as transcription factors by structure-based functional analysis. Science 286:2119–2125
12. Carroll K, Gomez C, Shapiro L (2004) Tubby proteins: the plot thickens. Nat Rev Mol Cell Biol 5:55–63
13. Castagnet P, Mavlyutov T, Cai Y et al (2003) RPGRIP1s with distinct neuronal localization and biochemical properties associate selectively with RanBP2 in amacrine neurons. Hum Mol Genet 12:1847–1863
14. Casteels I, Harris CM, Shawkat F et al (1992) Nystagmus in infancy. Br J Ophthalmol 76:434–437
15. Chacko DM, Das AV, Zhao X et al (2003) Transplantation of ocular stem cells: the role of injury in incorporation and differentiation of grafted cells in the retina. Vision Res 43:937–946
16. Chen S, Wang QL, Nie Z et al (1997) Crx, a novel Otx-like paired-homeodomain protein, binds to and transactivates photoreceptor cell-specific genes. Neuron 19:1017–1030
17. Coffey PJ, Girman S, Wang SM et al (2002) Long-term preservation of cortically dependent visual function in RCS rats by transplantation. Nat Neurosci 5:53–56
18. Cremers FP, van den Hurk JA, den Hollander AI (2002) Molecular genetics of Leber congenital amaurosis. Hum Mol Genet 11:1169–1176
19. D'Cruz PM, Yasumura D, Weir J et al (2000) Mutation of the receptor tyrosine kinase gene Mertk in the retinal dystrophic RCS rat. Hum Mol Genet 9:645–651
20. Dejneka NS, Surace EM, Aleman TS et al (2004) In utero gene therapy rescues vision in a murine model of congenital blindness. Mol Ther 9:182–188
21. Den Hollander AI, Davis J, van der Velde-Visser SD et al (2004) CRB1 mutation spectrum in inherited retinal dystrophies. Hum Mutat 24:355–369
22. Den Hollander AI, Ghiani M, de Kok YJ et al (2002) Isolation of Crb1, a mouse homologue of Drosophila crumbs, and analysis of its expression pattern in eye and brain. Mech Dev 110:203–207

23. Den Hollander AI, Heckenlively JR, van den Born LI et al (2001) Leber congenital amaurosis and retinitis pigmentosa with Coats-like exudative vasculopathy are associated with mutations in the crumbs homologue 1 (CRB1) gene. Am J Hum Genet 69:198–203
24. Dharmaraj S, Leroy BP, Sohocki MM et al (2004) The phenotype of Leber Congenital amaurosis in patients with AIPL1 mutations. Arch Ophthalmol 122:1029–1037
25. Dharmaraj SR, SilvaER, Pina AL et al (2000) Mutational analysis and clinical correlation in Leber congenital amaurosis. Ophthalmic Genet 21:135–150
26. Downes SM, Payne AM, Kelsell RE et al (2001) Autosomal dominant cone-rod dystrophy with mutations in the guanylate cyclase 2D gene encoding retinal guanylate cyclase-1. Arch Ophthalmol 119:1667–1673
27. Dryja TP, Adams SM, Grimsby JL et al (2001) Null RPGRIP1 alleles in patients with Leber congenital amaurosis. Am J Hum Genet 68:1295–1298
28. Elder MJ (1994) Leber congenital amaurosis and its association with keratoconus and keratoglobus. J Pediatr Ophthalmol Strabismus 31:38–40
29. Faktorovich EG, Steinberg RH, Yasumura D et al (1990) Photoreceptor degeneration in inherited retinal dystrophy delayed by basic fibroblast growth factor. Nature 347:83–86
30. Fillastre JP, Guenel J, Riberi P et al (1976) Senior-Loken syndrome (nephronophthisis and tapeto-retinal degeneration): a study of 8 cases from 5 families. Clin Nephrol 5:14–19
31. Foxman SG, Heckenlively JR, Bateman JB et al (1985) Classification of congenital and early onset retinitis pigmentosa. Arch Ophthalmol 103: 1502–1506
32. Franceschetti A, Dieterle P (1954) Diagnostic and prognostic importance of the electroretinogram in tapetoretinal degeneration with reduction of the visual field and hemeralopia. Confin Neurol 14:184–186
33. Francois J (1968) Leber's congenital tapetoretinal degeneration. Int Ophthalmol Clin 8:929–947
34. Freund CL, Gregory-Evans CY, Furukawa T et al (1997) Cone-rod dystrophy due to mutations in a novel photoreceptor-specific homeobox gene (CRX) essential for maintenance of the photoreceptor. Cell 91:543–553
35. Freund CL, Wang QL, Chen S et al (1998) De novo mutations in the CRX homeobox gene associated with Leber congenital amaurosis. Nat Genet 18: 311–312
36. Furukawa T, Morrow EM, Cepko CL (1997) Crx, a novel otx-like homeobox gene, shows photoreceptor-specific expression and regulates photoreceptor differentiation Cell 91:531–541
37. Furukawa T, Morrow EM, Li T et al (1999) Retinopathy and attenuated circadian entrainment in Crx-deficient mice. Nat Genet 23:466–470
38. Galvin JA, Fishman GA, Stone EM, Koenekoop RK (2005) Clinical phenotypes in carriers of Leber congenital amaurosis mutations. Ophthalmology 112:349–356
39. Gal A, Li Y, Thompson DA et al (2000) Mutations in MERTK, the human orthologue of the RCS rat retinal dystrophy gene, cause retinitis pigmentosa. Nat Genet 26:270–271
40. Gerber S, Perrault I, Hanein S et al (2001) Complete exon-intron structure of the RPGR-interacting protein (RPGRIP1) gene allows the identification of mutations underlying Leber congenital amaurosis. Eur J Hum Genet 9:561–571
41. Gollapalli DR, Maiti P, Rando RR (2003) RPE65 operates in the vertebrate visual cycle by stereospecifically binding all-trans-retinyl esters. Biochemistry (Mosc) 42:11824–11830
42. Gouras P, Kong J, Tsang SH (2002) Retinal degeneration and RPE transplantation in Rpe65(–/–) mice. Invest Ophthalmol Vis Sci 43:3307–3311
43. Gu S, Lennon A, Li Y et al (1998) Tubby-like protein-1 mutations in autosomal recessive retinitis pigmentosa. Lancet 351:1103–1104
44. Gu SM, Thompson DA, Srikumari CR et al (1997) Mutations in RPE65 cause autosomal recessive childhood-onset severe retinal dystrophy. Nat Genet 17:194–197
45. Haeseleer F, Jang GF, Imanishi Y et al (2002) Dual-substrate specificity short chain retinol dehydrogenases from the vertebrate retina. J Biol Chem 277:45537–45546
46. Hagstrom SA, Adamian M, Scimeca M et al (2001) A role for the Tubby-like protein 1 in rhodopsin transport. Invest Ophthalmol Vis Sci 42:1955–1962
47. Ham DI, Gentleman S, Chan CC et al (2002) RPE65 is highly uveitogenic in rats Invest Ophthalmol Vis Sci 43:2258–2263
48. Hanein S, Perrault I, Gerber S et al (2004) Leber congenital amaurosis: comprehensive survey of the genetic heterogeneity, refinement of the clinical definition, and genotype-phenotype correlations as a strategy for molecular diagnosis. Hum Mutat 23:306–317
49. Hanein S, Perrault I, Olsen P et al (2002) Evidence of a founder effect for the RETGC1 (GUCY2D) 2943DelG mutation in Leber congenital amaurosis pedigrees of Finnish origin. Hum Mutat 20: 322–323
50. Heckenlively JR, Foxman SG, Parelhoff ES (1988) Retinal dystrophy and macular coloboma. Doc Ophthalmol 68:257–271

51. Hong DH, Yue G, Adamian M et al (2001) Retinitis pigmentosa GTPase regulator (RPGRr)-interacting protein is stably associated with the photoreceptor ciliary axoneme and anchors RPGR to the connecting cilium. J Biol Chem 276:12091–12099
52. Ikeda S, He W, Ikeda A et al (1999) Cell-specific expression of tubby gene family members (tub, Tulp1, 2, and 3) in the retina. Invest Ophthalmol Vis Sci 40:2706–2712
53. Ikeda S, Shiva N, Ikeda A et al (2000) Retinal degeneration but not obesity is observed in null mutants of the tubby-like protein 1 gene. Hum Mol Genet 9:155–163
54. Jacobson SG, Cideciyan AV, Aleman TS et al (2003) Crumbs homolog 1 (CRB1) mutations result in a thick human retina with abnormal lamination. Hum Mol Genet 12:1073–1078
55. Jacobson SG, Cideciyan AV, Huang Y et al (1998) Retinal degenerations with truncation mutations in the cone-rod homeobox (CRX) gene. Invest Ophthalmol Vis Sci 39:2417–2426
56. Jacobson SG, Cideciyan AV, Huang Y et al (1998) Retinal degenerations with truncation mutations in the cone-rod homeobox (CRX) gene. Invest Ophthalmol Vis Sci 39:2417–2426
57. Jahng WJ, David C, Nesnas N et al (2003) A cleavable affinity biotinylating agent reveals a retinoid binding role for RPE65. Biochemistry (Mosc) 42:6159–6168
58. Janecke AR, Thompson DA, Utermann G et al (2004) Mutations in RDH12 encoding a photoreceptor cell retinol dehydrogenase cause childhood-onset severe retinal dystrophy. Nat Genet 36:850–854
59. Kanaya K, Sohocki MM, and Kamitani T (2004) Abolished interaction of NUB1 with mutant AIPL1 involved in Leber congenital amaurosis. Biochem Biophys Res Commun 317:768–773
60. Katz ML, Redmond TM (2001) Effect of Rpe65 knockout on accumulation of lipofuscin fluorophores in the retinal pigment epithelium. Invest Ophthalmol Vis Sci 42:3023–3030
61. Keegan DJ, Kenna P, Humphries MM et al (2003) Transplantation of syngeneic Schwann cells to the retina of the rhodopsin knockout (rho(−/−)) mouse. Invest Ophthalmol Vis Sci 44:3526–3532
62. Keen TJ, Mohamed MD, McKibbin M et al (2003) Identification of a locus (LCA9) for Leber's congenital amaurosis on chromosome 1p36. Eur J Hum Genet 11:420–423
63. Kirschner R, Rosenberg T, Schultz-Heienbrok R et al (1999) RPGR transcription studies in mouse and human tissues reveal a retina-specific isoform that is disrupted in a patient with X-linked retinitis pigmentosa. Hum Mol Genet 8:1571–1578
64. Klassen HJ, Ng TF, Kurimoto Y et al (2004) Multipotent retinal progenitors express developmental markers, differentiate into retinal neurons, and preserve light-mediated behavior. Invest Ophthalmol Vis Sci 45:4167–4173
65. Koenekoop RK (2004) An overview of Leber congenital amaurosis: a model to understand human retinal development. Surv Ophthalmol 49:379–398
66. Koenekoop RK, Loyer M, Dembinska O et al (2002) Visual improvement in Leber congenital amaurosis and the CRX genotype. Ophthalmic Genet 23:49–59
67. Kwan AS, Wang S, Lund RD (1999) Photoreceptor layer reconstruction in a rodent model of retinal degeneration. Exp Neurol 159:21–33
68. Lai CM., Yu MJ, Brankov M et al (2004) Recombinant adeno-associated virus type 2-mediated gene delivery into the Rpe65−/− knockout mouse eye results in limited rescue. Genet Vaccines Ther 2:3
69. Lawrence JM, Keegan DJ, Muir EM et al (2004) Transplantation of Schwann cell line clones secreting GDNF or BDNF into the retinas of dystrophic Royal College of Surgeons rats. Invest Ophthalmol Vis Sci 45:267–274
70. Lawrence JM, Sauve Y, Keegan DJ et al (2000) Schwann cell grafting into the retina of the dystrophic RCS rat limits functional deterioration. Royal College of Surgeons. Invest Ophthalmol Vis Sci 41:518–528
71. Leber T (1869) Ueber Retinitis Pigmentosa und angeborene Amaurose Graefes Arch Clin Exp Ophthalmol 15:1–25
72. Leveillard T, Mohand-Said S, Fintz AC et al (2004) The search for rod-dependent cone viability factors, secreted factors promoting cone viability. Novartis Found Symp 255:117–127
73. Leveillard T, Mohand-Said S, Lorentz O et al (2004) Identification and characterization of rod-derived cone viability factor. Nat Genet 36:755–759
74. Lewis CA, Batlle IR, Batlle KG et al (1999) Tubby-like protein 1 homozygous splice-site mutation causes early-onset severe retinal degeneration. Invest Ophthalmol Vis Sci 40:2106–2114
75. Livesey FJ, Furukawa T, Steffen MA et al (2000) Microarray analysis of the transcriptional network controlled by the photoreceptor homeobox gene Crx. Curr Biol 10:301–310
76. Lorenz B, Gampe E (2001) Analysis of 180 patients with sensory defect nystagmus (SDN) and congenital idiopathic nystagmus (CIN). Klin Monatsbl Augenheilkd 218:3–12
77. Lorenz B, Gyurus P, Preising M et al (2000) Early-onset severe rod-cone dystrophy in young children with RPE65 mutations. Invest Ophthalmol Vis Sci 41:2735–2742

78. Lorenz B, Wabbels B, Wegscheider E et al (2004) Lack of fundus autofluorescence to 488 nanometers from childhood on in patients with early-onset severe retinal dystrophy associated with mutations in RPE65. Ophthalmology 111:1585–1594
79. Lotery AJ, Jacobson SG, Fishman GA et al (2001) Mutations in the CRB1 gene cause Leber congenital amaurosis. Arch Ophthalmol 119:415–420
80. Lotery AJ, Namperumalsamy P, Jacobson SG et al (2000) Mutation analysis of 3 genes in patients with Leber congenital amaurosis. Arch Ophthalmol 118:538–543
81. Lu B, Kwan T, Kurimoto Y et al (2002) Transplantation of EGF-responsive neurospheres from GFP transgenic mice into the eyes of rd mice. Brain Res 943:292–300
82. Lund RD, Adamson P, Sauve Y et al (2001) Subretinal transplantation of genetically modified human cell lines attenuates loss of visual function in dystrophic rats. Proc Natl Acad Sci U S A 98: 9942–9947
83. Ma J, Zhang J, Othersen KL et al (2001) Expression, purification, and MALDI analysis of RPE65. Invest Ophthalmol Vis Sci 42:1429–1435
84. Marlhens F, Bareil C, Griffoin JM et al (1997) Mutations in RPE65 cause Leber's congenital amaurosis. Nat Genet 17:139–141
85. Mavlyutov TA, Zhao H, Ferreira PA (2002) Species-specific subcellular localization of RPGR and RPGRIP isoforms: implications for the phenotypic variability of congenital retinopathies among species. Hum Mol Genet 11:1899–1907
86. McGill TJ, Lund RD, Douglas RM et al (2004) Preservation of vision following cell-based therapies in a model of retinal degenerative disease. Vision Res 44:2559–2566
87. McHenry CL, Liu Y, Feng W et al (2004) MERTK arginine-844-cysteine in a patient with severe rod-cone dystrophy: loss of mutant protein function in transfected cells. Invest Ophthalmol Vis Sci 45:1456–1463
88. Mehalow AK, Kameya S, Smith RS et al (2003) CRB1 is essential for external limiting membrane integrity and photoreceptor morphogenesis in the mammalian retina. Hum Mol Genet 12:2179–2189
89. Meindl A, Dry K, Herrmann K et al (1996) A gene (RPGR) with homology to the RCC1 guanine nucleotide exchange factor is mutated in X-linked retinitis pigmentosa (RP3). Nat Genet 13:35–42
90. Michaelides M, Hunt DM, Moore AT (2004) The cone dysfunction syndromes. Br J Ophthalmol 88:291–297
91. Milam AH, Barakat MR, Gupta N et al (2003) Clinicopathologic effects of mutant GUCY2D in Leber congenital amaurosis. Ophthalmology 110: 549–558
92. Milam AH, Hendrickson AE, Xiao M et al (2000) Localization of tubby-like protein 1 in developing and adult human retinas. Invest Ophthalmol Vis Sci 41:2352–2356
93. Mohamed MD, Topping NC, Jafri H et al (2003) Progression of phenotype in Leber's congenital amaurosis with a mutation at the LCA5 locus. Br J Ophthalmol 87:473–475
94. Mohand-Said S, Hicks D, Dreyfus H et al (2000) Selective transplantation of rods delays cone loss in a retinitis pigmentosa model. Arch Ophthalmol 118:807–811
95. Morimura H, Fishman GA, Grover SA et al (1998) Mutations in the RPE65 gene in patients with autosomal recessive retinitis pigmentosa or Leber congenital amaurosis. Proc Natl Acad Sci U S A 95:3088–3093
96. Narfstrom K, Katz ML, Bragadottir R et al (2003) Functional and structural recovery of the retina after gene therapy in the RPE65 null mutation dog. Invest Ophthalmol Vis Sci 44:1663–1672
97. Narfstrom K, Katz ML, Ford M et al (2003) In vivo gene therapy in young and adult RPE65–/– dogs produces long-term visual improvement. J Hered 94:31–37
98. Otani A, Dorrell MI, Kinder K et al (2004) Rescue of retinal degeneration by intravitreally injected adult bone marrow-derived lineage-negative hematopoietic stem cells. J Clin Invest 114:765–774
99. Paunescu K, Wabbels B, Preising MN et al (2004) Longitudinal and cross-sectional study of patients with early-onset severe retinal dystrophy associated with RPE65 mutations. Graefes Arch Clin Exp Ophthalmol 243:417–426
100. Pellikka M, Tanentzapf G, Pinto M et al (2002) Crumbs, the Drosophila homologue of human CRB1/RP12, is essential for photoreceptor morphogenesis. Nature 416:143–149
101. Perrault I, Hanein S, Gerber S et al (2004) Retinal dehydrogenase 12 (RDH12) mutations in Leber congenital amaurosis. Am J Hum Genet 75:639–646
102. Perrault I, Hanein S, Gerber S et al (2003) Evidence of autosomal dominant Leber congenital amaurosis (LCA) underlain by a CRX heterozygous null allele. J Med Genet 40:e90
103. Perrault I, Rozet JM, Calvas P et al (1996) Retinal-specific guanylate cyclase gene mutations in Leber's congenital amaurosis. Nat Genet 14:461–464
104. Perrault I, Rozet JM, Gerber S et al (2000) Spectrum of retGC1 mutations in Leber's congenital amaurosis. Eur J Hum Genet 8:578–582

105. Perrault I, Rozet JM, Gerber S et al (1998) A retGC-1 mutation in autosomal dominant cone-rod dystrophy. Am J Hum Genet 63:651–654
106. Perrault I, Rozet JM, Ghazi I et al (1999) Different functional outcome of RetGC1 and RPE65 gene mutations in Leber congenital amaurosis. Am J Hum Genet 64:1225–1228
107. Porto FB, Perrault I., Hicks D et al (2002) Prenatal human ocular degeneration occurs in Leber's congenital amaurosis (LCA2). J Gene Med 4:390–396
108. Rahi JS, CableN (2003) Severe visual impairment and blindness in children in the UK. Lancet 362:1359–1365
109. Redmond TM, Yu S, Lee E et al (1998) Rpe65 is necessary for production of 11-cis-vitamin A in the retinal visual cycle. Nat Genet 20:344–351
110. Rex TS, Allocca M, Domenici L et al (2004) Systemic but not intraocular Epo gene transfer protects the retina from light-and genetic-induced Degeneration. Mol Ther 10:855–861
111. Rivolta C, Berson EL, Dryja TP (2001) Dominant Leber congenital amaurosis, cone-rod degeneration, and retinitis pigmentosa caused by mutant versions of the transcription factor CRX. Hum Mutat 18:488–498
112. Rivolta C, Peck NE, Fulton AB et al (2001) Novel frameshift mutations in CRX associated with Leber congenital amaurosis Hum Mutat 18:550–551
113. Roepman R, Bauer D, Rosenberg T et al (1996) Identification of a gene disrupted by a microdeletion in a patient with X-linked retinitis pigmentosa (XLRP). Hum Mol Genet 5:827–833
114. Roepman R, Bernoud-Hubac N, Schick DE et al (2000) The retinitis pigmentosa GTPase regulator (RPGR) interacts with novel transport-like proteins in the outer segments of rod photoreceptors. Hum Mol Genet 9:2095–2105
115. Rohrer B, Goletz P, Znoiko S et al (2003) Correlation of regenerable opsin with rod ERG signal in Rpe65-/- mice during development and aging. Invest Ophthalmol Vis Sci 44:310–315
116. Rozet JM, Perrault I, Gerber S et al (2001) Complete abolition of the retinal-specific guanylyl cyclase (retGC-1) catalytic ability consistently leads to Leber congenital amaurosis (LCA). Invest Ophthalmol Vis Sci 42:1190–1192
117. Russell-Eggitt, IM, Clayton PT, Coffey R et al (1998) Alstrom syndrome. Report of 22 cases and literature review. Ophthalmology 105:1274–1280
118. Schappert-Kimmijser J, Henkes HE, Van Den Bosch J (1959) Amaurosis congenita (Leber). AA Arch Opthalmol 61:211–218
119. Schuil J, Meire FM, Delleman JW (1998) Mental retardation in amaurosis congenita of Leber. Neuropediatrics 29:294–297
120. Silva E, Yang JM, Li Y et al (2000) A CRX null mutation is associated with both Leber congenital amaurosis and a normal ocular phenotype. Invest Ophthalmol Vis Sci 41:2076–2079
121. Simovich MJ, Miller B, Ezzeldin H et al (2001) Four novel mutations in the RPE65 gene in patients with Leber congenital amaurosis. Hum Mutat 18:164
122. Sitorus RS, Lorenz B, Preising MN (2003) Analysis of three genes in Leber congenital amaurosis in Indonesian patients. Vision Res 43:3087–3093
123. Sohocki MM, Bowne SJ, Sullivan LS et al (2000) Mutations in a new photoreceptor-pineal gene on 17p cause Leber congenital amaurosis. Nat Genet 24:79–83
124. Sohocki MM, Perrault I, Leroy BP et al (2000) Prevalence of AIPL1 mutations in inherited retinal degenerative disease. Mol Genet Metab 70:142–150
125. Sohocki MM, Sullivan LS, Mintz-Hittner HA et al (1998) A range of clinical phenotypes associated with mutations in CRX, a photoreceptor transcription-factor gene. Am J Hum Genet 63:1307–1315
126. Stockton DW, Lewis RA, Abboud EB et al (1998) A novel locus for Leber congenital amaurosis on chromosome 14q24. Hum Genet 103:328–333
1278.Swaroop A, Wang QL, Wu W et al (1999) Leber congenital amaurosis caused by a homozygous mutation (R90W) in the homeodomain of the retinal transcription factor CRX: direct evidence for the involvement of CRX in the development of photoreceptor function. Hum Mol Genet 8:299–305
128. Tabbara KF, Badr IA (1985) Changing pattern of childhood blindness in Saudi Arabia. Br J Ophthalmol 69:312–315
129. Tepass U, Theres C, Knust E (1990) Crumbs encodes an EGF-like protein expressed on apical membranes of Drosophila epithelial cells and required for organization of epithelia. Cell 61: 787–799
130. Thompson DA, Gyurus P, Fleischer LL et al (2000) Genetics and phenotypes of RPE65 mutations in inherited retinal degeneration. Invest Ophthalmol Vis Sci 41:4293–4299
131. Thompson DA, Li Y, McHenry CL et al (2001) Mutations in the gene encoding lecithin retinol acyltransferase are associated with early-onset severe retinal dystrophy. Nat Genet 28:123–124
133. Ticho B, Sieving PA (1989) Leber's congenital amaurosis with marbelized fundus and juvenile nephronophthisis. Am J Ophthalmol 107:426–428

133. Tschernutter M, Waseem NH, Perkins A, Bhattacharya SS, Holder GE, Jenkins SA, Bird AC, Ali, aRR Webster AR (2005) Detailed clinical characteristics of a family segregating a novel mutation in the MERTK gene. Invest Ophthalmol Vis Sci 46:537
134. Tucker CL, Woodcock SC, Kelsell RE et al (1999) Biochemical analysis of a dimerization domain mutation in RetGC-1 associated with dominant cone-rod dystrophy. Proc Natl Acad Sci U S A 96:9039–9044
135. Tzekov RT, Liu Y, Sohocki MM et al (2001) Autosomal dominant retinal degeneration and bone loss in patients with a 12-bp deletion in the CRX gene. Invest Ophthalmol Vis Sci 42:1319–1327
136. Van de Pavert SA, Kantardzhieva A, Malysheva A et al (2004) Crumbs homologue 1 is required for maintenance of photoreceptor cell polarization and adhesion during light exposure. J Cell Sci 117:4169–4177
137. Van der Spuy J, Chapple JP, Clark BJ et al (2002) The Leber congenital amaurosis gene product AIPL1 is localized exclusively in rod photoreceptors of the adult human retina. Hum Mol Genet 11:823–831
138. Van der Spuy J, Cheetham ME (2004) The Leber congenital amaurosis protein AIPL1 modulates the nuclear translocation of NUB1 and suppresses inclusion formation by NUB1 fragments. J Biol Chem 279:48038–48047
139. Van der Spuy J, Kim JH, Yu YS et al (2003) The expression of the Leber congenital amaurosis protein AIPL1 coincides with rod and cone photoreceptor development. Invest Ophthalmol Vis Sci 44:5396–5403
140. Van Hooser JP, Aleman TS, He YG et al (2000) Rapid restoration of visual pigment and function with oral retinoid in a mouse model of childhood blindness. Proc Natl Acad Sci U S A 97:8623–8628
141. Vervoort R, Lennon A, Bird AC et al (2000) Mutational hot spot within a new RPGR exon in X-linked retinitis pigmentosa Nat Genet 25: 462–466
142. Waardenburg PJ, Schappert-Kimmijser J (1963) On various recessive biotypes of Leber's congenital amaurosis. Acta Ophthalmol (Copenh) 41: 317–320
143. Wagner RS, Caputo AR, Nelson LB et al (1985) High hyperopia in Leber's congenital amaurosis. Arch Ophthalmol 103:1507–1509
144. Watanabe T, Miyatani S, Katoh I et al (2004) Expression of a novel secretory form (Crb1s) of mouse Crumbs homologue Crb1 in skin development. Biochem Biophys Res Commun 313:263–270
145. Wodarz A, Hinz U, Engelbert M et al (1995) Expression of crumbs confers apical character on plasma membrane domains of ectodermal epithelia of Drosophila. Cell 82:67–76
146. Wojciechowski AB, Englund U, Lundberg C et al (2002) Subretinal transplantation of brain-derived precursor cells to young RCS rats promotes photoreceptor cell survival. Exp Eye Res 75:23–37
147. Woodruff ML, Wang Z, Chung HY et al (2003) Spontaneous activity of opsin apoprotein is a cause of Leber congenital amaurosis. Nat Genet 35:158–164
148. Xue L, Gollapalli DR, Maiti P et al (2004) A palmitoylation switch mechanism in the regulation of the visual cycle. Cell 117:761–771
149. Zhao Y, Hong DH, Pawlyk B et al (2003) The retinitis pigmentosa GTPase regulator (RPGR)-interacting protein: subserving RPGR function and participating in disk morphogenesis. Proc Natl Acad Sci U S A 100:3965–3970
150. Moiseyev G, Chen Y, Takahashi Y, Wu BX, Ma JX (2005) RPE65 is the isomerohydrolase in the retinoid visual cycle. Proc Natl Acad Sci U S A 102:12413–12418
151. Ramamurthy V, Roberts M, van den AF, Niemi G, Reh TA, Hurley JB (2003) AIPL1, a protein implicated in Leber's congenital amaurosis, interacts with and aids in processing of farnesylated proteins. Proc Natl Acad Sci U S A 100:12630–12635

Childhood Stationary Retinal Dysfunction Syndromes

11

Michel Michaelides, Anthony T. Moore

Core Messages

- The stationary retinal dysfunction syndromes represent an important cause of childhood visual impairment
- This heterogeneous group of disorders are inherited as autosomal recessive, autosomal dominant or X-linked (XL) recessive traits
- They can be usefully divided into rod dysfunction syndromes (congenital stationary night blindness, Oguchi disease, fundus albipunctatus) and cone dysfunction syndromes (complete achromatopsia, incomplete achromatopsia, blue cone monochromatism, oligocone trichromacy and XL cone dysfunction with dichromacy)
- Presentation is at birth or in early infancy, often associated with nystagmus
- Rod dysfunction syndromes usually, but not always, have symptomatic night blindness. Central visual function is variably affected. Rod-specific ERGs are absent/reduced, with variable less severe abnormalities of the cone ERG
- Cone dysfunction syndromes usually present with photophobia, reduced visual acuity and colour vision disturbance. Cone ERGs are abnormal with normal rod responses
- The underlying molecular genetic basis of the majority of the retinal dysfunction syndromes is now well characterised, allowing molecular genetic diagnosis and the potential for future treatment strategies.

11.1 Introduction

The inherited retinal disorders can be classified according to their natural history (stationary or progressive), the mode of inheritance (autosomal dominant (AD), autosomal recessive (AR), X-linked recessive (XL), or mitochondrial) and principal site of dysfunction within the retina (retinal pigment epithelium, rod or cone photoreceptor, or inner retina). This classification is undertaken by careful clinical history and examination, and with the assistance of detailed psychophysical and electrophysiological assessment.

Major advances have been made in the field of retinal molecular genetics in the last decade, with identification of the causative genes underlying most inherited retinal disorders, especially those associated with the stationary dysfunction syndromes. At present routine molecular diagnostic testing is only available for a few disorders but the numbers will increase as advances are made in the technology of genetic analysis.

This chapter aims to discuss the stationary dysfunction syndromes and for convenience they have been divided into those conditions characterised principally by either rod or cone photoreceptor dysfunction. The phenotypes identified within these two groups will be described and an outline of our current understanding of the molecular biology underpinning their pathogenesis will be provided.

Table 11.1. Summary of the rod dysfunction syndromes

Rod dysfunction syndrome	Subtype	Mode of inheritance	Visual acuity	Refractive error	Nystagmus	Cone function	Fundi	Mutated gene(s)
Congenital stationary night blindness (AR CSNB)		Autosomal recessive	6/12–6/60	Often myopia	Present	Reduced	Usually normal or myopic	*GRM6*
Congenital stationary night blindness (AD CSNB)		Autosomal dominant	Normal	–	Absent	Normal	Usually normal	*RHO* *GNAT1* *PDE6B*
Congenital stationary night blindness (XL CSNB)	Complete CSNB (absent rod-specific ERG)	X-linked	6/12–6/60	Often myopia	Present	Reduced	Usually normal or myopic	*NYX*
	Incomplete CSNB (detectable rod-specific ERG)	X-linked	6/18–6/60	Often myopia	Present	Markedly reduced	Usually normal or myopic	*CACNA1F*
Oguchi disease		Autosomal recessive	Often normal or mild reduction	–	Absent	Normal	Mizuo–Nakamura phenomenon	*GRK1* *SAG*
Fundus albipunctatus	Without cone dystrophy	Autosomal recessive	Often normal	–	Absent	Normal	Multiple white dots scattered throughout the retina at the level of the RPE	*RDH5*
	With cone dystrophy	Autosomal recessive	Often normal	–	Absent	Reduced	Multiple white dots scattered throughout the retina at the level of the RPE	*RDH5*

AR autosomal recessive, *AD* autosomal dominant, *XL* X-linked

Table 11.2. Summary of the cone dysfunction syndromes

Cone dysfunction syndrome	Alternative names	Mode of inheritance	Visual acuity	Refractive error	Nystagmus	Colour vision	Fundi	Mutated gene(s) or chromosome locus
Complete achromatopsia	Rod monochromatism	Autosomal recessive	6/36–6/60	Often hypermetropia	Present	Absent	Usually normal	*CNGA3* *CNGB3* *GNAT2*
	Typical achromatopsia							Chromosome 14
Incomplete achromatopsia	Atypical achromatopsia	Autosomal recessive	6/24–6/36	Often hypermetropia	Present	Residual	Usually normal	*CNGA3*
Blue cone monochromatism	X-linked atypical achromatopsia	X-linked	6/24–6/36	Often myopia	Present	Residual tritan discrimination	Usually normal	(a) Deletion of the LCR
	X-linked incomplete achromatopsia							(b) Single inactivated L/M hybrid gene
Oligocone trichromacy	Oligocone syndrome	Autosomal recessive	6/12–6/24	Equal incidence of myopia and hypermetropia	Usually absent	Normal	Normal	–
X-linked cone dysfunction syndrome with dichromacy and myopia	Bornholm eye disease	X-linked	6/12–6/36	Moderate to high myopia with astigmatism	Absent	Deuteranopia or protanopia	Myopic	Xq28

LCR Locus control region

11.2 Stationary Retinal Dysfunction Syndromes

These disorders are subdivided on the basis of whether rod or cone photoreceptors are predominantly involved. These conditions are summarised in Tables 11.1 and 11.2.

11.2.1 Rod Dysfunction Syndromes (Stationary Night Blindness)

Three forms of stationary night blindness are recognised: congenital stationary night blindness (CSNB), fundus albipunctatus and Oguchi disease.

11.2.1.1 Congenital Stationary Night Blindness

Clinical Features and Electrophysiology

CSNB is characterised by night blindness, variable visual loss and usually normal fundi, although some patients have pale or tilted optic discs. CSNB may be inherited as an AD, AR or XL disorder; with XL inheritance being most common. Patients with AD CSNB usually present with nyctalopia and have normal visual acuity [36]; whereas in XL and AR, CSNB presentation is usually in infancy with nystagmus, moderate to high myopia, strabismus, reduced central vision, and in some cases paradoxical pupil responses (pupillary dilatation to bright light) [34].

XL CSNB is further subdivided into the complete and incomplete forms. Patients with complete CSNB are myopic and have more pronounced night blindness. Both complete and incomplete CSNB show a negative type of ERG, in that the photoreceptor derived a-wave in the maximal response is usually normal, but there is selective reduction in the inner nuclear derived b-wave so that it is smaller than the a-wave. In complete CSNB, the rod-specific ERG is more severely affected and is often nonrecordable [2]. Cone ERGs show mild abnormalities reflecting ON- bipolar pathway dysfunction. In contrast, there is always a detectable rod-specific ERG in incomplete CSNB and cone ERGs are much more abnormal than in complete CSNB, reflecting involvement of both ON- and OFF- bipolar pathways.

AR CSNB is phenotypically very similar to XLCSNB, both clinically and on ERG testing. In most families with AD CSNB, affected individuals show attenuated rod responses but normal cone responses on ERG testing, without evidence of a negative waveform on maximal response testing. Inner retinal dysfunction has been reported in a few cases.

Molecular Biology

AD CSNB

Consistent with clinical and electrophysiological findings, mutations in genes encoding three components of the rod-specific phototransduction cascade have been reported in association with AD CSNB: namely rhodopsin [10], the α-subunit of rod transducin [11] and the rod cGMP phosphodiesterase β-subunit [15].

XL CSNB

Two genes (*CACNA1F* and *NYX*) have been implicated in XL CSNB. Incomplete CSNB is associated with mutation in *CACNA1F*, which encodes the retina-specific α_{1F}-subunit of the voltage-gated L-type calcium channel expressed in the outer nuclear layer, inner nuclear layer, and ganglion cell layer [5, 38]. The majority of the mutations reported are inactivating truncation sequence variants. The loss of functional channels impairs the calcium flux into rod and cone photoreceptors required to sustain tonic neurotransmitter release from presynaptic terminals. This may result in the inability to maintain the normal transmembrane potential of bipolar cells, such that the retina remains in a partially light-stimulated state, unable to respond to changes in light levels. Although most patients with XL CSNB have nonprogressive disease, two brothers with a mutation in *CACNA1F* have been described who showed progressive decline in visual function and eventually had a nonrecordable rod and cone ERG [29].

Complete CSNB is associated with mutation in *NYX*, the gene encoding the leucine-rich proteoglycan nyctalopin [6, 35]. Leucine-rich repeats are believed to be important for protein interactions and the described mutations frequently involve these regions. It has been suggested that nyctalopin plays a role in the development and function of the ON- pathway within the retina, consistent with observed electrophysiological findings.

AR CSNB

Mutations in *GRM6*, the gene encoding the glutamate receptor mGluR6, have been identified in patients with AR CSNB [12]. This neurotransmitter receptor is present in the synapses of ON- bipolar cell dendrites, mediating synaptic transmission from rod and cone photoreceptors to these second-order neurones.

11.2.1.2 Oguchi Disease

Clinical Features and Electrophysiology

This rare AR form of stationary night blindness was first described in Japanese patients but has been subsequently reported in Europeans [22] and African-Americans [41]. Most patients present with poor night vision. Visual acuity is usually normal or only mildly reduced and photopic visual fields and colour vision are normal. In Oguchi disease, a characteristic greyish or green-yellow discolouration of the fundus is seen, which reverts to normal on prolonged dark adaptation (Mizuo–Nakamura phenomenon) [22]. The abnormal appearance may be confined to the posterior pole or extend beyond the vascular arcades. Most patients with Oguchi disease have a negative waveform maximal ERG, confirming the site of dysfunction to be post-phototransduction, as observed in XL and AR CSNB. In direct contrast to fundus albipunctatus, the ERG remains abnormal even after prolonged dark adaptation.

Molecular Biology

Nonsense mutations have been identified in two rod phototransduction proteins, arrestin [14] and rhodopsin kinase (RK) [44], both involved in terminating activation of the phototransduction cascade and thereby restoring photoreceptor sensitivity after exposure to light. In Oguchi disease the rods therefore behave as if they are light adapted and thus unresponsive to light at low levels of illumination. The key function, of both rhodopsin kinase and arrestin, in the normal deactivation and recovery of the photoreceptor after exposure to light, is entirely consistent with the delayed recovery seen in Oguchi disease. Evidence from knock-out mice models suggests that patients with RK or arrestin mutations may be more susceptible to light-induced retinal damage; it may therefore be advisable to encourage patients to wear tinted spectacles, thereby restricting excessive light exposure [8, 9].

11.2.1.3 Fundus Albipunctatus

Clinical Features and Electrophysiology

Fundus albipunctatus (FA) has an AR mode of inheritance with a highly characteristic fundus appearance with multiple white dots scattered throughout the retina at the level of the RPE (Fig. 11.1). The white deposits are most numerous in the mid-periphery and are usually absent from the macula. Patients either present with night blindness or because the abnormal retinal appearance is noted on routine ophthalmoscopy. Visual acuity is usually normal and the condition is nonprogressive in the majority of affected individuals. The rod-specific ERG is undetectable under standard conditions, but becomes normal following prolonged dark adaptation, in direct contrast to Oguchi disease. Two forms of FA have been described, the common form in which cone ERGs are normal, and a second type described as FA with cone dystrophy and negative ERG [28].

Molecular Biology

Mutations in *RDH5*, the gene encoding 11-cis retinol dehydrogenase, a component of the visual cycle involved in recycling the chromophore 11-cis retinal, have been identified in FA with or without cone dystrophy [43]. The function of the protein product of *RDH5* is consistent with the delay in the regeneration of photopigments characteristic of the disorder.

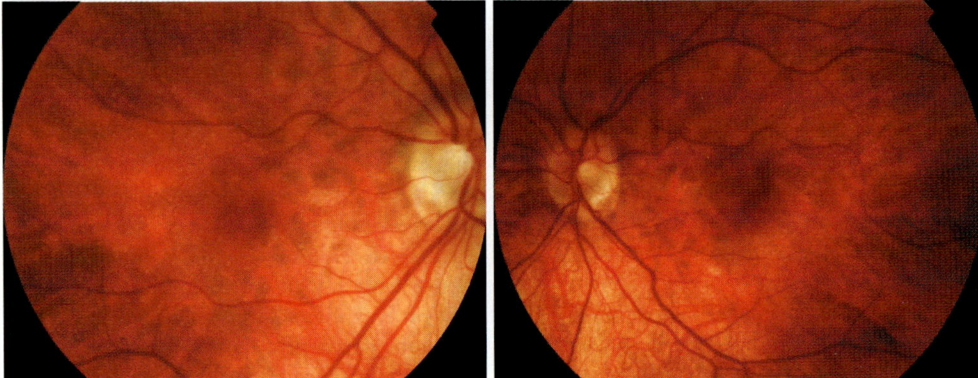

Fig. 11.1. Fundus albipunctatus. Characteristic fundus appearance with multiple white dots scattered throughout the retina at the level of the RPE

11.2.2 Cone Dysfunction Syndromes

These different syndromes encompass a wide range of clinical, electrophysiological and psychophysical findings [25]. Presentation is in infancy or at birth, usually with photophobia, nystagmus, reduced central vision, and normal rod function. The cone dysfunction syndromes include complete and incomplete achromatopsia, blue cone monochromatism, oligocone trichromacy, and XL cone dysfunction with dichromacy.

11.2.2.1 Achromatopsia – Complete and Incomplete

Achromatopsia refers to a genetically heterogeneous group of autosomal recessive stationary retinal disorders in which there is an absence of functioning cones in the retina [25]. They are characterised by reduced central vision, poor colour vision, photophobia, pendular nystagmus and usually normal fundi, and may occur in complete (typical) and incomplete (atypical) forms.

Clinical Features and Electrophysiology

Complete achromatopsia (previously known as rod monochromatism), has an incidence of approximately 1 in 30,000, is inherited as an autosomal recessive trait and results in impaired vision and complete colour blindness. The usual presentation is with reduced vision (6/36–6/60), nystagmus and marked photophobia in infancy. Vision is usually better in mesopic conditions. Pupil reactions are sluggish or may show paradoxical pupil responses. Hypermetropic refractive errors are common and fundus examination is generally normal. The nystagmus, although marked in infancy, may improve with age, as can the photophobia. Rod-specific ERGs are normal but there are no detectable cone-derived responses.

Incomplete achromatopsia is less common than the complete subtype and has a milder phenotype. The presentation and clinical findings of incomplete achromatopsia in infancy are similar to complete achromatopsia, but visual acuity is usually in the range 6/24 to 6/36 and there often is some residual colour perception.

Molecular Biology

Three achromatopsia genes have been identified, *CNGA3*, *CNGB3*, and *GNAT2*; which all encode components of the cone-specific phototransduction cascade. Mutations in all three genes have been reported in association with complete achromatopsia, whereas only mutations in *CNGA3* have been identified in incomplete achromatopsia.

CNGA3 and *CNGB3*, code for the α- and β-subunits of the cGMP-gated (CNG) cation channel in cone cells. In the dark, cGMP levels are high in cone photoreceptors, therefore enabling cGMP to bind to the α- and β-subunits of CNG channels, resulting in them adopting an open conformation and permitting an influx of cations, with consequent cone depolarisation. On exposure to light, activated photopigment initiates a cascade culminating in increased cGMP-phosphodiesterase activity, thereby lowering the concentration of cGMP in the photoreceptor, which results in closure of CNG cation channels and consequent cone hyperpolarization.

More than 50 disease-causing mutations in *CNGA3* have been identified in patients with achromatopsia [21, 42], with the majority being missense sequence variants, indicating that there is little tolerance for substitutions with respect to functional and structural integrity of the channel polypeptide. Four mutations (Arg277Cys, Arg283Trp, Arg436Trp and Phe547Leu) account for approximately 40% of all mutant *CNGA3* alleles [42]. By comparison, approximately only 12 mutations have been identified in *CNGB3* [17, 19, 39], with the majority being nonsense variants. The most frequent mutation of *CNGB3* identified to date is the 1-base-pair frameshift deletion, 1148delC (Thr383 fs), which accounts for up to 80% of *CNGB3* mutant disease chromosomes [17, 19]. It is currently proposed that approximately 25% of achromatopsia results from mutations of *CNGA3* [42] and 40–50% from mutations of *CNGB3* [17, 19].

Mutations within a third gene, *GNAT2*, which encodes the α-subunit of cone transducin, have also been shown to cause achromatopsia [1, 20]. In cone cells, light activated photopigment interacts with transducin, a three subunit guanine nucleotide binding protein, stimulating the exchange of bound GDP for GTP. All the *GNAT2* mutations identified to date result in premature translation termination and in protein-truncation at the carboxy-terminus. Mutations in this gene are thought to be responsible for less than 2% of patients affected with this disorder, suggesting the presence of further genetic heterogeneity in achromatopsia.

The phenotype associated with mutations in the two cation channel protein genes appears to be in keeping with previous clinical descriptions of achromatopsia [17, 19, 21, 39, 42]. The phenotype of a large consanguineous family with *GNAT2* inactivation has been reported [23]. The findings of note were clinical evidence of progressive deterioration in older affected individuals, residual colour vision, and relative preservation of S-cone ERGs in all subjects.

11.2.2.2 Blue Cone Monochromatism (S-Cone Monochromatism)

Clinical Features and Electrophysiology

Blue cone monochromatism (BCM) is an XL recessive disorder, affecting fewer than 1 in 100,000 individuals, in which affected males have normal rod and blue (S) cone function but lack red (L) and green (M) cone function. The clinical features are similar to incomplete achromatopsia. Affected infants are photophobic and develop fine rapid nystagmus in early infancy. In keeping with achromatopsia, the nystagmus often reduces with time. They are usually myopic (a common finding in XL retinal disorders), with a visual acuity of 6/24–6/36. By comparison, subjects with achromatopsia more commonly have a hypermetropic refractive error. Fundi are usually normal in BCM or have changes consistent with myopia. Female carriers of BCM may have abnormal cone ERGs and mild anomalies of colour vision.

Achromatopsia and BCM may be differentiated by the mode of inheritance, findings on psychophysical and electrophysiological testing, and via molecular genetic analysis. In contrast to achromatopsia, there is some preservation of the single flash photopic ERG in BCM and normal S-cone function can be demonstrated using specialised spectral ERG techniques. On colour vision testing, good residual tritan discrimination is consistent with BCM, with the Farnsworth 100-Hue test, Berson plates, Hardy, Rand and Rittler plates all having been used successfully.

BCM is generally a stationary disorder but progressive deterioration, with or without the development of macular pigmentary changes, has been reported in some patients [3, 13, 27, 30].

Molecular Biology

The underlying molecular genetic basis of BCM involves inactivation of the L- and M-opsin genes located at Xq28 [3, 4, 27, 30, 31]. The mutations in the L- and M- pigment gene array causing BCM fall into two classes:

1. In the first class, a normal L- and M- pigment gene array is inactivated by a deletion in the locus control region (LCR), located upstream of the L- pigment gene. A deletion in this region abolishes transcription of all genes in the pigment gene array and therefore inactivates both L- and M- cones.
2. In the second class of mutations, the LCR is preserved but changes within the L- and M-pigment gene array lead to loss of functional pigment production. The most common genotype in this class consists of a single inactivated L/M hybrid gene. The first step in this second mechanism is unequal crossing over reducing the number of genes in the array to one, followed in the second step by a mutation that inactivates the remaining gene. The most frequent inactivating mutation that has been described is a thymine-to-cytosine transition at nucleotide 648, which results in a cysteine-to-arginine substitution at codon 203 (Cys203Arg), a mutation known to disrupt the folding of cone opsin molecules.

Approximately 40 % of blue cone monochromat genotypes are a result of a one-step mutational pathway that leads to deletion of the LCR, with the remaining 60 % comprising a heterogeneous group of multi-step pathways [3, 4, 27, 30, 31]. Nevertheless, a significant minority of subjects are not found to have disease-causing alterations to the opsin array [3, 31], suggesting genetic heterogeneity yet to be identified in BCM. Patients with a progressive phenotype have not been found to have a particular genotype to account for the progression [3, 4, 27, 31].

11.2.2.3 Oligocone Trichromacy

Clinical Features and Electrophysiology

Oligocone trichromacy is an unusual cone dysfunction syndrome in which patients are believed to have a reduced number of normal functioning cone photoreceptors (oligocone syndrome), with preservation of the three cone types in the normal proportions, thereby permitting trichromacy [18, 40].

The disorder is characterised by reduced visual acuity from infancy (6/12 to 6/24), mild photophobia, normal fundi, and abnormal cone ERGs, but normal colour vision [18, 24, 32, 40]. Normal colour vision is a unique finding in the cone dysfunction syndromes. Rod-specific ERGs are normal. Patients usually have no nystagmus. On detailed psychophysical testing, some subjects have slightly elevated colour discrimination thresholds, compatible with a reduction in cone numbers [18, 24].

Cone ERG findings in patients with oligocone trichromacy were found to be poorly concordant in a recent case series [24]. Cone 30-Hz flicker ERG responses were absent or markedly reduced in two siblings, who additionally showed a photopic b-wave of shortened implicit time; suggesting some preservation of the cone OFF- pathway, as the implicit time of the OFF- response in normal subjects is similar to that in these patients. Other patients showed clearly present, but delayed and reduced cone 30-Hz flicker ERGs, with some showing a mildly electronegative maximal response, suggestive of inner retinal abnormality. Cone system implicit time changes are not expected in restricted disease, and in addition are more usually associated with generalised dysfunction, rather than loss of function related to a reduction in photoreceptor numbers [24]. This phenotypic heterogeneity suggests that there may be more than one disease mechanism and therefore more than one disease-causing gene associated with the oligocone phenotype. It has previously been proposed that these patients have a reduced number of retinal cones that function normally. That may apply to central cones, but recent electrophysiological data suggest that remaining peripheral cones do not function normally [24].

Previous reports have suggested this disorder to be stationary, but there is clinical evidence of progression in one family that has been investigated, consisting of two affected brothers whose grandmother had evidence of bull's-eye maculopathy and abnormal cone ERGs with normal rod responses [24]. However, until molecular genetic data become available it can not be proven that the grandmother's cone dysfunction is the same disorder as that of the two brothers.

Molecular Biology

Oligocone trichromacy is likely to be inherited as an autosomal recessive trait, but the molecular genetic basis of the disorder is unknown. Since oligocone trichromacy may have a developmental component, genes involved in retinal photoreceptor differentiation, when cone numbers are being determined, may represent good candidate genes. Since electrophysiological testing suggests that the site of abnormality may not be exclusively at the level of the photoreceptor, genes expressed preferentially in the inner retina may represent alternative candidates.

11.2.2.4 X-Linked Cone Dysfunction Syndrome with Dichromacy and Myopia

Clinical Features and Electrophysiology

A stationary XL cone dysfunction syndrome has been described consisting of moderate to high myopia, astigmatism, moderately reduced acuity (6/12 to 6/36), dichromacy (deuteranopia or protanopia), normal or myopic fundi (Fig. 11.2) and abnormal cone ERGs but normal rod responses [16, 26, 45]. Nystagmus is not observed in affected subjects. This disorder was first reported in a large five-generation Danish family that had its origins on the Danish island of Bornholm. The syndrome was therefore named Bornholm eye disease (BED) [16]. Affected members in that family were found to be deuteranopes on detailed colour vision testing. Subsequently, further families have been identified with similar characteristics and with either deuteranopia or protanopia [26, 45, unpublished data].

Molecular Biology

Linkage analysis performed in the original BED family has mapped the locus to Xq28, in the same chromosomal region as the L-/M- opsin gene array [37]. The association of protanopia or deuteranopia with cone dysfunction indi-

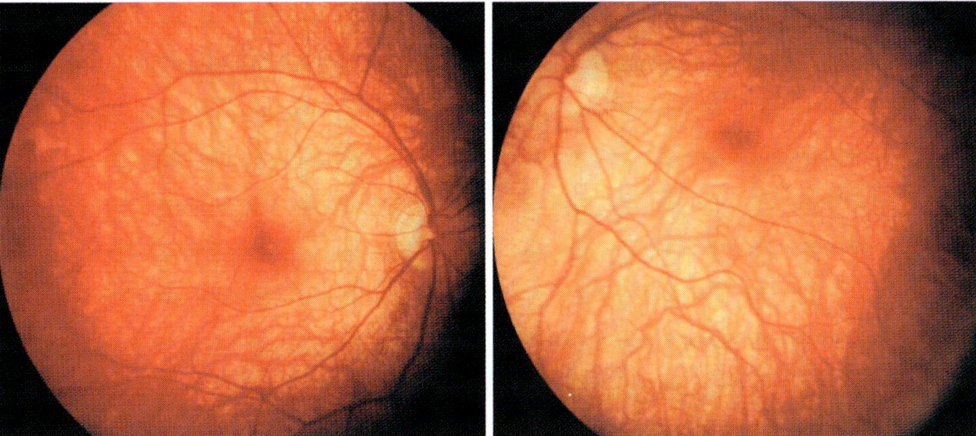

Fig. 11.2. X-linked cone dysfunction syndrome with dichromacy and myopia. Myopic fundi with tilted optic discs

cates a potential role for opsin gene mutations in the aetiology of this disorder. However, molecular analysis of the opsin gene array, whilst revealing changes that are consistent with the colour vision defects associated with this syndrome (dichromacy), failed to identify alterations that also potentially account for the cone dysfunction [26, 45].

It is therefore possible that rearrangements within the opsin gene array account for the colour vision findings, whilst the cone dysfunction component of the disorder may be ascribed to mutation within an adjacent but separate locus. To date however, the only cone dystrophy (COD2) that maps to an adjacent region (Xq27), displays a different phenotype [7]. Nevertheless, it is becoming increasingly well recognised in retinal molecular genetics that disparate phenotypes can be caused by both different mutations in the same gene, and even the same mutation in the same gene.

It is of note that a similar XL cone dysfunction syndrome without dichromacy has not been described, so it would appear that this form of cone dysfunction is only seen in association with dichromacy. This observation may suggest that the cone dysfunction arises from a mutation in a gene that only causes cone dysfunction when expressed in dichromats.

11.3 Management of Stationary Retinal Dysfunction Syndromes

The stationary retinal dysfunction syndromes are currently not amenable to any form of treatment. However, all patients and their families benefit from genetic counselling, educational and occupational advice, and supportive measures such as the provision of appropriate spectacle correction and low vision aids, and the treatment of concurrent ocular problems such as myopia or cataracts.

Photophobia is often a prominent symptom in the cone disorders and therefore tinted spectacles or contact lenses may be beneficial to patients, in terms of both improved comfort and vision. For example, red contact lenses have been suggested to successfully alleviate photophobia in patients with cone disorders [33].

Advances in molecular biology have led to the identification of many of the causative genetic mutations, which should offer new therapeutic prospects. In the stationary retinal dysfunction syndromes, histopathological or high resolution in vivo microscopy data are often not yet available; however, the evidence to date suggests that photoreceptor cells remain present in these disorders, and could therefore potentially be targeted in the future with directed gene therapy.

11.4 Conclusions

The stationary retinal dysfunction syndromes presenting in childhood comprise a group of disorders that are both clinically and genetically heterogeneous. Their clinical, psychophysical and electrophysiological phenotypic features are now well characterised, and in most cases the causative genes have been identified. Perhaps not surprisingly these genes mainly encode proteins involved in either the cone or rod phototransduction pathway. Gene therapy treatment trials will be shortly commencing for the rod–cone dystrophy Leber congenital amaurosis (see Chap. 10); if successful, we may be at the beginning of an exciting time when these stationary retinal dysfunction syndromes, which represent an important cause of childhood blindness, may finally be treatable.

Summary for the Clinician

- See Tables 11.1 and 11.2

References

1. Aligianis IA, Forshew T, Johnson S et al (2002) Mapping of a novel locus for achromatopsia (*ACHM4*) to 1p and identification of a germline mutation in the α-subunit of cone transducin (*GNAT2*). J Med Genet 39:656–660
2. Allen LE, Zito I, Bradshaw K et al (2003) Genotype-phenotype correlation in British families with X linked congenital stationary night blindness. Br J Ophthalmol 87:1413–1420
3. Ayyagari R, Kakuk LE, Bingham EL et al (2000) Spectrum of color gene deletions and phenotype in patients with blue cone monochromacy. Hum Genet 107:75–82
4. Ayyagari R, Kakuk LE, Coats EL et al (1999) Bilateral macular atrophy in blue cone monochromacy (BCM) with loss of the locus control region (LCR) and part of the red pigment gene. Mol Vis 5:13–18
5. Bech-Hansen NT, Naylor MJ, Maybaum TA et al (1998) Loss-of-function mutations in a calcium-channel alpha1-subunit gene in Xp11.23 cause incomplete X-linked congenital stationary night blindness. Nat Genet 19:264–267
6. Bech-Hansen NT, Naylor MJ, Maybaum TA et al (2000) Mutations in *NYX*, encoding the leucine-rich proteoglycan nyctalopin, cause X-linked complete congenital stationary night blindness. Nat Genet 26:319–323
7. Bergen AA, Pinckers AJ (1997) Localization of a novel X-linked progressive cone dystrophy gene to Xq27: evidence for genetic heterogeneity. Am J Hum Genet 60:1468–1473
8. Chen CK, Burns ME, Spencer M et al (1999) Abnormal photoresponses andlight-induced apoptosis in rods lacking rhodopsin kinase. Proc Natl Acad Sci U S A 96:3718–3722
9. Chen J, Simon MI, Matthes MT, Yasumura D, LaVail MM (1999) Increased susceptibility to light damage in an arrestin knockout mouse model of Oguchi disease (stationary night blindness). Invest Ophthalmol Vis Sci 40:2978–2982
10. Dryja TP, Berson EL, Rao VR, Oprian DD (1993) Heterozygous missense mutation in the rhodopsin gene as a cause of congenital stationary night blindness. Nature Genet 4:280–283
11. Dryja TP, Hahn LB, Reboul T, Arnaud B (1996) Missense mutation in the gene encoding the alpha subunit of rod transducin in the Nougaret form of congenital stationary night blindness. Nat Genet 13:358–360
12. Dryja TP, McGee TL, Berson EL et al (2005) Night blindness and abnormal cone electroretinogram ON responses in patients with mutations in the GRM6 gene encoding mGluR6. Proc Natl Acad Sci U S A 102:4884–4889
13. Fleischman JA, O'Donnell FE Jr (1981) Congenital X-linked incomplete achromatopsia. Evidence for slow progression, carrier fundus findings, and possible genetic linkage with glucose-6-phosphate dehydrogenase locus. Arch Ophthalmol 99:468–472
14. Fuchs S, Nakazawa M, Maw M et al (1995) A homozygous 1 base pair deletion in the arrestin gene is a frequent cause of Oguchi's disease in Japanese. Nature Genet 10:360–362
15. Gal A, Orth U, Baehr W et al (1994) Heterozygous missense mutation in the rod cGMP phosphodiesterase beta subunit gene in autosomal dominant stationary night blindness. Nature Genet 7:64–68
16. Haim M, Fledelius HC, Skarsholm D (1988) X-linked myopia in a Danish family. Acta Ophthalmol (Copenh) 66:450–456
17. Johnson S, Michaelides M, Aligianis IA et al (2003) Achromatopsia caused by novel mutations in both *CNGA3* and *CNGB3*. J Med Genet 41:e20
18. Keunen JEE, De Brabandere SRS, Liem ATA (1995) Foveal densitometry and color matching in oligocone trichromacy. In: Drum B (ed) 12th IRGCVD Symposium, Colour Vision Deficiencies XII, Kluwer, pp 203–210
19. Kohl S, Baumann B, Broghammer M et al (2000) Mutations in the *CNGB3* gene encoding the beta-subunit of the cone photoreceptor cGMP-gated channel are responsible for achromatopsia (*ACHM3*) linked to chromosome 8q21. Hum Mol Genet 9:2107–2116
20. Kohl S, Baumann B, Rosenberg T et al (2002) Mutations in the cone photoreceptor G-protein alpha-subunit gene *GNAT2* in patients with achromatopsia. Am J Hum Genet 71:422–425
21. Kohl S, Marx T, Giddings I et al (1998) Total colour-blindness is caused by mutations in the gene encoding the alpha-subunit of the cone photoreceptor cGMP-gated cation channel. Nat Genet 19:257–259
22. Krill AE (1977) Congenital stationary night-blindness. In: Krill AE (ed) Hereditary retinal and choroidal disease, vol. II. Harper & Row, London, pp 391–417
23. Michaelides M, Aligianis IA, Holder GE et al (2003) Cone dystrophy phenotype associated with a frameshift mutation (M280fsX291) in the α-subunit of cone-specific transducin (*GNAT2*). Br J Ophthalmol 87:1317–1320
24. Michaelides M, Holder GE, Bradshaw K et al (2004) Oligocone trichromacy: a rare and unusual cone dysfunction syndrome. Br J Ophthalmol 88:497–500
25. Michaelides M, Hunt DM, Moore AT (2004) The cone dysfunction syndromes. Br J Ophthalmol 88:291–297

26. Michaelides M, Johnson S, Bradshaw K et al (2005) X-linked cone dysfunction syndrome with myopia and protanopia. Ophthalmology 112:1448–1454
27. Michaelides M, Johnson S, Simunovic MP et al (2005) Blue cone monochromatism: a phenotype and genotype assessment with evidence of progressive loss of cone function in older individuals. Eye 19:2–10
28. Miyake Y, Shiroyama N, Sugita S, Horiguchi M, Yagasaki K (1992) Fundus albipunctatus associated with cone dystrophy. Br J Ophthalmol 76:375–379
29. Nakamura M, Ito S, Piao CH, Terasaki H, Miyake Y (2003) Retinal and optic disc atrophy associated with a *CACNA1F* mutation in a Japanese family. Arch Ophthalmol 121:1028–1033
30. Nathans J, Davenport CM, Maumenee IH et al (1989) Molecular genetics of human blue cone monochromacy. Science 245:831–838
31. Nathans J, Maumenee IH, Zrenner E et al (1993) Genetic heterogeneity among blue-cone monochromats. Am J Hum Genet 53:987–1000
32. Neuhann T, Krastel H, Jaeger W (1978) Differential diagnosis of typical and atypical congenital achromatopsia. Analysis of a progressive foveal dystrophy and a nonprogressive oligo-cone trichromacy (general cone dysfunction without achromatopsia), both of which at first had been diagnosed as achromatopsia. Albrecht Von Graefes Arch Klin Exp Ophthalmol 209:19–28
33. Park WL, Sunness JS (2004) Red contact lenses for alleviation of photophobia in patients with cone disorders. Am J Ophthalmol 137:774–775
34. Price MJ, Judisch GF, Thompson HS (1988) X-linked congenital stationary night blindness with myopia and nystagmus without clinical complaints of nyctalopia. J Pediatr Ophthalmol Strabismus 25:33–36
35. Pusch CM, Zeitz C, Brandau O et al (2000) The complete form of X-linked congenital stationary night blindness is caused by mutations in a gene encoding a leucine-rich repeat protein. Nat Genet 26:324–327
36. Rosenberg T, Haim M, Piczenik Y et al (1991) Autosomal dominant stationary night blindness. A large family rediscovered. Acta Ophthalmol 69:694–703
37. Schwartz M, Haim M, Skarsholm D (1990) X-linked myopia: Bornholm Eye Disease. Linkage to DNA markers on the distal part of Xq. Clin Genet 38:281–286
38. Strom TM, Nyakatura G, Apfelstedt-Sylla E et al (1998) An L-type calcium-channel gene mutated in incomplete X-linked congenital stationary night blindness. Nat Genet 19:260–263
39. Sundin OH, Yang J-M, Li Y et al (2000) Genetic basis of total colour-blindness among the Pingelapese islanders. Nat Genet 25:289–293
40. van Lith GHM (1973) General cone dysfunction without achromatopsia. In: Pearlman JT (ed) 10th ISCERG Symposium. Doc Ophthalmol Proc Ser 2:175–180
41. Winn S, Tasman W, Spaeth G, McDonald PR, Justice J Jr (1969) Oguchi's disease in Negroes. Arch Ophthalmol 81:501–507
42. Wissinger B, Gamer D, Jägle H et al (2001) *CNGA3* mutations in hereditary cone photoreceptor disorders. Am J Hum Genet 69:722–737
43. Yamamoto H, Simon A, Eriksson U et al (1999) Mutations in the gene encoding 11-cis retinol dehydrogenase cause delayed dark adaptation and fundus albipunctatus. Nat Genet 22:188–191
44. Yamamoto S, Sippel KC, Berson EL, Dryja TP (1997) Defects in the rhodopsin kinase gene in the Oguchi form of stationary night blindness. Nat Genet 15:175–178
45. Young TL, Deeb SS, Ronan SM et al (2004) X-linked high myopia associated with cone dysfunction. Arch Ophthalmol 122:897–908

Childhood Retinal Detachment

Arabella V. Poulson, Martin P. Snead

Core Messages

- Retinal detachment in childhood is uncommon and has a different range of aetiologies from adult retinal detachment
- It often presents late or with involvement of the fellow eye
- High myopia, particularly if congenital, usually indicates an underlying abnormality
- Retinal dialysis is not associated with posterior vitreous detachment
- Giant retinal tear is usually associated with abnormal gel and an underlying hereditary vitreoretinopathy and should be differentiated from dialysis because it has a different prognosis and requires different management
- Stickler syndrome is the commonest inherited cause of retinal detachment with a lifetime risk of more than 60 %
- Stickler syndrome may have no systemic features and can be diagnosed purely on the vitreous phenotype
- Many causes of retinal detachment in childhood are associated with an underlying developmental abnormality which may limit the prognosis for good vision
- There is a real case for offering prophylactic treatment to prevent retinal detachment where there is a familial risk of giant retinal tear

12.1 Introduction

Retinal detachment in is uncommon in childhood, accounting for between 1.7 % and 5.7 % of all retinal detachment [4, 34]. In a study of 45,000 army recruits, it has been calculated that the age-related annual incidence of retinal detachment in patients aged 10–19 years is 2.9 per 100,000 [32].

Young children and infants do not complain of visual loss and retinal detachment in children frequently presents late or with fellow eye involvement; 22–38 % may present with proliferative vitreoretinopathy of grade C or D [2].

Many studies have identified trauma and myopia as predisposing causes of retinal detachment in children. Emphasis is now also placed on the importance of inherited disorders, such as Stickler syndrome, which is associated with a high risk of giant retinal tear and the recognition that myopia, especially congenital myopia, is likely to be an indication of other ophthalmic or systemic abnormalities. Retinal detachment may complicate developmental abnormalities, including colobomata, congenital cataract, congenital glaucoma and retinopathy of prematurity. Congenital retinal detachment, or congenital nonattachment of the retina, is now recognized as part of the spectrum of vitreoretinal dysplasia. Retinoblastoma or other tumours may give rise to a "solid" detachment. Retinal detachment may also result from intraocular infection or inflammation.

When considering the aetiology, family history and examination of relatives and, in particular, examination of the vitreous can give valuable information. Children may need careful examination under anaesthesia to determine the cause of the retinal detachment and whether it is rhegmatogenous, tractional or exudative.

The range of underlying causes of retinal detachment in children is different from that in adults. The association with complex intraocular pathology and the additional problems of amblyopia in young children means that they often present a formidable challenge to treatment. Where possible, therefore, serious consideration should be given to prophylaxis against retinal detachment.

12.2 Trauma

Trauma has been reported as the cause in 27–51% of cases of childhood retinal detachment [47]. Traumatic retinal detachment is seen most commonly in older children and is usually caused by blunt trauma. Retinal tears may be found in approximately 2–5% [9]. Penetrating injuries and retained intraocular foreign bodies are less frequent causes but are associated with severe proliferative vitreoretinopathy.

12.2.1 Blunt Ocular Trauma

Retinal detachment due to blunt trauma is almost always rhegmatogenous and most commonly caused by a disinsertion at the ora serrata (dialysis) (Fig. 12.1A), usually occurring in older children. Bilateral retinal detachment due to traumatic dialysis has been described as a rare presenting feature of nonaccidental injury [14]. Sudden antero-posterior compression associated with a corresponding coronal expansion typically causes avulsion of the pars plana epithelium, which can be seen as a characteristic irregular ribbon within the vitreous cavity (Fig. 12.1B). The superior quadrant is more often involved in contrast to the usual lower temporal quadrant involvement in nontraumatic dialysis [17, 33]. The disinsertion may involve more than 90° of the circumference and superficially resemble a giant retinal tear. However, the vitreous gel remains attached to the posterior flap so that there is no independent mobility characteristic of a giant retinal tear. Further distinguishing features are the absence of radial extensions, which frequently occur at the apices of giant retinal tears and the normal compact healthy vitreous gel architecture. Giant tears in childhood are typically associated with abnormal gel and inherited vitreoretinopathies. Recruitment of subretinal fluid is typically slow in a dialysis so that unless the ora serrata is routinely examined after blunt trauma, the diagnosis may be delayed by several weeks until the macular becomes involved [22]. Dialyses respond well to repair with scleral buckling techniques.

Ragged impact necrosis breaks account for about one-fifth of retinal breaks seen in blunt

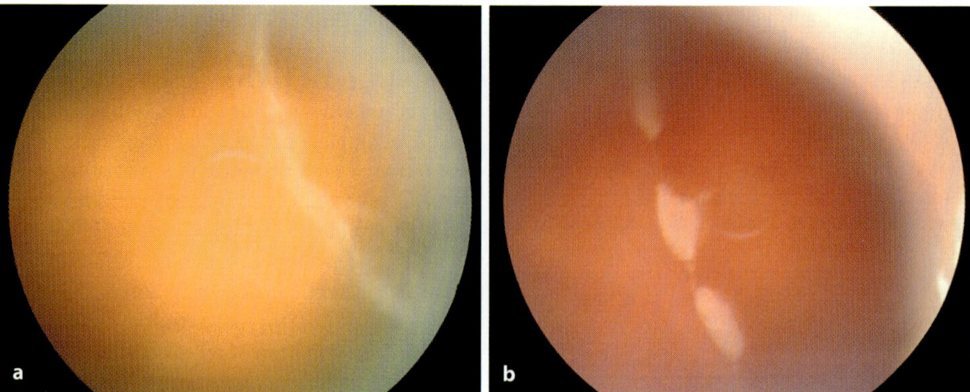

Fig. 12.1. **a** Retinal detachment due to traumatic retinal dialysis. **b** Avulsed pars plana epithelium in the vitreous cavity following blunt trauma

trauma [22]. Retinal vessel and retinal pigment epithelial disruption may be confirmed on fundus fluorescein angiography. The retinal detachment usually presents soon after the injury. These breaks are often large, irregular and posterior to the equator and therefore need an internal approach with vitrectomy for effective repair. Giant retinal tears account for a minority of retinal breaks due to blunt trauma. They respond well to vitrectomy and internal tamponade, although the visual prognosis is often limited by associated ocular damage.

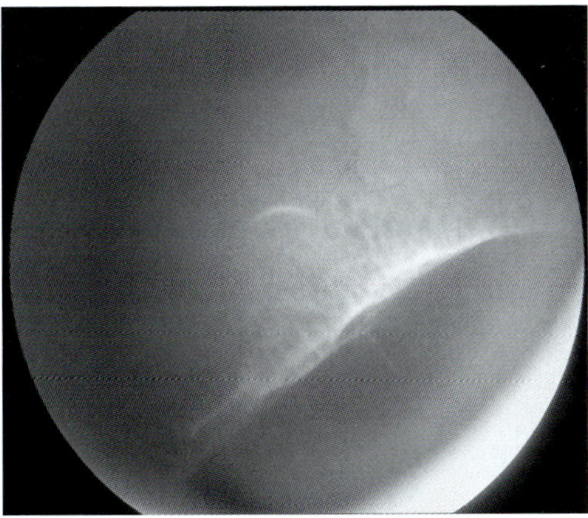

Fig. 12.2. Retinal detachment due to nontraumatic retinal dialysis

12.2.2 Penetrating Ocular Trauma

Retinal perforation or incarceration from penetrating trauma rarely causes acute rhegmatogenous retinal detachment. The associated corneoscleral wound provides access for extrinsic fibroblasts so that combined tractional and rhegmatogenous retinal detachment presents sometimes much later. Vitrectomy and internal tamponade with or without relieving retinectomy may be required as severe proliferative vitreoretinopathy commonly occurs. Traumatic giant retinal tears have been reported to occur in 22% of open globe injuries [34].

12.3 Nontraumatic Retinal Dialysis

Nontraumatic retinal dialysis (Fig. 12.2) accounts for approximately 10% of all juvenile retinal detachment [17, 43]. The male-to-female ratio is 3:2 [43] and the majority of patients are hypermetropic or emmetropic [17, 33, 36]. In 97% of cases, the dialysis affects the inferotemporal quadrant but multiple dialyses occur in one-third and 37% may be bilateral [43]. Detachments associated with dialyses progress slowly, have a low incidence of PVR and characteristically present either as an incidental finding or when the macula becomes detached. They can be managed routinely with buckling techniques and the use of a small (typically 3-mm) circumferential sponge reduces the likelihood of postoperative motility problems. Although the anatomical success rate of surgery is high, visual recovery may remain poor if there has been chronic macular involvement. Examination of the fellow eye under anaesthesia is also important, as retinal dialysis may be bilateral and oral abnormalities, in the form of a "frill" or flat dialysis, are found in the fellow eye in up to 30% of cases.

Summary for the Clinician

- **Retinal dialysis**
  - **May or may not be caused by trauma**
  - **Is not associated with posterior vitreous detachment**
- **Giant retinal tear**
  - **Is usually associated with abnormal gel and an underlying hereditary vitreoretinopathy**
  - **Should be differentiated from dialysis because it has a different prognosis and requires different management**
  - **Results from posterior vitreous detachment and can be recognized by independent mobility of the posterior flap and may develop radial extensions because of this**
  - **Can involve less than 90° of circumference**

Table 12.1. Inherited disorders associated with retinal detachment

Disorder	Symbol	Locus	Gene	Protein	McKusick No
Stickler syndrome type 1	STL1	12q13.2	COL2A1	Type II collagen	108300
Stickler syndrome type 2	STL2	1p21	COL11A1	Type XI collagen	604841
Kniest dysplasia	–	12q13.11–13.2	COL2A1	Type II collagen	156550
Spondyloepiphyseal dysplasia congenita	SEDC	12q13.11–13.2	COL2A1	Type II collagen	183900
Spondyloepimetaphyseal dysplasia (Strudwick type)	SMED	12q13.11–13.2	COL2A1	Type II collagen	184250
VPED[a]	–	12q13.11–13.2	COL2A1	Type II collagen	–
Ehlers–Danlos type VI	EDS VI	1p36.3-p36.2	PLOD1	lysine hydroxylase	225400
Marfan syndrome	MFS	15q21.1	FBN1	Fibrillin	154700
Wagner vitreoretinopathy	WGN1	5q14.3	–	–	143200
Smith–Magenis	SMS	17p11.2	RAI1	–	182290
Norrie's disease	ND	Xp11.4	NDP	Norrin	310600
Familial exudative vitreo-retinopathy (FEVR)	EVR1	11q13–23	FZD4	Frizzled-4 receptor	133780
	EVR1	11q13.4	LRP5	LRP5[b]	603506
	EVR2	Xp11.4	NDP	Norrin	310600
	EVR3	11p12–13	–	–	605750
Incontinentia pigmenti	IP2	Xq28	NEMO	–	308300
Juvenile X-linked retinoschisis	RS1	Xp22.2–22.1	RS	–	312700
Knobloch syndrome	KNO	21q22.3	COL18A1	Type XVIII collagen	267750

[a] Vitreoretinopathy associated with phalangeal epiphyseal dysplasia, [b]LRP5 low-density lipoprotein receptor-5

12.4 Familial Retinal Detachment

Rhegmatogenous retinal detachment can occur in a number of inherited disorders (see Table 12.1), the most common being the Stickler syndromes due to mutations in the genes for type II and type XI collagens, constituents of both vitreous and cartilage. High myopia and retinal detachment are also seen in Marfan syndrome, Ehlers–Danlos syndrome, Smith–Magenis syndrome, Kniest syndrome and spondyloepiphyseal dysplasia congenita. The detachments are often complex and frequently caused by giant retinal tear. In familial exudative vitreoretinopathy (FEVR), Norrie disease and incontinentia pigmenti, there is an underlying retinovascular abnormality and tractional retinal detachment. Rarely retinal detachment may complicate juvenile X-linked retinoschisis.

12.4.1 The Stickler Syndromes

12.4.1.1 Type 1 Stickler Syndrome

Stickler initially described a family with a dominantly inherited pattern of high myopia, a high incidence of retinal detachment and abnormal epiphyseal development with premature degenerative changes in various joints. Subsequent analysis of this and other families linked the disorder to *COL2A1*, the gene for type II col-

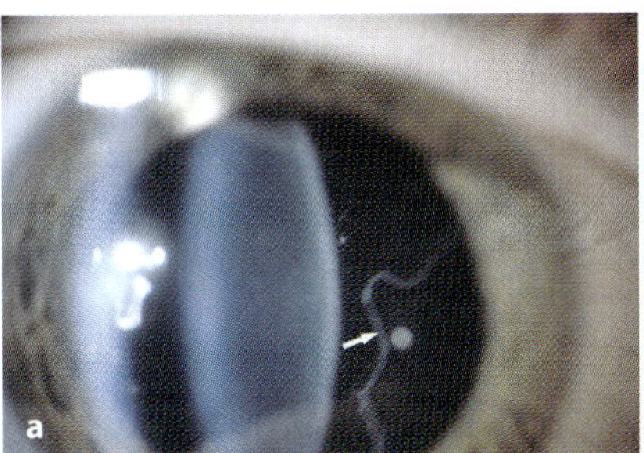

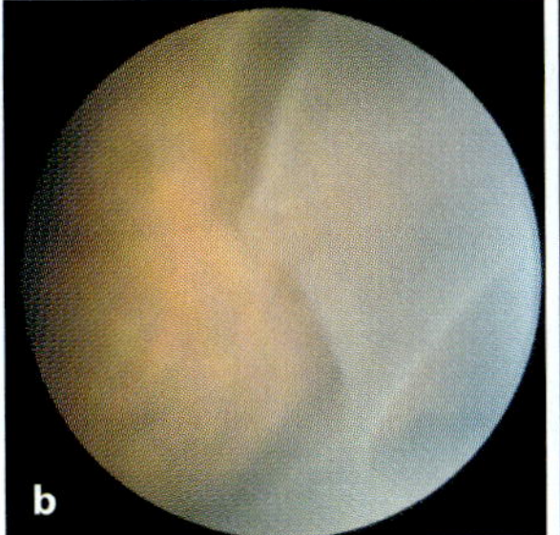

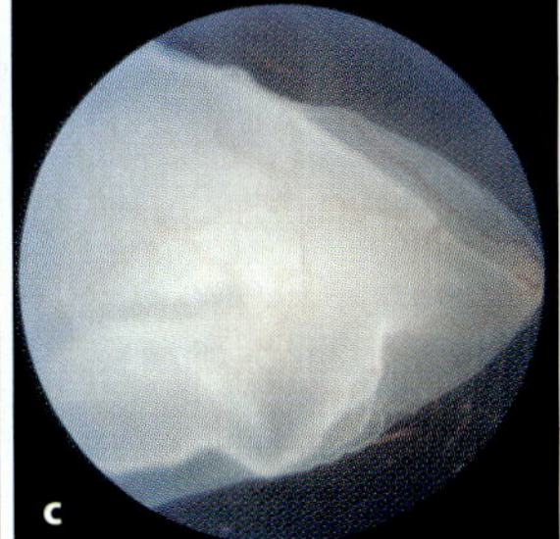

Fig. 12.3. **a** Type 1 (membranous) vitreous anomaly (*arrow*) seen in type 1 Stickler syndrome. **b** Giant retinal tear with radial extensions. **c** Total retinal detachment due to 360° giant retinal tear

lagen on chromosome 12. Stickler syndrome is therefore on the mild end of a spectrum of chondrodysplasias, which include spondyloepiphyseal dysplasia congenita, spondyloepimetaphyseal dysplasia and Kniest dysplasia.

Ophthalmic Features

Eighty percent of patients with type 1 Stickler syndrome are myopic. The myopia is congenital and usually of high degree. The 20% who are emmetropic, or even hypermetropic, do in fact have an increased axial length which is refractively compensated by cornea plana. The term "congenital megalophthalmos" or "cryptomyopia" has been used to encompass both states. Lens opacities, often wedge-shaped cortical opacities peculiar to Stickler syndrome, may be seen. Pigmented radial paravascular lattice is a characteristic feature but the fundus appearances can be deceptively normal. The vitreous phenotype, however, is pathognomonic. A vestigial amount of gel behind the lens is bordered by a distinct folded membrane, termed the membranous or type 1 vitreous anomaly (Fig. 12.3A) [39]. This membrane is congenital and should not be confused with the posterior hyaloid membrane, which differs in its position, its movement and the degree of surface crinkling. The lifetime risk of retinal detachment, particularly due to giant retinal tear (Fig. 12.3B, C), and which can occur at any age, is at least 60% [38].

Facial Features

Classically, patients have a flat midface with a depressed nasal bridge, anteverted nares, and a small, recessed chin. These findings are usually most evident in children, becoming less obvious in adults. Facial features are so variable that in isolation they are unreliable for making a diagnosis. Many patients have some degree of midline clefting ranging from the extreme of the Pierre-Robin sequence, through clefting of the hard or soft palate, to the mildest manifestation of bifid uvula.

Hearing

Patients with Stickler syndrome may suffer hearing difficulties for two reasons. Firstly, the association with cleft and high arched palate leads to an increased incidence of serous otitis media causing a conductive hearing deficit. In some patients, a mild conductive element persists, despite treatment, because of ossicle defects or tympanic membrane abnormalities. Secondly, there can be an associated high tone sensorineural hearing loss that may be so subtle that many patients are unaware of the deficit. Baseline audiometry therefore has an important diagnostic role to reveal subtle asymptomatic high tone loss.

Joints

Children with Stickler syndrome classically have hypermobile joints (Fig. 12.4). Joint mobility can be assessed objectively using the Beighton scoring system to allow comparison with an age, sex, and race matched population.

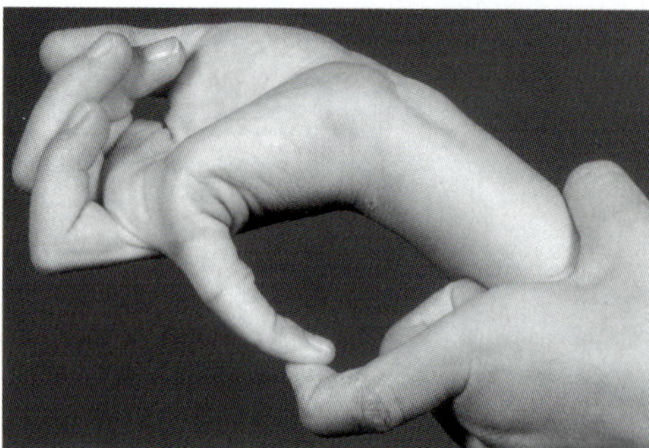

Fig. 12.4. Joint hypermobility in Stickler syndrome

With increasing age, the hypermobility is lost and a degenerative arthropathy of variable severity may develop by the third or fourth decade. Typical radiological changes show irregularity of articular contour and loss of joint space. By middle age, some patients require joint replacement surgery for hips or knees.

Other Features

Patients are of normal height and often have slender extremities and long fingers. They are of normal intellect. Early reports of increased mitral valve prolapse have not been substantiated by recent studies which show that it is no more frequent than in the general population [1].

Ocular Only Stickler Syndrome

A subgroup of type 1 Stickler syndrome has been identified without systemic skeletal or auditory involvement. One mechanism explaining this is a mutation in exon 2 of the COL2A1 gene. Exon 2 is principally expressed in the eye and spliced out of cartilage, resulting in a predominantly ocular form of Stickler syndrome with minimal or absent systemic involvement [27]. Because of the absent systemic features, this group are at particular high risk of missed diagnosis, emphasising the importance of the ophthalmic examination in the diagnosis of Stickler syndrome.

12.4.1.2 Type 2 Stickler Syndrome

Although most patients with Stickler syndrome were found to have the type 1 vitreous phenotype, it became clear that a minority of pedigrees had the same classical systemic features and the same risk of retinal detachment but had a different vitreous phenotype. The vitreous was also highly abnormal but instead of the classical membranous anomaly, sparse, irregularly thickened, "beaded" fibrils were seen throughout an otherwise empty-looking gel (type 2 vitreous phenotype). Linkage to *COL2A1* was excluded. Mutations in the gene encoding the α1 chain of type XI collagen (*COL11A1*) on chromosome 1 have been found in seven families [23, 31, 40] and these are, to date, the only mutations associated with the type 2 vitreous phenotype. These pedigrees have a similarly high risk of detachment and giant retinal tear but appear to have a higher prevalence of sensorineural deafness than the type 1 Stickler families [26].

12.4.1.3 Molecular Genetics

Types II and XI are fibrillar collagens and are found in both vitreous and cartilage. Collagens consist of three polypeptide chains (α chains), which are folded into triple helical molecules to form fibrils. Collagen II is a homotrimer, each α chain being the product of the COL2A1 gene. Collagen XI is a heterotrimer with each α chain being the product of a different gene. In vitreous, the three genes are *COL11A1*, *COL5A2* and *COL2A1* and in cartilage *COL11A2* on chromosome 6 replaces *COL5A2*. Mutations of *COL11A2* may thus cause systemic features of Stickler syndrome without eye involvement (type 3 Stickler syndrome).

The difference in severity of clinical features between the type II collagenopathies can be explained in part by the fact that in Stickler syndrome many different mutations in *COL2A1* cause premature termination codons. These result in haploinsufficiency where normal, but half-quantity, collagen is produced. Mutations in the more severe conditions have a dominant negative effect, where normal and mutant collagen are available to co-assemble, with consequent adverse effect on trimer assembly.

Some families have neither of the two vitreoretinal phenotypes and linkage to the known loci has been excluded so there is at least one further locus to be discovered.

12.4.1.4 Management

Once the diagnosis of Stickler syndrome has been established, a coordinated multidisciplinary approach may be needed to manage myopia and retinal detachment, combined conductive and sensorineural deafness, cleft palate and joint problems. Although intelligence is normal, patients of school age may face considerable educational difficulties because of combined visual, hearing and speech impairment. Prophylactic retinopexy should be offered to reduce the risk of retinal detachment [38] and because of the lifetime risk of detachment, all patients require long-term follow-up. Parents and other siblings should also be examined so that affected members of the family are identified, offered prophylaxis and genetic advice.

Summary for the Clinician

- **The Stickler syndromes are dominantly inherited disorders of collagen connective tissue and the commonest inherited cause of rhegmatogenous retinal detachment in childhood**
- **Type 1 Stickler syndrome is caused by mutations in *COL2A1*, the gene for type II collagen**
- **The diagnosis can reliably be made by examination of the vitreous phenotype**
- **Type 2 Stickler syndrome is caused by mutations in *COL11A1*, a gene for type XI collagen and has a different "beaded" vitreous phenotype**
- **Other variable features include cleft palate, deafness and arthropathy**
- **The risk of retinal detachment is extremely high and frequently due to giant retinal tear**
- **The diagnosis should be considered in:**
  - **Neonates with Pierre-Robin sequence or midline cleft**
  - **Infants with spondyloepiphyseal dysplasia associated with myopia or deafness**
  - **Patients with a family history of rhegmatogenous retinal detachment**
  - **Sporadic cases of retinal detachment associated with joint hypermobility, midline clefting, or deafness.**

12.4.2 Kniest Syndrome

Kniest syndrome is an autosomal dominant disorder that shares many similarities with Stickler syndrome. Mutations are found in the same gene as for Type 1 Stickler syndrome (*COL2A1*), but result in dominant-negative effects rather than haploinsufficiency with consequently more severe arthropathy. It typically presents at birth with shortened trunk and limbs, congenital megalophthalmos and flattened nasal bridge. The joints are often large at birth and the fingers long and knobbly. Motor milestones can be delayed because of joint deformities and muscle atrophy may result from disuse. Both conductive and sensorineural hearing loss may be present as with the Stickler syndromes. The intellect is normal and myopia, retinal detachment and giant retinal tear are the major ophthalmic complications.

12.4.3 Spondyloepiphyseal Dysplasia Congenita

Spondyloepiphyseal dysplasia congenita (SEDC) presents at birth with shortening of the trunk and to a lesser extent the extremities. It is inherited as an autosomal dominant disorder and characteristically results from dominant-negative mutations in the gene for type II collagen (*COL2A1*). Patients classically develop a barrel-shaped chest associated with an exaggerated lumbar lordosis which may compromise respiratory function. Odontoid hypoplasia may be present predisposing to cervico-medullary instability and imaging of the cervical spine should be considered prior to general anaesthesia. The limb shortening is disproportionate, affecting mainly the proximal limbs with hands and feet appearing relatively normal. Myopia, retinal detachment and giant retinal tear are the major ophthalmic complications and, as with the other type II collagenopathies, both conductive and sensorineural hearing loss may be present.

12.4.4 Spondyloepimetaphyseal Dysplasia (Strudwick Type)

Spondyloepimetaphyseal dysplasia (SEMD) also forms part of the clinical spectrum of dominantly inherited type II collagenopathies. The features include severe dwarfism, pectus carinatum and scoliosis which are usually marked. Cleft palate and retinal detachment are frequently associated, as with SEDC. Disproportionately short limbs and delayed epiphyseal maturation are present at birth. Radiologically, the disorder is indistinguishable from SEDC during infancy but a characteristic mottled appearance created by alternating zones of osteosclerosis and osteopaenia develops during early childhood.

12.4.5 Vitreoretinopathy Associated with Phalangeal Epiphyseal Dysplasia

Richards [29] reported a large family with dominantly inherited rhegmatogenous retinal detachment, premature arthropathy and development of phalangeal epiphyseal dysplasia, resulting in brachydactyly. The phenotype appears distinct form other type II collagenopathies, but sequencing identified a novel mutation in the C-propeptide region of *COL2A1*. The glycine to aspartic acid change occurred in a region that is highly conserved in all fibrillar collagen molecules.

12.4.6 Dominant Rhegmatogenous Retinal Detachment

Rhegmatogenous retinal detachment without systemic involvement can occur as a dominantly inherited trait. Recent work [28, 30] has identified a number of novel missense mutations in *COL2A1*, some of which have resulted in vitreous phenotypes similar to those seen in isolated cases of rhegmatogenous detachment rather than those seen in Stickler syndrome. Dominant rhegmatogenous retinal detachment (DRRD) is a more appropriate description for this subtype.

12.4.7 Marfan Syndrome

Marfan syndrome is a dominantly inherited disorder of fibrillin production with a prevalence of approximately one in 20,000 and features skeletal, cardiovascular and ocular abnormalities. The fibrillins are high-molecular-weight extracellular glycoproteins, and mutations in the fibrillin gene on chromosome 15 (FBN1) cause Marfan syndrome and dominant ectopia lentis. Fibrillin has been found to be widespread in lens capsule, zonules, iris, ciliary body, choroid and sclera [45]. In a study to correlate genotype with phenotype [35], it was noted that, whereas large-joint hypermobility is more common in those with premature termination codon mutations, lens dislocation and retinal detachment are less common. The association of rhegmatogenous retinal detachment with Marfan syndrome is well recognized and approximately 75% occur below 20 years of age [24]. Retinal detachment due to giant retinal tear formation is reported to occur in 11% [37]. Although there is a significant association with myopia, this is characteristically developmental in contrast to the congenital, nonprogressive myopia found in type 1 Stickler syndrome. In Marfan syndrome the pupils characteristically dilate poorly because of a structural iris abnormality and, when combined with lens subluxation and thin sclera, retinal detachment repair can be particularly difficult. Pars plana lensectomy and internal tamponade are often required.

12.4.8 Ehlers–Danlos Syndrome

The Ehlers–Danlos syndromes are a heterogeneous group of inherited connective tissue disorders that are characterized by joint hypermobility and skin fragility and hyperextensibility. Patients with the autosomal recessive type VI variant of the Ehlers–Danlos syndromes (EDS VI), also classified as the kyphoscoliotic type, are clinically characterized by neonatal kyphoscoliosis, generalized joint laxity, skin fragility, and severe muscle hypotonia at birth. EDS VI results from mutations in the lysyl hydroxylase 1 gene (*PLOD1*) causing a deficiency of lysyl hydroxylase. This enzyme hydroxylates specific lysine residues in the collagen molecule to form hydroxylysines, important in collagen cross-linking, which gives collagen its tensile strength. Ocular involvement in EDS VI includes myopia, thin sclera, microcornea and rhegmatogenous retinal detachment. Retinal detachment repair may be complicated by susceptibility to suprachoroidal haemorrhage because of vascular fragility.

12.4.9 Wagner Vitreoretinopathy

Wagner described 13 affected individuals in a three-generation pedigree with autosomal dominant inheritance, low myopia, fluid vitreous, cortical cataract, and variably affected dark adaptation. The cardinal features noted were the complete absence of the normal vitreal scaffolding and preretinal, equatorial, and avascular greyish-white membranes. Rhegmatogenous retinal detachment was not originally reported. There are no associated systemic features. Twenty-eight members of the original pedigree have been examined [16] and four patients had a history of a rhegmatogenous retinal detachment in one eye at a median age of 20 years and 55% of patients older than 45 years had peripheral tractional retinal detachments. Chorioretinal atrophy and cataract increased with the patients' age. Several families with Wagner syndrome, including the original pedigree, have been linked to 5q14.3.

12.4.10 X-Linked Retinoschisis

X-linked retinoschisis is an uncommon cause of retinal detachment in childhood accounting for 2.5–5% of all paediatric retinal detachments. Most affected children have a characteristic foveal schisis and peripheral retinoschisis is seen in 70% (Fig. 12.5) [12]. Highly elevated, bullous retinoschisis involving the macula may occur in infancy and eventually reattach spontaneously, leaving pigment demarcation lines [11]. Haemorrhage may occur within the schisis cavity or the vitreous. Retinal detachment may occur in up to 16% [12]. A full thickness retinal break occurring de novo or a communication between outer and inner leaf defects in the schisis wall may lead to rhegmatogenous retinal detachment. Full thickness breaks may be effectively managed by scleral buckling procedures. Where communication exists between inner and outer leaf breaks, an internal approach may be required. The gene causing X-linked retinoschisis has now been identified and molecular genetic diagnosis in affected males and carrier females is now possible.

12.4.11 Familial Exudative Vitreoretinopathy

Familial exudative vitreoretinopathy (FEVR) is a bilateral, clinically and genetically heterogeneous condition that is characterized by a failure of peripheral retinal vascularisation. It has a remarkable similarity to retinopathy of prematurity but occurs in full-term infants who are otherwise healthy and have not been treated with oxygen in the neonatal period. The changes may be mild with a peripheral retinal avascular zone, detectable with certainty only by fluorescein angiography, or may slowly progress to cause peripheral neovascularisation and exudative or tractional retinal detachment and vitreous haemorrhage. Rhegmatogenous retinal detachment may also occur. Progression of fundus changes and threat to vision is rare after age 20 years. There is a high incidence of myopia, anisometropia and amblyopia, especially in asymmetric disease. Progressive disease may be treated with peripheral photocoagulation or cryotherapy. Vitreoretinal surgery may be challenging because of adherent posterior hyaloid membrane [20]. Since the original description in 1969 [7] demonstrating autosomal dominant inheritance, many more reports

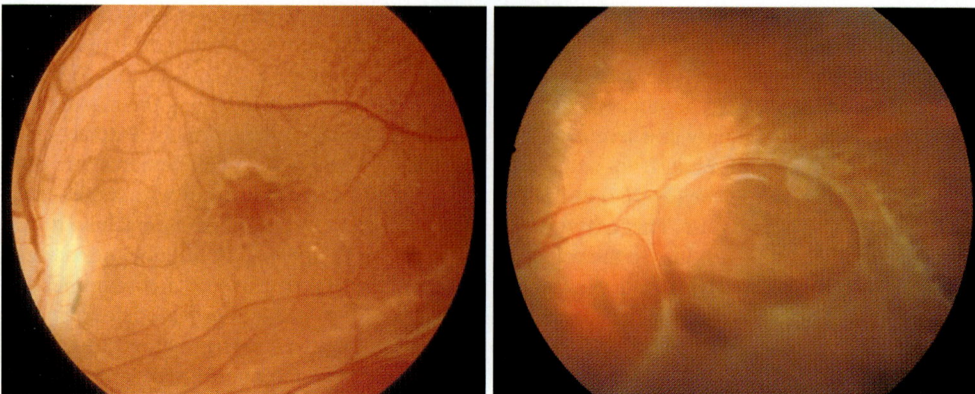

Fig. 12.5. Characteristic foveal and peripheral features of X-linked retinoschisis

have confirmed autosomal dominant, X-linked and even autosomal recessive forms.

The autosomal dominant form (EVR1) can be caused by mutations in the frizzled-4 gene (*FZD4*) on chromosome 11q13-q23 and also by mutations in the LRP5 (low-density lipoprotein receptor-related protein-5) gene, which maps to 11q13.4. The X-linked form (EVR2) can be caused by mutations of the Norrie disease gene (*NDP*), which has been mapped to Xp11.4. The gene products are proteins important in Wnt signalling pathways that regulate vascular development in the eye [41, 46]. The gene underlying EVR3 which has been mapped to 11p12–13 has yet to be identified. Mutations in the LRP5 gene have been suggested to cause autosomal recessive as well as autosomal dominant FEVR [21].

12.4.12 Norrie Disease

Norrie disease is an X-linked recessive syndrome of blindness, deafness, and mental retardation.

Affected males are blind at birth or early infancy. About 25% are mentally retarded and about one-third develop progressive sensorineural hearing loss, with onset at any time from infancy to adult life, which may lead to profound deafness. The ocular findings include abnormal vascularization of the peripheral retina, bilateral retinal folds, traction retinal detachment, vitreous haemorrhage and bilateral retrolental masses. The retinal detachments are usually of early onset and have been diagnosed in utero. Most cases progress to an extensive vitreoretinal mass and bilateral blindness. The gene for Norrie disease has been identified on Xp11.4. Norrin, the product of the Norrie disease gene, is a secreted protein important for normal retinal vascularization and regression of hyaloid vessels and also regulates the interaction of the cochlea with its vasculature.

12.4.13 Incontinentia Pigmenti

Incontinentia pigmenti is an X-linked dominantly inherited disorder usually lethal in males, affecting skin, bones, teeth, the central nervous system and eyes. The characteristic skin lesion begins soon after birth, with a linear eruption of bullae, which resolve to leave a linear pattern of hyperpigmentation. Ocular features are usually apparent within the 1st year of life can occur in up to 77% [18]. The main abnormalities are peripheral vascular abnormalities and retinal pigment epithelial defects. Macular vasculopathy with progressive capillary closure has also been described [13]. The affected eye is often microphthalmic and complications can arise from late tractional retinal detachment in up to half of those with eye involvement [18]. Prophylactic cryotherapy or photocoagulation to the peripheral avascular retina has been reported to arrest vascular proliferation and prevent late tractional detachment. Familial incontinentia pigmenti is caused by mutations in the NEMO gene and is referred to as IP2, or classical incontinentia pigmenti. Sporadic incontinentia pigmenti, the so-called IP1, which maps to Xp11, is categorized as hypomelanosis of Ito.

12.5 Retinal Detachment Complicating Developmental Abnormalities

Paediatric rhegmatogenous retinal detachment has been found to be associated with a developmental abnormality in 41% [44]. These include retinopathy of prematurity, persistent fetal vasculature (persistent hyperplastic primary vitreous), buphthalmos, coloboma, microspherophakia and retinoblastoma.

12.5.1 Congenital Cataract

Retinal detachment complicating surgery for isolated congenital cataract has been reported to occur in 5% of cases with an average interval of 22 years. Detachment may occur during childhood in a minority [10]. Whether this is as a result of cataract surgery or related to an intrinsic abnormality is not entirely clear, although a long delay and retinal detachment also occurring in unoperated eyes would suggest the latter.

12.5.2 Ocular Coloboma

Eyes with ocular colobomas are at a significantly increased risk of detachment and account for approximately 0.5% of paediatric retinal detachments [25]. Giant retinal tears are seen in association with lens colobomas [19] and rhegmatogenous detachment may develop in eyes with choroidal coloboma, when small retinal breaks may be found in the hypoplastic retina overlying the coloboma. Assessment of vision can be difficult and the diagnosis of detachment can be further impaired by nystagmus, microphthalmos and cataract. Retinal breaks occurring away from the colobomatous area may be managed by conventional buckling techniques, provided the sclera is of sufficient quality for suturing and the break can be adequately closed. More usually, the retinal break overlies the colobomatous area. Breaks are often small and may be multiple, and their localization can be aided peroperatively by the identification of "schlieren" during internal drainage. Argon laser photocoagulation may be applied around the border of the colobomatous area and, where this includes the papillomacular bundle, this may be applied prior to retinal reattachment to minimize associated thermal damage to the nerve fibre layer. Both retinal pigment epithelium and Müller cells are vestigial or absent within the coloboma so that to be effective, retinopexy needs to be applied outside the margin. Recurrent detachment is common [15], so permanent internal tamponade is often required.

12.5.3 Optic Disc Pits and Serous Macular Detachment

The association of serous macular detachment and optic disc pits is well recognized and similar findings with the morning glory disc abnormality indicate that these two conditions are variations of the same basic abnormality. Serous macular detachment may occur in 30–50% and usually in patients too young to have a posterior vitreous detachment. Spontaneous resolution is reported to occur in up to 25%, although permanent visual loss may result if macular detachment is prolonged or recurrent. The origin of the subretinal fluid is more likely to be cerebrospinal fluid rather than vitreous, although the evidence is not conclusive. The combination of argon laser photocoagulation with internal tamponade either with or without vitrectomy appears to offer greater chance of successful retinal reattachment. Attempts at internal drainage have suggested that there is no rhegmatogenous element and fluid is displaced by gas tamponade until it is reabsorbed and recurrence is prevented by formation of a chorioretinal adhesion at the disc margin.

12.5.4 Retinopathy of Prematurity

The incidence of early retinal detachment following advanced retinopathy of prematurity (ROP) has been substantially reduced by better screening and prophylactic cryotherapy or photocoagulation. However, the visual results following vitreoretinal surgery for those which do progress to retinal detachment have been very disappointing. The major, and often multiple, surgical challenges need to be carefully weighed against a partial and spontaneous retinal reattachment in up to 10% of cases. Lens-sparing techniques have been advocated for pathology confined posterior to the equator [5]. Preserving the lens whilst gaining surgical access to the vitreous base in the neonatal eye is technically demanding and requires adequate visualization of the pars plicata by using the operating indirect ophthalmoscope or wide-angle viewing systems.

Late retinal detachment following treated or untreated retinopathy of prematurity is well-recognized and is more commonly rhegmatogenous, but may be tractional or a combination of the two. Retinal changes, which may be an indication of regressed ROP, include myopic changes, displacement of macula and retinal vessels, retinal folds, pigmentary changes, incompletely vascularized peripheral retina, abnormal branching and tortuous and telangiectatic vessels. Repair of late retinal detachment is frequently possible with vitreoretinal surgery and the prognosis relates more to the pre-existing visual potential prior to retinal detachment. A recent report reviewed 29 patients with late rhegmatogenous retinal detachment following regressed, untreated ROP [42]. Sixty-three per cent presented between 8 and 20 years and 90% were myopic. The majority of breaks were found in the temporal retina, mainly superotemporal. There was a 69% success after initial surgery with scleral buckling or vitrectomy and, with repeated surgery, a final reattachment rate of 97%.

12.6 Other

12.6.1 Inflammatory or Infectious

In one series, 15% of 34 children with rhegmatogenous retinal detachment had a history of inflammatory or infectious disease in the eye with the detachment [44]. Acute retinal necrosis, characterized by anterior uveitis, occlusive retinal vasculitis and progressive peripheral retinal necrosis, occurs primarily in nonimmunocompromised adults as a result of reactivated herpes simplex or varicella zoster virus infection. The risk of retinal detachment is high, reported to be between 25% and 75% and due to retinal breaks, usually following posterior vitreous detachment after the acute phase is over. Although less common, it has been reported to occur in children [6].

Ocular involvement in paediatric AIDS patients has been reported in 50%, 33% having CMV retinitis and 17% retinal detachment [3].

Although uncommon, bilateral serous retinal detachment in Vogt-Koyanagi-Harada may affect young children, and has been reported in children as young as 4 years old [8].

Ocular toxocariasis is a rare cause of retinal detachment, usually tractional, associated with a peripheral granuloma.

12.6.2 Exudative Retinal Detachment

Exudative retinal detachment is uncommon but has a wide variety of causes in childhood, including Coat's disease, retinoblastoma, choroidal haemangioma, capillary haemangioma, posterior scleritis and Harada's disease. If there is doubt about the diagnosis, computed tomographic (CT) scan or ultrasound, or a careful examination under anaesthesia should be carried out in order to rule out retinoblastoma.

12.7 Prophylaxis in Rhegmatogenous Retinal Detachment

In contrast to most other paediatric blinding retinal disorders, blindness through retinal detachment is in most cases potentially avoidable if a rationale for the prediction and prevention of retinal detachment could be developed. This goal has been frustrated by a lack of understanding of the factors influencing retinal detachment even in high-risk groups, which are only now beginning to be unravelled.

Factors traditionally associated with retinal detachment include refractive error, a positive family history, visible lattice retinopathy and fellow eye involvement, but the nature of these associations is poorly understood. The prevalence of myopia varies enormously and even in Stickler syndrome up to 20 % patients may have no significant refractive error. Many patients with retinal detachment have none of the accepted risk features such as lattice retinopathy and, in those that do, retinal tear formation frequently occurs in areas remote from such pathology, so that the associations with accepted risk factors requires refinement.

In Stickler syndrome there is a high risk of giant retinal tear (GRT) which is often bilateral and a frequent cause of blindness. The rationale for offering prophylaxis in such high-risk cases is to prevent progression of GRT to detachment by applying treatment to the post-oral retina at the site of giant tear development.

A study investigating the role of prophylactic 360° cryotherapy in type 1 Stickler syndrome has recently been completed. Although there were significant differences between the ages of the control and study groups, the risk of retinal detachment in 204 patients with type 1 Stickler syndrome reduced from 62 % to between 3 % and 10 % [38].

References

1. Ahmad N, Richards AJ, Murfett HC et al (2003) Prevalence of mitral valve prolapse in Stickler syndrome. Am J Med Genet 116A:234–237
2. Akabane N, Yamamoto S, Tsukahara I et al (2001) Surgical outcomes in juvenile retinal detachment. Jpn J Ophthalmol 45:409–411
3. Biswas J, Kumar AA, George AE et al (2000) Ocular and systemic lesions in children with HIV. Indian J Pediatr 67:721–724
4. Butler TK, Kiel AW, Orr GM (2001) Anatomical and visual outcome of retinal detachment surgery in children. Br J Ophthalmol 85:1437–1439
5. Capone A Jr, Trese MT (2001) Lens-sparing vitreous surgery for tractional stage 4A retinopathy of prematurity retinal detachments. Ophthalmology 108:2068–2070
6. Chen S, Weinberg GA (2002) Acute retinal necrosis syndrome in a child. Pediatr Infect Dis J 21:78–80
7. Criswick VG, Schepens CL (1969) Familial exudative vitreoretinopathy. Am J Ophthalmol 68:578–594
8. Cunningham ET Jr, Demetrius R, Frieden IJ et al (1995) Vogt-Koyanagi-Harada syndrome in a 4-year old child. Am J Ophthalmol 120:675–677
9. Eagling EM (1974) Ocular damage after blunt trauma to the eye. Its relationship to the nature of the injury. Br J Ophthalmol 58:126–140
10. Francis PJ, Ionides A, Berry V et al (2001) Visual outcome in patients with isolated autosomal dominant congenital cataract. Ophthalmology 108:1104–1108
11. George ND, Yates JR, Bradshaw K et al (1995) Infantile presentation of X linked retinoschisis. Br J Ophthalmol 79:653–657
12. George ND, Yates JR, Moore AT (1996) Clinical features in affected males with X-linked retinoschisis. Arch Ophthalmol 114:274–280
13. Goldberg MF (1998) Macular vasculopathy and its evolution in incontinentia pigmenti. Trans Am Ophthalmol Soc 96:55–65
14. Gonzales CA, Scott IU, Chaudry NA et al (1999) Bilateral rhegmatogenous retinal detachments with unilateral vitreous base avulsion as the presenting signs of child abuse. Am J Ophthalmol 127:475–477
15. Gopal L, Badrinath SS, Sharma T et al (1998) Surgical management of retinal detachments related to coloboma of the choroid. Ophthalmology 105:804–809
16. Graemiger RA, Niemeyer G, Schneeberger SA et al (1995) Wagner vitreoretinal degeneration. Follow-up of the original pedigree. Ophthalmology 102:1830–1839

17. Hagler WS (1980) Retinal dialysis: a statistical and genetic study to determine pathogenic factors. Trans Am Ophthalmol Soc 78:686–733
18. Holmstrom G, Thoren K (2000) Ocular manifestations of incontinentia pigmenti. Acta Ophthalmol Scand 78:348–353
19. Hovland KR, Schepens CL, Freeman HM (1968) Developmental giant retinal tears associated with lens coloboma. Arch Ophthalmol 80:325–331
20. Ikeda T, Fujikado T, Tano Y et al (1999) Vitrectomy for rhegmatogenous or tractional retinal detachment with familial exudative vitreoretinopathy. Ophthalmology 106:1081–1085
21. Jiao X, Ventruto V, Trese MT et al (2004) Autosomal recessive familial exudative vitreoretinopathy is associated with mutations in LRP5. Am J Hum Genet 75:878–884
22. Johnston PB (1991) Traumatic retinal detachment. Br J Ophthalmol 75:18–21
23. Martin S, Richards AJ, Yates JR et al (1999) Stickler syndrome: further mutations in COL11A1 and evidence for additional locus heterogeneity. Eur J Hum Genet 7:807–814
24. Maumenee IH (1981) The eye in the Marfan syndrome. Trans Am Ophthalmol Soc 79:684–733
25. McDonald HR, Lewis H, Brown G et al (1991) Vitreous surgery for retinal detachment associated with choroidal coloboma. Arch Ophthalmol 109:1399–1402
26. Poulson AV, Hooymans JM, Richards AJ et al (2004) Clinical features of type 2 Stickler syndrome. J Med Genet 41:e107
27. Richards AJ, Martin S, Yates JR et al (2000) COL2A1 exon 2 mutations: relevance to the Stickler and Wagner syndromes. Br J Ophthalmol 84:364–371
28. Richards AJ, Meredith S, Poulson AV et al (2004) A novel mutation of COL2A1 resulting in dominantly inherited rhegmatogenous retinal detachment. Invest Ophthalmol Vis Sci 46:663–668
29. Richards AJ, Morgan J, Bearcroft PW et al (2002) Vitreoretinopathy with phalangeal epiphyseal dysplasia, a type II collagenopathy resulting from a novel mutation in the C-propeptide region of the molecule. J Med Genet 39:661–665
30. Richards AJ, Scott JD, Snead MP (2002) Molecular genetics of rhegmatogenous retinal detachment. Eye 16:388–392
31. Richards AJ, Yates JR, Williams R et al (1996) A family with Stickler syndrome type 2 has a mutation in the COL11A1 gene resulting in the substitution of glycine 97 by valine in alpha 1 (XI) collagen. Hum Mol Genet 5:1339–1343
32. Rosner M, Treister G, Belkin M (1987) Epidemiology of retinal detachment in childhood and adolescence. J Pediatr Ophthalmol Strabismus 24:42–44
33. Ross WH (1991) Retinal dialysis: lack of evidence for a genetic cause. Can J Ophthalmol 26:309–312
34. Sarrazin L, Averbukh E, Halpert M et al (2004) Traumatic pediatric retinal detachment: a comparison between open and closed globe injuries. Am J Ophthalmol 137:1042–1049
35. Schrijver I, Liu W, Odom R et al (2002) Premature termination mutations in FBN1: distinct effects on differential allelic expression and on protein and clinical phenotypes. Am J Hum Genet 71: 223–237
36. Scott JD (1977) Retinal dialysis. Trans Ophthalmol Soc U K 97:33–35
37. Sharma T, Gopal L, Shanmugam MP et al (2002) Retinal detachment in Marfan syndrome: clinical characteristics and surgical outcome. Retina 22: 423–428
38. Snead MP, Goodburn S, Poulson AV et al (2004) Retinal detachment in Stickler syndrome. XXIV Meeting Club Jules Gonin, 2004
39. Snead MP, Payne SJ, Barton DE et al (1994) Stickler syndrome: correlation between vitreoretinal phenotypes and linkage to COL 2A1. Eye 8:609–614
40. Snead MP, Yates JR (1999) Clinical and molecular genetics of Stickler syndrome. J Med Genet 36: 353–359
41. Toomes C, Bottomley HM, Jackson RM et al (2004) Mutations in LRP5 or FZD4 underlie the common familial exudative vitreoretinopathy locus on chromosome 11q. Am J Hum Genet 74:721–730
42. Tufail A, Singh AJ, Haynes RJ et al (2004) Late onset vitreoretinal complications of regressed retinopathy of prematurity. Br J Ophthalmol 88:243–246
43. Verdaguer J (1982) Juvenile retinal detachment. Pan American Association of Ophthalmology and American Journal of Ophthalmology Lecture. Am J Ophthalmol 93:145–156
44. Weinberg DV, Lyon AT, Greenwald MJ et al (2003) Rhegmatogenous retinal detachments in children: risk factors and surgical outcomes. Ophthalmology 110:1708–1713
45. Wheatley HM, Traboulsi EI, Flowers BE et al (1995) Immunohistochemical localization of fibrillin in human ocular tissues. Relevance to the Marfan syndrome. Arch Ophthalmol 113:103–109
46. Xu Q, Wang Y, Dabdoub A et al (2004) Vascular development in the retina and inner ear: control by Norrin and Frizzled-4, a high-affinity ligand-receptor pair. Cell 116:883–895
47. Yokoyama T, Kato T, Minamoto A et al (2004) Characteristics and surgical outcomes of paediatric retinal detachment. Eye 18:889–892

Eye Manifestations of Intrauterine Infections

13

Marilyn Baird Mets, Ashima Verma Kumar

13.1 Introduction

The most common congenital infections are summarized by the mnemonic TORCH: *Toxoplasma gondii*, Others, Rubella, Cytomegalovirus, and Herpes simplex virus. "Others" includes treponema pallidum, varicella-zoster virus, Epstein–Barr virus, human immunodeficiency virus, and lymphocytic choriomeningitis virus. There is an additional "other," namely West Nile virus.

These are all agents that produce a relatively mild illness in the mother. More virulent agents result in a spontaneous abortion or stillbirth. They are transmitted transplacentally, and have a direct toxic effect. Additionally, in the first trimester, when the fetus has immature, developing organs, there may be a teratogenic effect. Diagnosis can be made by elevated levels of IgM and IgA antibodies, and if the fetus is unable to eliminate the organism, this may lead to chronic infection and immune tolerance.

13.2 Toxoplasma gondii

13.2.1 Agent and Epidemiology

Toxoplasma gondii derives from the Greek, *toxon* meaning bow (the shape of the proliferative form), and *gondii*, for a rodent (*Ctenodactylus gundi*) indigenous to North Africa from which the organism was first isolated [55]. *Toxoplasma gondii* is an obligate intracellular parasite, which probably evolved from a unicellular alga since it has an organelle similar to a chloroplast. It has a life cycle that has three forms, an oocyst (found in the gut of cats), a tissue cyst, and an active, or proliferative form. The source to humans includes cat feces, in which the oocyst may be infective for up to 1 year in warm, moist soil, and raw meat, in which the tissue cysts are viable. The prevalence in humans varies with age, under 5 years, the antibodies are found in less than 5% of the population, while over 80 years, they are present in 60%.

Seventy percent of the obstetric population have negative antibodies, and is at risk for transmission to the fetus [40]. The risk of passage to the fetus and the severity of the infection are affected by the gestational age at the time of maternal infection. Transmission to the fetus is 25% in the first trimester, 75% in the third trimester, and over 90% in the last few weeks of pregnancy. The severity of the fetal infection is inversely related to gestational age, with the earlier infections being the most severe [23, 61].

13.2.2 Diagnosis

The diagnosis is made by multiple methods including ELIZA for IgM and IgA. It is important to test undiluted samples, because the serum levels may be very low in eye disease. The work-up includes a CBC, with differential and platelet levels, and a CT scan looking for hydrocephalus and intracranial calcifications especially in the periventricular regions.

13.2.3 Systemic Manifestations

The systemic manifestations are the classic triad of chorioretinitis, hydrocephalus, and intracranial calcifications. Ninety percent of neonates are asymptomatic; however, they can show a continuous clinical spectrum including: abnormal cerebrospinal fluid, anemia, seizures, intracranial calcifications, jaundice, fever, hepato splenomegaly, hydrocephalus, microcephalus, retardation, vomiting, and diarrhea [42, 70].

13.2.4 Eye Manifestations

Eighty-five percent of patients with subclinical congenital infections are reported to develop chorioretinitis [70]. The eye manifestations of congenital toxoplasmosis found in a large study are summarized in Table 13.1 [48].

Anterior Segment. Microcornea was seen in 19% of patients and cataracts in 10% [49]. It should be noted that these were never isolated findings and that they were always seen in association with posterior segment disease.

Retina. The most common eye finding in patients with congenital toxoplasmosis is chorioretinal scars, which were present in 79% of the patients. The classic location is the macula (Fig. 13.1); however, the most common location was in the periphery (64%). If you consider the total surface area of the retina, there was a predisposition for the macular area (58%). In addition, active retinitis was seen in 11% and retinal detachment in 10% [49].

Optic Nerve. Optic atrophy was present in 20% of patients with congenital toxoplasmosis [49].

Microphthalmia and Phthisis. Microphthalmia and phthisis were reported in 13% and 4%, respectively [49].

Visual acuity ranges from 20/20 to 20/400 in the presence of macular lesions, the better vision being unexpected [49]. Therefore, pre-

Table 13.1. Ophthalmology manifestations of congenital toxoplasmosis

Diagnoses of patients checked	Percentage of patients with findings
Chorioretinal scars	79 (74)
Macular	58 (52/89)
Juxtapapillary	52 (46/89)
Peripheral	64 (57/89)
Strabismus	33 (31)
Nystagmus	27 (25)
Optic atrophy	20 (19)
Microcornea	19 (18)
Microphthalmos	13 (12)
Retinitis (active)	11 (10)
Cataract	10 (9)
Retinal detachment	10 (9)
Vitreitis (active)	5 (5)
Phthisis	4 (4)

Numerator represents number of patients with finding; denominator is the total number, unless otherwise specified. Patients with bilateral retinal detachment in whom the location of scars was not possible were excluded from the denominator. Number in parentheses is total number of patients with findings

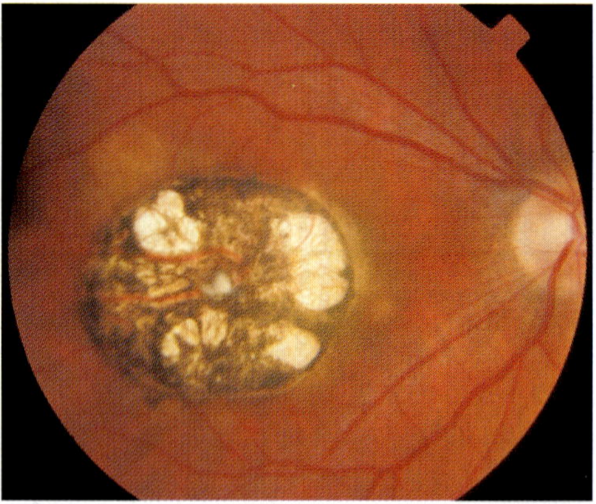

Fig. 13.1. The right eye of a 25-year-old white male with a history of congenital toxoplasmosis. Vision recorded at this exam was 20/80. The slide shows a characteristic "toxo" lesion of the macula with areas of significant atrophy in which both choroidal vessels and sclera are visible

dicting future vision in a preverbal child should be done with caution. Of the patients followed from the newborn period and treated, 29% had bilateral visual impairment with the vision in the better eye being less than 20/40. Causes for this visual impairment in eyes with quiescent lesions included macular scars, dragging of the macula secondary to a peripheral lesion, retinal detachment, optic atrophy, cataract, amblyopia, and phthisis. Recurrences were seen in 13% of treated patients, and 44% of untreated historical patients, and occurred contiguous to old scars, but also in previously uninvolved retina. This latter finding is consistent with the fact that toxoplasmosis cysts have been demonstrated in mouse retinas, with no disturbance of the retinal structure, thus on ophthalmologic examination would appear normal [10]. Recurrent infection can result in further loss of vision, especially if they occur in the macular area.

13.2.5 Treatment

Treatment is triple therapy with pyramethamine, sulfadiazine, and leukovorin [47]. Leukovorin (folinic acid) should always be administered in conjunction with pyramethamine to provide for the synthesis of nucleic acids by the human cells. Monitoring by CBC and platelet counts weekly is required because of the possible, reversible bone marrow suppression from the pyramethamine. In spite of these required precautions, this therapy can be used safely in very young infants for extended periods of time.

13.2.6 Prevention

Prevention includes avoidance of raw meat and cat feces (changing cat litter boxes and gardening) during pregnancy. If a pregnant woman is known to contract toxoplasmosis during her pregnancy, treatment with spiramycin decreases the possibility of passage of the organism to the fetus [17, 22, 23]. Spiramycin has no known teratogenic effect. Later in gestation, if the fetus is known to be infected, treatment with pyramethamine and sulfadiazine is appropriate [17–19, 36].

13.3 Rubella Virus

13.3.1 Agent and Epidemiology

The rubella virus is a member of the Togaviridae family in which the virus contains a single-stranded RNA surrounded by a lipid envelope, or "toga." The congenital form was first described by an ophthalmologist, Sir Norman McAlister Gregg in 1941. He practiced in Sydney, Australia, where he reported several cases of congenital cataracts, congenital heart disease, and deafness associated with rubell a during pregnancy [31]. This represents the first demonstration of teratogenicity secondary to a viral agent. Rubella has worldwide distribution, and is a major cause of blindness in developing countries. However, it is rare in the United States since its epidemic pattern was interrupted in 1969 by widespread use of the vaccine [3].

13.3.2 Transmission

Transplacental infection occurs during the viremic phase in the mother, resulting in fetal viremia. The incidence of congenital infection is dependent on the month of gestation during exposure, with it being 90% in the first 11 weeks, 50% during weeks 11–20, 37% during weeks 20–35, and 100% during the last month of pregnancy. However, the rate of congenital defects is 100% in the first 11 weeks, 30% in weeks 11–20, and none after that. Interestingly, cataracts and glaucoma are observed when the exposure is in the first 2 months, and retinopathy during the first 5 months [52, 63]. Virus may persist for months to years after birth, so appropriate precautions should be taken.

13.3.3 Diagnosis

The presence of IgM antibodies to rubella in cord blood confirms the diagnosis. Also, viral throat culture may be performed, or serum sampling, for serially rising IgG titers.

13.3.4 Systemic Manifestations

The most common finding is hearing loss, seen in 44% of cases [39]. Other abnormalities include intrauterine growth retardation, heart disease (atrial and ventricular septal defects, and patent ductus arteriosus), microcephaly, and mental retardation. Hepatitis and hepatomegaly may also be seen, and, in the perinatal period, petechiae secondary to thrombocytopenia.

13.3.5 Eye Manifestations

Cornea. The cornea may be edematous either from endotheliopathy (secondary to live virus in the aqueous), or glaucoma [71, 72].

Iris and Ciliary Body. These structures may be poorly developed if the virus was contracted early (first trimester), resulting in iris hypoplasia. In addition, a chronic, granulomatous iridocyclitis may persist with focal necrosis and vacuolization of the pigment epithelium of the iris and ciliary body.

Lens. Virus infection during the first trimester effects lens development and results in cataract formation, usually in the form of a nuclear cataract, but may be total. Live virus persists for years and appropriate precautions should be taken during cataract extraction to minimize exposure to cortical material. A robust inflammatory reaction may follow surgery and systemic steroids may be required.

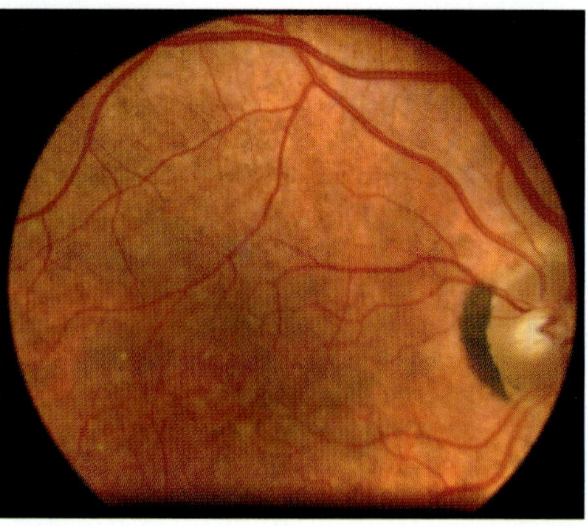

Fig. 13.2. The right fundus of a 32-year-old Black woman with a history of congenital rubella syndrome. The patient was deaf and mute, and showed some developmental delay. Vision in this eye was 20/25. Salt-and-pepper background retinopathy can be seen throughout the slide but especially in the macular area

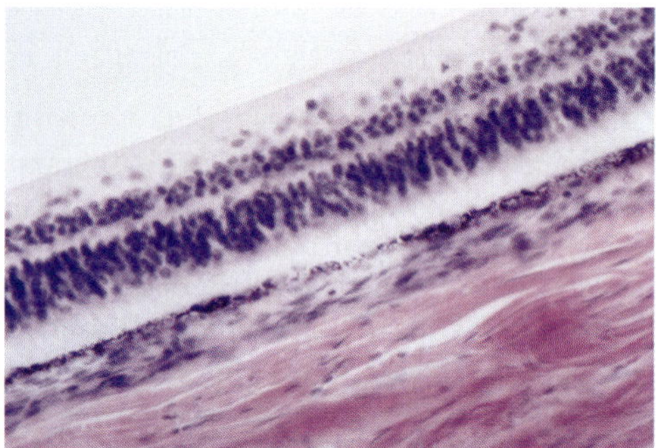

Fig. 13.3. A light micrograph of hematoxylin-eosin stained retina of a child with congenital rubella syndrome. Between the neuroretina above and the choroid below lies the retinal pigment epithelium (see *arrow*). It can be seen that the normal palisade of even pigmentation is disrupted. This variability in RPE pigmentation is the cause for the salt-and-pepper appearance in the retinopathy of rubella syndrome

Retina. The classic retinal finding is described as "salt and pepper" retinopathy, and was described in 22% of patients in a large study. (Fig. 13.2) [21]. It corresponds to a histopathologic depigmentation of the retinal pigment epithelium without associated inflammation

(Fig. 13.3). The distribution of this finding varies greatly and is associated with a normal ERG.

Glaucoma. Glaucoma is reported in 10% of children with congenital rubella syndrome [71]. The pathogenesis varies from abnormal development of the angle similar to primary congenital glaucoma, to glaucoma secondary to chronic iridocyclitis, to angle closure secondary to a large cataractous lens.

Microphthalmos. Microphthalmos and/or microcornea have been described in 10% of patients [71]. Microphthalmos is often associated with cataract, and it is postulated that it reflects the growth retardation effect of the virus on developing tissues paralleling the systemic growth retardation [74].

13.3.6 Treatment

Therapy is supportive.

13.3.7 Prevention

Use of the vaccine RA-27 has had an enormous impact on the incidence of congenital rubella, with the last major outbreak in the United States being in 1964 [3].

13.4 Cytomegalovirus

13.4.1 Agent and Epidemiology

Cytomegalovirus is a member of the herpesvirus group, and was first described in the late nineteenth century as a rare cause of "cytomegalic inclusion disease" of the fetus and newborn [35]. It is the cause for the most common intrauterine infection, with reported rates ranging from 0.5% to 2.4% of live births [24]. Infection is usually subclinical. The prevalence of latent infections in young adults varies with age and geography, increasing with age, and being more prevalent in developing countries [43, 67].

13.4.2 Transmission

Prenatal transmission is thought to occur during maternal viremia secondary to a primary infection (most serious damage to the fetus), reinfection, or reactivation of a latent maternal infection [27]. Natal transmission may occur secondary to exposure to genital secretions at the time of delivery. Also, neonatal transmission may occur from ingestion of breast milk.

13.4.3 Diagnosis

Specific IgM antibody in the neonate is strong presumptive evidence. Isolation of virus from the infant within the first 3 weeks definitively makes the diagnosis, and virus has been recovered from urine, cerebrospinal fluid, saliva, buffy coat, aqueous, biopsy, and postmortem tissue [26]. PCR analysis is also promising [64].

13.4.4 Systemic Manifestations

Most neonates with congenital cytomegalovirus infection, 90–95%, are asymptomatic during the neonatal period [67]. Clinical manifestations include intrauterine growth retardation, thrombocytopenic purpura, microcephaly, (periventricular calcifications), hepatosplenomegaly, jaundice, pneumonia, and sensorineural deafness [21].

13.4.5 Eye Manifestations

Anterior Segment. Corneal opacities have been described in pathology specimens [56]. Bilateral anterior polar cataracts were seen in 1 of 42 symptomatic patients studied by Coats [16].

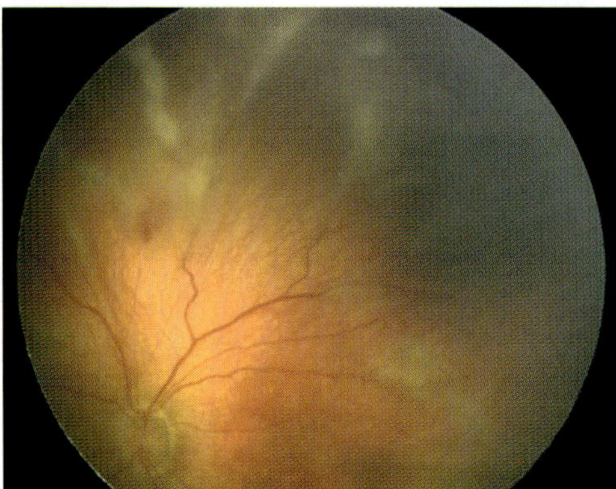

Fig. 13.4. The left fundus of a 6-month-old female child with congenital cytomegalovirus (demonstrating CMV retinitis). The superior vessels are sheathed

Retina. The retinal disease is a chorioretinitis, resulting in a chorioretinal scar similar to that of toxoplasmosis. Dobbins reported 15 % of patients showed retinal disease, and a later study by Coats had 22 % of symptomatic patients with retinal disease (7 % macular and 14 % peripheral scars) [16, 24]. The retinitis usually develops in patients with clinically apparent cytomegalic inclusion disease, but has been reported as the only manifestation of congenital CMV infection. (Fig. 13.4) [66]. In addition, it has been reported that retinal disease developed several weeks after birth [56]. The histopathology has been reported as "many inclusion bodies in the retina and a few in the choroid, accompanied by extensive chorioretinitis. Accumulation of inclusion bodies in the retina results in focal destruction and gave rise to the development of pseudocolobomas" [51].

Optic Nerve. Optic nerve hypoplasia and optic nerve coloboma have been described in association with cytomegalic inclusion disease [34]. These findings are consistent with the teratogenic effect on the central nervous system seen in this infection, which results in faulty organogenesis. In a large study by Coats, 7 % of 42 symptomatic patients had bilateral optic atrophy [24].

Other. Cyclopia and anophthalmia have also been reported, and further support the evidence for a teratogenic effect [12, 28].

13.4.6 Treatment

Ganciclovir and foscarnet delivered intravenously are being used and studied; however, trials of both show that viruria returns to pretreatment levels after the cessation of the drug [4, 62, 68]. Intravitreal therapy with ganciclovir implants has also been used for the eye disease.

13.4.7 Prevention

Pregnant women who are seronegative should practice good hygiene when they are around young children either at home or in group child-care settings [21].

13.5 Herpes Simplex Virus

13.5.1 Agent and Epidemiology

Herpes simplex virus (HSV) is a double-stranded DNA virus. HSV infections were first described by the Greeks, and Hippocrates used the word "herpes," which means to creep or crawl to describe the spreading of the lesion [69]. There are two types of Herpes simplex virus (HSV), HSV type 1 and type 2. HSV-1 is the oral strain, and is responsible for mouth lesions, eye infections, and encephalitis, while HSV-2 is the genital strain, and produces genital infection [26, 69]. The latter is transmitted venereally, the former is not.

13.5.2 Transmission

Of herpes infections seen in the neonatal period, 4 % are congenital, 86 % natal, and 10 % postnatal [69]. Therefore, this is most often a neonatal disease, and not a congenital disease. It is thought that the congenital infection occurs during maternal leukocyte-associated viremia with transplacental transmission. The natal transmission is due to aspiration of infected vaginal secretions on passage through the birth canal. Other possible entry sites include eyes, scalp, skin, and umbilical cord [54, 68, 69].

13.5.3 Diagnosis

The diagnosis can be made definitively by isolation of the virus from vesicular fluid, nasal secretions, conjunctival secretions, buffy coat of blood, and cerebral spinal fluid of the infant [29].

13.5.4 Systemic Manifestations

Systemic manifestations reported in 30 patients with congenital HSV include low birth weight, small for gestational age, microcephaly, seizures, diffuse brain damage, intracranial calcifications, scars on skin or digits, pneumonitis, and hepatomegaly [38]. Infants with natal or postnatal herpes commonly present 5–15 days postnatally and resemble bacterial sepsis: alterations in temperature, lethargy, respiratory distress, anorexia, vomiting, and cyanosis. The overall mortality rate from untreated, neonatal HSV infection is 49% and only 26% of survivors develop normally [26].

13.5.5 Eye Manifestations

Thirteen percent of neonates with HSV have eye manifestations [26]. It is difficult to separate congenital and neonatal cases in the literature.

Anterior Segment. Conjunctivitis, keratitis, iridocyclitis, iris atrophy, posterior synechiae, and cataract have been described in congenital and neonatal herpes [53].

Retina. Retinitis, chorioretinitis, chorioretinal scarring, and white vitreous masses have been described. (Fig. 13.5) [41, 53, 58].

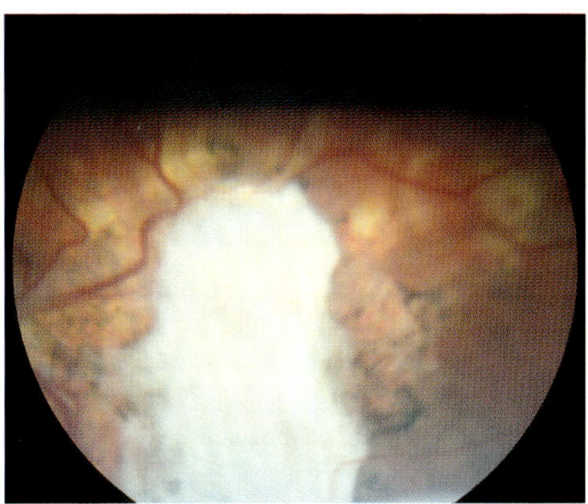

Fig. 13.5. The left fundus of a 13-year-old boy with a diagnosis of congenital herpes simplex virus infection. Centrally, there is a large white gliotic scar overlying the macular area. In the background there are areas of migration of the pigment of the retinal pigment epithelium

Optic Nerve. There have been cases of optic neuritis and optic atrophy [41, 53].

Microphthalmia. Microcornea and microphthalmia have been described in a patient with associated intrauterine growth retardation and microcephaly, suggesting a teratogenic effect of early intrauterine herpes [41].

13.5.6 Treatment

For disseminated herpes infections, acyclovir is the drug of choice, delivered intravenously at a dose of 30 mg/kg per day for 10 days to 4 weeks [55]. The major side effect is renal toxicity. Vidarabine is also administered as a single IV infusion of 15 mg/kg per day over 12 h. Hepatic toxicity and bone marrow suppression are potential side effects.

Topical antivirals (vidarabine, trifluorothymidine, and idoxuridine) are used to treat the epithelial keratitis along with debridement.

13.5.7 Prevention

Perinatal screening and neonatal treatment may be helpful for the neonatal and postnatal forms.

13.6 Lymphocytic Choriomeningitis Virus

This agent is in the "other" category, but will be discussed more extensively because the author feels it is greatly underdiagnosed due to lack of knowledge.

13.6.1 Agent and Epidemiology

Lymphocytic choriomeningitis virus (LCMV) is an arena virus that was discovered in 1933 but not classified until the late 1960s, when it was placed in the newly formed arena virus family of single-stranded RNA viruses with rodent reservoirs [2, 59]. *Mus musculus*, the common house mouse, is both the natural host and reservoir for the virus, which is transferred vertically within the mouse population by intrauterine infection [57, 59]. A nationwide outbreak in the 1970s provided evidence that pet (Syrian) hamsters may be competent alternative reservoirs [8, 20, 33, 60, 65]. Infections from house mice are associated with substandard housing, such as trailer parks and inner city dwellings [57]. Outbreaks have also been attributed to laboratory mice and hamsters; laboratory workers, especially those handling mice or hamsters, have a higher risk of infection [6, 25, 37]. Transmission is thought to be airborne; from contamination of food by infected mouse urine, feces, and saliva [37] or, possibly, from the bites of infected rodents [57]. The first case of congenital LCMV in the United States was reported in 1993 [45].

13.6.2 Transmission

Transmission to the fetus is thought to occur during maternal viremia. Most likely, as with the other agents, the earlier in gestation, the more serious the sequelae.

13.6.3 Diagnosis

Although complement fixation (CF) tests for LCMV are widely available, CF antibodies are short-lived; the test is insensitive and should not be utilized. Immunofluorescent antibody (IFA) tests and Western blot assays are sensitive, detect both IgM and IgG antibody, and are available both commercially as well as at the Centers for Disease Control (CDC). Enzyme-linked immunosorbent assay (ELISA) is also a sensitive diagnostic modality, but it is performed only at the CDC.

13.6.4 Systemic Manifestations

A recent publication identified 26 cases of congenital LCMV in the world literature between 1955 and 1996 and summarized the ten cases reported in the United States [73]. The most common systemic, neonatal findings among these cases were macrocephaly and microcephaly. A subsequent report summarizing 49 cases in the world literature states that 17 of 19 infants in whom imaging was reported showed hydrocephalus or intracranial calcifications [5]. Evidently, systemic signs suggesting congenital infection are infrequent though neonatal meningitis, hepatosplenomegaly, and congenital heart disease have been reported [5, 50, 73]. As development progresses, neurologic abnormalities become more obvious, including cerebral palsy, mental retardation, and seizures [5]. There have been two cases reported in which the eye findings were the only manifestation [11].

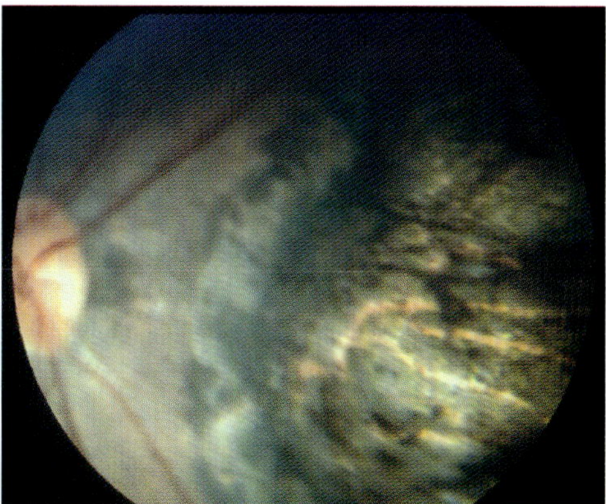

Fig. 13.6. The left eye of a 3-year-old child with a diagnosis of congenital lymphocytic choriomeningitis virus (LCMV). A large chorioretinal scar is visible filling the nasal retina. There are also some irregularities of the retinal pigment epithelium just nasal to the disc at the 9 and 11 o'clock positions. There appears to be some straightening of the nasal arcade vessels secondary to the scarring

Table 13.2. Eye findings described in congenital LCMV

Finding	
Chorioretinal scars	
Generalized	71% (20)
Macula	36% (10)
Optic atrophy	21% (6)
Nystagmus	10% (3)
Esotropia	4% (1)
Microphthalmos	4% (1)
Cataract	4% (1)
Retinitis	4% (1)

Total number of eyes described in the literature is 28. Each eye may have more than one finding, therefore the percentages do not add up to 100%

13.6.5 Eye Manifestations

The eye findings of LCMV described in the US literature (17 cases), 14 with eye findings described (28 eyes), are listed in Table 13.2 [50]. The most common finding is chorioretinal scars in the periphery (20 eyes) (Fig. 13.6). Macular chorioretinal scars were the second most prevalent findings (ten eyes) and in five of these eyes there was also peripheral scarring. Optic atrophy was seen bilaterally in three patients, but always in association with extensive chorioretinal scars and therefore it may be secondary to the scarring. Nystagmus was present in three cases, but that along with esotropia and exotropia, each in one patient, is probably secondary to the visual loss due to the chorioretinal scarring. The cataract and microphthalmia were seen in the same eye.

13.6.6 Treatment

Treatment is supportive.

13.6.7 Prevention

Pregnant women should be informed to avoid mice and hamsters.

13.7 Others

13.7.1 Treponema Pallidum

The eye manifestations of congenital syphilis include corneal opacities, scarring from uveitis, cataract, glaucoma, pigmentary retinopathy (salt and pepper), and optic atrophy [46].

13.7.2 Varicella-Zoster Virus

The ocular manifestations described in the congenital varicella syndrome include chorioretinitis, both atrophy and hypoplasia of the optic nerve, congenital cataract, and Horner's syndrome [44].

13.7.3 Human Immunodeficiency Virus

The incidence of children with congenital HIV is decreasing dramatically with the advent of new drugs. Both CMV retinitis and toxoplasmic chorioretinitis have been described in this patient population [7, 9].

13.7.4 Epstein–Barr Virus

Congenital Epstein–Barr virus infection (infectious mononucleosis) has been reported associated with congenital cataracts in two of five cases [29].

These agents produce a relatively mild illness in the mother and are transmitted transplacentally to the fetus and have both a direct toxic and a teratogenic effect. Often, because of immunologic immaturity, the infant is unable to eliminate the organisms and immune tolerance and chronic infection results.

13.8 West Nile Virus

13.8.1 Agent and Epidemiology

West Nile virus (WNV) was first isolated from a febrile patient in the West Nile district of Uganda in 1937. From 1937 to the early 1990s, human outbreaks, manifesting as mild febrile illnesses, were rarely reported in Israel and Africa. Since 1996, there have been outbreaks involving thousands of people in Romania, Russia, Israel, and the United States and Canada. More than 4,000 people were affected in the Ohio and Mississippi River basins in 2002. Eighty-five percent of human infections occur in August and September, consistent with the bird-mosquito-bird cycle. Increased age is a risk factor for mortality.

West Nile virus is a single-stranded RNA flavivirus belonging to the Japanese encephalitis virus antigenic complex. This complex contains several viruses that cause encephalitis in humans: St. Louis encephalitis virus in the Americas, Japanese encephalitis virus in East Asia, and Murray Valley encephalitis virus and Kunjin virus in Australia. Two lineages of WNV exist. Only lineage 1 viruses cause human disease. The virus has minimally evolved genetically since being isolated in 1999 [30].

13.8.2 Transmission

WNV is transmitted in a bird-mosquito-bird cycle with passerine birds serving as the primary host and mosquitoes from the genus *Culex* serving as the primary vectors. The virus, however, has been isolated from 29 mosquito species in the United States alone [13, 30]. Almost all human infections with WNV have been caused by mosquito bites. However, in 2002, there were several cases reporting transmission via other modalities, including one baby transplacentally, one baby via breast milk, two laboratory workers via percutaneous inoculation, four recipients of organs from a single donor, and 23 recipients of transfused platelets, red blood cells, or fresh frozen plasma [30].

13.8.3 Diagnosis

Diagnosis is made by detecting the IgM antibody in serum or CSF using the IgM antibody-capture enzyme-linked immunosorbent assay (MAC-ELISA). Of patients presenting with meningoencephalitis, 90% will demonstrate IgM antibody in the CSF within 8 days of onset of clinical symptoms. Because IgM antibody may persist in serum for more than 500 days, a fourfold or higher increase in WNV-specific neutralizing antibody titer in serum samples is considered confirmatory of acute infection. A set of other flaviviruses should be included in the assay for comparison [13].

13.8.4 Systemic and Eye Manifestations

There has only been one case report of transplacental transmission. This infant presented with bilateral chorioretinitis, clear vitreous, and severe neurologic impairment [1, 14, 30].

13.8.5 Treatment

All patients should be hospitalized for observation and supportive care, and to rule out treatable CNS conditions. There is no vaccine. Antiviral agents, including ribavirin, interferon alpha, and human immunoglobulin, have not proven effective [13, 14].

13.8.6 Prevention

Pregnant women should avoid mosquito bites by wearing protective clothing and using repellants containing N,N-diethyl-m-toluamide (DEET) [14].

Summary for the Clinician

- The eye finding most characteristic of a prenatal, and therefore, congenital infection is a chorioretinal scar or an active chorioretinitis as can be seen in congenital toxoplasmosis, cytomegalovirus, herpes simplex, lymphocytic choriomeningitis virus, varicella-zoster infections, and most recently West Nile virus. Congenital cataracts are suggestive, but less specific for congenital infection. They may be a relatively isolated finding in rubella, syphilis, varicella-zoster, and Epstein–Barr virus infections. When they are present in congenital toxoplasmosis, herpes simplex, and cytomegalovirus, they are associated with extensive eye involvement. Other manifestations are less common, as discussed above. The mechanism of action of these agents appears to be both a direct toxic and a teratogenic effect.

Acknowledgements. This paper is supported in part by grants to Dr. Mets from the Guild Fund of the Children's Memorial Hospital, and Research to Prevent Blindness (unrestricted grant), Chicago, Illinois.

References

1. Alpert SG, Fergerson J, Noel LP (2003) Intrauterine West Nile Virus: ocular and systemic findings. Am J Ophthalmol 136:733–735
2. Armstrong C, Lillie R (1934) Experimental lymphocytic choriomeningitis of monkeys and mice produced by a virus encountered in studies of the 1933 St. Louis encephalitis epidemic. Public Health Rep (Wash) 49:1019–1027
3. Bart KJ, Orenstein WA, Preblud SR et al (1985) Elimination of rubella and congenital rubella from the United States. Pediatr Infect Dis J 4:14–21
4. Bartlett JG (1997) The Johns Hopkins Hospital guide to medical care of patients with HIV infection. Williams and Wilkins, Baltimore
5. Barton LL, Mets M (2001) Congenital lymphocytic choriomeningitis virus infection: decade of rediscovery (Erratum in: Clin Infect Dis (2001) 33:1445). Clin Infect Dis 33:370–374
6. Baum S, Lewis A, Rowe W, Huebner R (1966) Epidemic non-meningitic lymphocytic-choriomeningitis infection: an outbreak in a population of laboratory personnel. N Engl J Med 274: 934–936
7. Baumal C, Levin A, Read S (1999) Cytomegalovirus retinitis in immunosuppressed children. Am J Ophthalmol 127:550–557
8. Biggar R, Woodall J, Walter P, Haughie G (1975) Lymphocytic choriomeningitis outbreak associated with pet hampsters: fifty-seven cases from New York state. JAMA 232:494–500
9. Bremond-Gignac D, Aron-Rosa D, Rohrlich P, Deplus S, Faye A, Vilmer E (1995) Cytomegalovirus retinitis in children with AIDS acquired through maternal-fetal transmission. J Fr Ophtalmol 18: 91–95
10. Brezin AP, Kasner L, Thulliez P, Li Q, Daffos F, Nussenblatt RB, Chan CC (1994) Ocular toxoplasmosis in the fetus. Retina 14:19–26
11. Brezin AP, Thulliez P, Cisneros B, Mets MB, Saron M (2000) Lymphocytic choriomeningitis virus chorioretinitis mimicking ocular toxoplasmosis in two otherwise normal children [In Process Citation]. Am J Ophthalmol 130:245–247
12. Byrne PJ, Silver MM, Gilbert JM, Cadera W, Tanswell AK (1987) Cyclopia and congenital cytomegalovirus infection. Am J Med Genet 28:61–65

13. Campbell GL, Marfin AA, Lanciotti RS, Gubler DJ (2002) West Nile virus. The Lancet Infectious Diseases 2:519–529
14. Centers for Disease Control and Prevention (2002) Provisional surveillance summary of the West Nile Virus Epidemic: United States, January-November 2002. Morbidity and Mortality Weekly Report 51:1129–1146
15. Childs J, Glass G, Korch G, Ksiazek T, Leduc J (1992) Lymphocytic choriomeningitis virus infection and house mouse (MUS musculus) distribution in urban Baltimore. Am J Trop Med Hyg 47:27–34
16. Coats DK, Demmler GJ, Paysse EA, Du LT, Libby C (2000) Ophthalmologic findings in children with congenital cytomegalovirus infection. J AAPOS 4:110–116
17. Couvreur J, Desmonts G, Thiulliez P (1988) Prophylaxis of congenital toxoplasmosis. Effects of spiramycin on placental infection. J Antimicrobial Chemother 22:193–200
18. Couvreur J, Thulliez P, Daffos F et al (1993) In utero treatment of toxoplasmic fetopathy with the combination pyramethamine-sulfadiazine. Fetal Diagn Ther 8:45–50
19. Daffos F, Forestier F, Capella-Pavlovsky M et al (1988) Prenatal management of 746 pregnancies at risk for congenital toxoplasmosis. N Eng J Med 318:271–275
20. Deibel R, Woodall J, Decher W, Schryver G (1975) Lymphocytic choriomeningitis virus in man: serologic evidence of association with pet hamsters. JAMA232:501–504
21. Demmler GJ (1996) Congenital cytomegalovirus infection and disease. Advances in Pediatr Dis 11:135–162
22. Desmonts G, Couvreur J (1974) Congenital toxoplasmosis. A prospective study of 378 pregnancies. N Eng J Med 290:1110–1116
23. Desmonts G, Couvreur J (1984) Congenital toxoplasmosis. Prospective study of the outcome of pregnancy in 542 women with toxoplasmosis acquired during pregnancy. Ann Pediatr (Paris) 31:805–809
24. Dobbins J, Stewart J, demmler G. Surveillance of congenital cytomegalovirus disease, 1990–1991: collaborating Registry Group. *MMWR CDC Surveill Summ.* 1992;41:35–39
25. Dykewicz C, Dato V, Fisher-Hoch S, Howarth M, Perez-Oronoa G, Ostrof S, Gar H, Schonberge L, McCormick J (1992) Lymphocytic choriomengitis outbreak associated with nude mice in a research institute. JAMA 267:1349–1353
26. Feigin R, Cherry J (1998) Textbook of pediatric infectious disease, 4th edn., vol. 1. WB Saunders, Philadelphia
27. Fowler KB, Stagno S, Pass RF, Britt WJ, Boll TJ, Alford CA (1992) The outcome of congenital cytomegalovirus infection in relation to maternal antibody status [see comments]. N Engl J Med 326:663–667
28. Frenkel LD, Keys MP, Hefferen SJ, Rola-Pleszczynski M, Bellanti JA (1980) Unusual eye abnormalities associated with congenital cytomegalovirus infection. Pediatrics 66:763–766
29. Goldberg G, Fulginiti V, Ray G, Ferry P, Jones J, Cross H, Minnich L (1981) In utero Epstein-Barr virus (infectious mononucleosis) infection. JAMA 246:1579–1581
30. Petersen LR, Marfin AA, Gubler DJ (2003) West Nile Virus. JAMA 290:524–528
31. Gregg NM (1941) Congenital cataract following German measles in the mother. Trans Ophthalmol Soc Aust 3:35
32. Guyton TB, Ehrlich F, Blanc WA et al (1957) New observations in generalized cytomegalic-inclusion disease of the newborn: report of a case with chorioretinitis. N Engl J Med 257:803–807
33. Hirsch M, Moellering R, Pope H, Poskanzer D (1974) Lymphocytic-choriomeningitis-virus infection traced to a pet hamster. N Engl J Med 291:610–612
34. Hittner HM, Speer ME, Rudolph AJ (1981) Examination of the anterior vascular capsule of the lens: III. Abnormalities in infants with congenital infection. J Pediatr Ophthalmol Strabismus 18: 55–60
35. Ho M (1991) History of cytomegalovirus. In: Ho M (ed) Cytomegalovirus: biology and infection. Plenum, New York, pp 1–10, 57–60, 189–203
36. Hohlfeld P, Daffos F, Thulliez P et al (1989) Fetal toxoplasmosis: outcome of pregnancy and infant follow-up after in utero treatment. J Pediatr 115: 765–769
37. Hotchin J (1971) The contamination of laboratory animals with lymphocytic choriomeningitis virus. Am J Pathol 64:747–769
38. Hutto C, Arvin A, Jacob R et al (1987) Intrauterine herpes simplex virus infections. J Pediatr 110: 97–101
39. Keir E (1965) Results of rubella in pregnancy. II. Hearing defects. Med J Austral 2:691–698
40. Kimball A, Kean B, Fuchs F (1971) Congenital toxoplasmosis: a prospective study of 4,048 obstetric patients. Am J Obstet Gynecol 111:211–218
41. Komorous JM, Wheeler CE, Birggaman RA, Caro I (1977) Intrauterine herpes simplex infections. Arch Dermatol 113:918–922
42. Koppe JG, Loewer-Sieger D, de Roever-Bonnet H (1986) Results of 20-year follow-up of congenital toxoplasmosis. Lancet 1:254–256

43. Krech U (1973) Complement-fixing antibodies against cytomegalovirus in different parts of the world. Bull World Health Organ 49:103–106
44. Lambert SR, Taylor D, Kriss A, Holzel H, Heard S (1989) Ocular manifestations of the congenital varicella syndrome. Arch Ophthalmol 107:52–56
45. Larsen P, Chartrand S, Tomashek K, Hauser L, Ksiazek T (1993) Hydrocephalus complicating lymphocytic choriomeningitis virus infection. Pediatr Infect Dis J 12:528–531
46. Margo CE, Hamed LM (1992) Ocular syphilis. Surv Ophthalmol 37:203–220
47. McCauley J, Boyer K, Patel D, et al (1994) Early and longitudinal evaluation of treated infants and children and untreated historical patients with congenital toxoplasmosis: the Chicago collaborative treatment trial. Clin Infectious Dis 18:38–72
48. Mets MB, Holfels E, Boyer KM, Swisher CN, Roizen N, Stein L, Stein M, Hopkins J, Withers S, Mack D, Luciano R, Patel D, Remington JS, Meier P, McLeod R (1996) Eye manifestations of congenital toxoplasmosis. Am J Ophthalmol 122:309–324
49. Mets MB, Holfels E, Boyer KM, Swisher CN, Roizen N, Stein L, Stein M, Hopkins J, Withers S, Mack D, Luciano R, Patel D, Remington JS, Meier P, McLeod R (1997) Eye manifestations of congenital toxoplasmosis. Am J Ophthalmol 123:1–16
50. Mets MB, Barton LL, Khan AS, Ksiazek TG (2000) Lymphocytic choriomeningitis virus: an underdiagnosed cause of congenital chorioretinitis. Am J Ophthalmol 130:209–215
51. Miklos G, Orban T (1964) Ophthalmic lesions due to cytomegalic inclusion disease. Ophthalmologica 148:98–106
52. Miller E, Cradock-Watson JE, Pollack TM (1982) Consequences of confirmed maternal rubella at successive stages of pregnancy. Lancet 2:781–784
53. Nahmias AJ, Visintine AM, Caldwell DR, Wilson LA (1976) Eye infections with herpes simplex virus in neonates. Surv Ophthalmol 21:100–105
54. Overall JC (1985) Herpes simplex simples virus infection of the fetus and newborn. Pediatr Ann 23:131–136
55. Pepose J, Holland G, Wilhelmus K (1996) Ocular infection and immunity1st edn. Mosby, St. Louis
56. Perlman JM, Argyle C (1992) Lethal cytomegalovirus infection in preterm infants: clinical, radiological, and neuropathological findings. Ann Neurol 31:64–68
57. Peters C, Johnson K (1995) Lymphocytic choriomeningitis virus, Lassa virus, and other arenaviruses. In: Mandell G, Bennet J, Dolin R (eds) Infectious diseases and their etiologic agents, 4th edn., vol. 2. Churchill Livingstone, New York, pp 1572–1579
58. Reynolds JD, Griebel M, Mallory S, Steele R (1986) Congenital herpes simplex retinitis. Am J Ophthalmol 102:33–36
59. Rowe W, Murphy P, Bergold G, Casals J, Hotchin J, Johnson K, Lehmann-Grube F, Mims C, Traub E, Webb P (1970) Arena viruses: proposed name for a newly defined virus group. J Virol 5:651–652
60. Smadel J, Wall M (1942) Lymphocytic choriomeningitis in the Syrian hampster. J Exp Med 75:581–591
61. Stray-Pedersen B, Jenum P (1992) Current status of toxoplasmosis in pregnancy in Norway. Scand J Infect Dis Suppl 84:80–83
62. Trang J, Kidd L, Gruber W et al (1993) Linear single-dose pharmacokinetics of gangcyclovir in newborns with congenital cytomegalovirus infection. Clin Pharm Ther 53:15–23
63. Ueda K, Nishida Y, Oshima K et al (1979) Congenital rubella syndrome: correlation of gestational age at time of maternal rubella with type of defect. J Pediatr 94:763–765
64. Van der Meer JT, Drew WL, Bowden RA, Galasso GJ, Griffiths PD, Jabs DA, Katlama C, Spector SA, Whitley RJ (1996) Summary of the International Consensus Symposium on Advances in the Diagnosis, Treatment and Prophylaxis and Cytomegalovirus Infection. Antiviral Res 32:119–140
65. Volkert M, Larsen J (1965) Studies on immunological tolerance to LCM virus. 5. The induction of tolerance to the virus. Acta Path Microbiol Scand 63:161–171
66. Weller T, Hanshaw J (1962) Virologic and clinical manifestations of cytomegalic inclusion disease. N Engl J Med 266:1233–1244
67. Wentworth BB, Alexander ER (1971) Seroepidemiology of infections due to members of the herpesvirus group. Am J Eidemiol 94:496–507
68. Whitley RJ, Arvin A, Prober C et al (1991) A controlled trial comparing vidarabine with acyclovir in neonatal herpes simplex virus infection. N Eng J Med 324:444–449
69. Whitley RJ, Kimberlin DW, Roizman B (1998) Herpes simplex viruses. Clin Infectious Dis 26:541–555
70. Wilson CB, Remington JS, Stagno S, Reynolds DW (1980) Development of adverse sequelae in children born with subclinical congenital Toxoplasma infection. Pediatrics 66:767–774
71. Wolff SM (1973) The ocular manifestations of congenital rubella: a prospective study of 328 cases of congenital rubella. J Ped Ophthalmol 10:101
72. Wolff S (1985) Rubella syndrome. In: Viral diseases of the eye. Lea & Febiger, Philadelphia

73. Wright R, Johnson D, Neumann M, Ksiazek T, Rollin P, Keech R, Bonthius D, Hitchon P, Grose C, Bell W, Bale J (1997) Congenital lymphocytic choriomeningitis virus syndrome: a disease that mimics congenital toxoplasmosis of cytomegalovirus infection. Pediatrics 100:126–127

74. Zimmerman L (1958) Histopathologic basis for ocular manifestations of congenital rubella syndrome. Am J Ophthalmol 65:837

Nonaccidental Injury. The Pediatric Ophthalmologist's Role

Alex V. Levin

Core Messages

- Ophthalmologists are mandated reporters of suspected child abuse
- Report suspected abuse. Abuse need not be proven by the ophthalmologist
- Any injury to the eye may have been the result of abuse
- The eye may be involved with all forms of abuse: physical abuse, sexual abuse, neglect, and emotional abuse
- The ophthalmologist may look for signs of abuse on other parts of the body when an eye finding raises this suspicion
- An inconsistent or changing history or physical findings of trauma in the absence of a history of trauma should raise concern about possible abuse
- Always consider an appropriate differential diagnosis before reporting abuse, but as long as abuse is in the differential diagnosis one must ensure that the child is in a safe environment. Timely evaluation to rule out other disorders is essential but should not delay reporting if the suspicion of abuse is strong

14.1 Introduction

14.1.1 Basics

Child abuse has been part of the human condition since ancient times. In 1962, Kempe published his landmark paper entitled, "The Battered Child Syndrome" [10], which brought child abuse to the forefront of the medical field and eventually led to a worldwide increase in recognition, reporting and intervention, perhaps resulting in the improvement if not saving of thousands of children's lives. Child abuse continues to be a worldwide endemic reality. Virtually every pediatric ophthalmologist will at some time be faced with a child who has been a victim.

Child abuse is traditionally divided into four subtypes: physical abuse, sexual abuse, neglect, and emotional abuse. Each form of abuse may be associated with ocular signs.

14.1.2 Reporting

Almost every country in the developed world has some form of mandatory reporting which is based on the principle of an obligation for professionals who work with children, which would of course include the pediatric ophthalmologist, to report their *suspicion* that a child is a victim of abuse. The ophthalmologist is not a police officer, judge, or jury. These roles exist for the purpose of providing information which might assist in making a confirmed diagnosis of abuse as well as adjudicating who abused the child. When an ophthalmologist is confronted with a situation in which he or she suspects possible child abuse, there is an obligation to either report directly to child protective services or seek consultation from another physician or team with expertise in the field of abuse who may confirm that the suspicion is appropriate and initiate reporting on behalf of the ophthalmologist. Child abuse teams are usually multidisciplinary and may include nurses, child abuse pediatricians, social workers, psychologists and other professionals. However, if the ophthalmologist believes they have a justified suspicion and the child abuse experts do not agree, then the ophthalmologist would still be mandated to report.

Although any individual who works with children in any professional capacity is a mandated reporter, anyone, even a lay neighbor reporting anonymously, can initiate a report. Unfortunately, physicians are the most believed reporters when a case is evaluated by child protective agencies, yet physicians are also the least consistent in their reporting behaviors. Some physicians cite many excuses that lead to their failure to report, including a fear that they will be called to testify in court, they will lose patients (and income), they have an unsure diagnosis, the parents will go to jail, the child will be taken from the family, the family will take action (physical or legal) against them, or the system just will not work well on behalf of the child. In reality, in less than 1% of cases will the ophthalmologist be asked to go to court, as many cases are settled or do not involve criminal charges, and when the case does go to court, the ophthalmologist is often not called to testify as other child abuse experts may be able to testify to the eye findings on behalf of the ophthalmologist. There is no obligation that the physician be correct in his or her suspicion. In most countries, physicians are protected from being successfully prosecuted for reporting incorrectly unless they have reported with malicious intent. Reporting does not necessarily mean that the parents will go to jail or the child will be separated from them. The primary interest of most child protection agencies is to preserve family unity wherever possible, as long as the child is safe. When separation must occur, all attempts will be made to rehabilitate a parent perpetrator so that the family can be reunified. I am unaware of any case in which physical harm came to a physician for reporting. Although the system is not perfect, and some children are returned to unsafe environments or are abused in foster care, the only way to improve the system is by continuing to use it.

When physicians do report abuse, there is evidence that over-reporting occurs for visible minorities and those from low socioeconomic groups, and under-reporting occurs with Caucasians and families from higher income groups [9, 12]. In fact, child abuse occurs in every racial group, country, religious group and socioeconomic group [33]. It is recommended that physicians be open with families when they are reporting and avoid accusations. Rather, it can be suggested that someone may have injured the child and that the parents and ophthalmologist must work as a team to be sure whether this did or did not occur and ensure that if the child has been abused, that it will not occur again. Very few parents will not be willing to openly agree with such a stance. Even if it is patently obvious that the child was abused and the most likely perpetrator is in the room, the ophthalmologist must come to grips with their own emotions and realize that to help the child they must work together with the family, taking a similar approach without confrontation. Although physical discipline of children is accepted in many communities (and not endorsed by this author), perpetrators of abuse rarely injure children (with the exception of sexual abuse, see below) purposely and specifically with the intent to harm to a degree that will need medical attention. In the 10% that purposely cause significantly bodily harm, psychiatric disease is usually a factor. Most perpetrators regret their actions and will accept help. However, they rely on the reporter's initiative to be identified so that their child can be protected.

14.1.3 Testifying

The ophthalmologist may occasionally be called to court as either a fact witness or an expert witness. In the former, the witness is being asked only to report what they witnessed, which in the case of an ophthalmologist would be limited to observations made during the eye examination and any other communications related to the care of the patient. The ophthalmologist will likely be asked to detail the nature of the eye examination and the findings. If called as an expert witness, whether or not the ophthalmologist has examined the child, the ophthalmologist will then be asked to give opinions regarding the interpretation of the physical findings, perhaps extending into areas such as pathophysiology, mechanisms of injury, differential diagnosis, and prognosis.

Much has been written to help the physician prepare for their role as an expert witness and there has been much concern about irresponsible expert testimony [3, 19]. In general, it serves the ophthalmologist well to remember a few basic principles

1. Testify for the facts and your interpretation of the facts rather than what the prosecution or the defense wants you to say.
2. Remember that you are not on trial, even when it seems that an attorney is trying to challenge and discredit you.
3. Do not testify in areas that you are not truly expert.
4. Say you do not know when you do not know.
5. Remember that you are there to educate the court, not to prove a point.

Although testifying is not enjoyed by many physicians, it is a professional role that in the context of abuse is part of the physician's duty as an advocate for the abused child.

14.2 Physical Abuse

Any physical injury to the eye could be caused by abuse. The key to making a diagnosis of physical abuse lies in recognizing patterns of injury that are not consistent with a given history from the caretakers. Likewise, certain ophthalmic findings indicate trauma (e.g., avulsion of the vitreous base, commotio retinae, ruptured globe) and in the absence of a history of trauma, should raise a suspicion of abuse. Other concerning red flags include a history which is changed each time it is offered, a history of multiple or recurrent injuries without adequate explanation, and high-risk social situations such as a parent who presents inebriated or exhibiting violent tendencies towards the child in the waiting room (e.g., "If you don't shut up I will beat you with this belt"). Physical abuse may occur as part of what the perpetrator perceived as acceptable discipline. In most jurisdictions, even those which allow for spanking, any visible injury as a result of discipline is considered indicative that the perpetrator has lost control and entered the realm of abusive behavior. It is important that the ophthalmologist conduct a complete body examination (or refer to another physician specifically for this purpose) when abusive eye injury is suspected as there may be other signs of abuse elsewhere (Fig. 14.1).

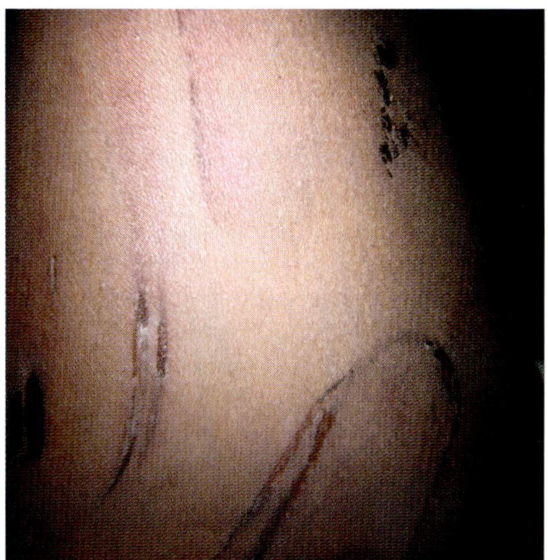

Fig. 14.1. Lacerations and ecchymosis in the pattern of a looped chord which was used to abusively beat this child. These injuries could not be accidental

14.2.1 Blunt Trauma

The multitudes of injuries that can be caused by blunt trauma are well beyond the scope of this chapter. However, a few deserve special mention.

Periorbital ecchymosis is a not uncommon result of blunt trauma. However, the presence of bilateral involvement does not prove abuse. A blunt injury (accidental or nonaccidental) to the forehead can result in bilateral periocular ecchymosis. Bilateral ecchymosis can also result from systemic disease such as neuroblastoma.

Abuse should never be reported on the basis of bruising or bleeding alone unless appropriate history and testing has been conducted to rule out coagulopathy. A basic panel should include at least a complete blood count with differential and platelet count, prothrombin time, partial thromboplastin time, and perhaps tests to rule out factor deficiencies or INR and von Willebrand disease. Bruising of the skin is difficult to date and particularly unreliable when located in the loose periocular and eyelid skin, which can allow for excessive accumulation of blood, thus changing color-related dating patterns. It is probably best not to attempt dating of periocular ecchymosis.

This author has now observed eight cases in which a child's eye was injured "accidentally" during a beating with a belt directed at other parts of the body. All sustained hyphema, one also had commotio of the macula, one required enucleation, and another resulted in a permanently legally blind eye. In each case, the diagnosis was made by history obtained from the parent or the child. Indeed, children may be interviewed directly by the physician. It may be helpful when suspicion arises to ask the child if they would like to speak to the ophthalmologist alone or to make an encouraging statement such as "I sometimes see children who have injuries like this because someone has hurt them. I can help make it so that they don't get hurt like this again. Might someone have hurt you?" Despite the parent's remorse and lack of intent to injure the eye, these cases do require reporting to child protective services to help the parent learn alternative means of discipline and prevent another episode where control is lost resulting in such serious injury.

Summary for the Clinician

- **Dating of periocular ecchymosis is imprecise and should be avoided**
- **Accidental forehead injury (with ecchymosis), coagulopathy and neuroblastoma are part of the differential diagnosis of unilateral or bilateral periorbital ecchymosis**
- **Unintended eye injury that occurs during discipline is a measure of the caretaker's loss of control and should be reported as suspected physical abuse**

14.2.2 Shaken Baby Syndrome

Shaken baby syndrome (SBS) is a form of child physical abuse in which a perpetrator subjects a child to repeated acceleration-deceleration forces with or without impact of the head. Alternate terminology has been suggested, including shaken impact syndrome, abusive head trauma, and inflicted neurotrauma. Herein, the term SBS will be used, understanding that the classic "shaking," for example when a perpetrator grasps a child by the thorax, is but one way in which abuse can cause the findings. But regardless of the terminology used, the syndrome findings are well recognized and share in common the presence of characteristic central nervous system injury, fractures, and/or retinal hemorrhages. Some physicians and biomechanists, most of whom are not clinically active in caring for abused children, have argued that it is impossible for a human being to shake a child hard enough to cause serious injury or death [7]. Unfortunately, such arguments fail to recognize that much lower levels of force are needed to incite the cascade of events that lead to cell injury and death than those that would be calculated to actually injure or kill the cell outright. There is overwhelming evidence that this syndrome is real, including the confessions of perpetrators [29], experiments with animal [24] and mechanical [5] models, the absence of similar physical findings following witnessed accidental injury [16], and the failure of alternative proposed pathophysiologic mechanisms to explain the observed findings [26]. The syndrome is well recognized by virtually every major professional organization, including the American Academy of Ophthalmology and the American Association of Pediatric Ophthalmology and Strabismus, and is described throughout the world. Excellent reviews are available [25].

The infant head is relatively big and poorly supported by weak cervical musculature. Acceleration–deceleration forces may lead to cervical and neck injury. There is relatively more room for the immature incompletely myelinated infant brain to move within the cranial vault. It is for these reason, and the progressive inability for adults to apply sufficient force to bigger children, that SBS occurs most frequently in the 1st year of life and decreases steadily in frequency over the next 3–4 years. Characteristic brain injuries include subdural hemorrhage, subarachnoid hemorrhage, brain contusion, and secondary cerebral edema with evidence of shearing injury to the parenchyma, including diffuse axonal injury on histology. The edema may be so severe as to result in auto-infarction of major cerebral blood vessels, including the distribution to the occipital lobes. The most common cause of visual loss and blindness following SBS is cortical visual impairment. Of the two-thirds of patients who survive, approximately one-half have permanent physical sequelae, which not uncommonly include vision deficits. Neuroimaging should be conducted in all cases where SBS is considered.

Fractures may occur either from the perpetrator grasping the rib cage, resulting in characteristic and often multiple posterior or posterolateral rib fractures, or the extremities, resulting in typical chip fractures to the metaphyses and/or periosteal stripping with subperiosteal hemorrhage. Evidence of blunt head trauma, which significantly increases the magnitude of acceleration-deceleration force [6], may result in fracture of the skull. Skull fractures that are comminuted, depressed, or crossing sutures in the absence of a history of severe accidental injury are particularly worrisome and should raise a suspicion of abuse. In SBS, fractures are less common than eye and brain injury, and are not required for diagnosis.

The retinal hemorrhages that characterize SBS are perhaps the most common reason that ophthalmologists will become involved with abused children. This topic is reviewed elsewhere in great detail [15, 16, 31]. It is essential to remember that not all retinal hemorrhages are the same and although characteristic patterns may help to diagnose abuse, a small number of intraretinal hemorrhages confined to the posterior pole is a nonspecific picture that can be seen in many disorders (Fig. 14.2). Approximately two-thirds of children with retinal hemorrhage as a result of SBS will show too numerous to count retinal hemorrhages, including preretinal, superficial nerve fiber layer, intraretinal dot/blot hemorrhage, and subretinal hemorrhage extending to the ora serrata [17–19] (Fig. 14.3). With the exception of hemorrhages following normal birth, this is a picture that is rarely seen in any other clinical entity. Although one isolated case report has suggested that such a finding can be seen as a result of crush injury to the head [14], we were unable to demonstrate such findings in our own clinical and pathologic case series. Of course, crush injury to the head

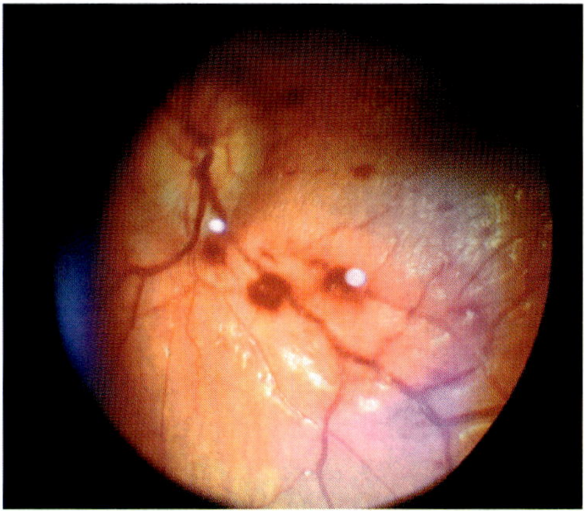

Fig. 14.2. Mild nonspecific pattern of preretinal and intraretinal hemorrhages confined to the posterior pole and peripapillary area

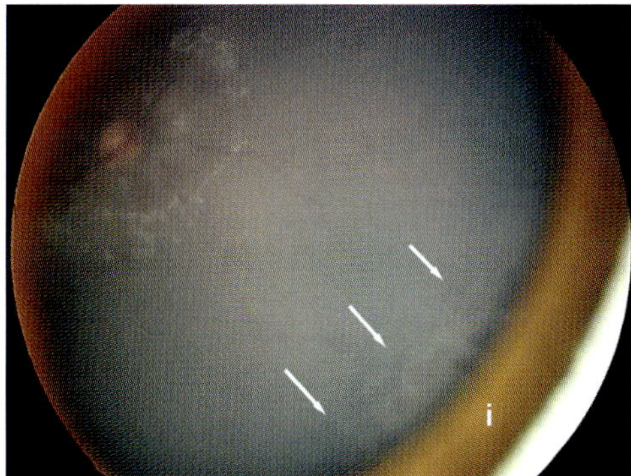

Fig. 14.3. Transpupillary view of retina showing retinal hemorrhage in posterior pole and peripherally approaching ora serrata (*arrows*) with relative sparing of the equatorial retina. This 3 years old child was a victim of shaken baby syndrome in which the father gave a detailed account of shaking the child

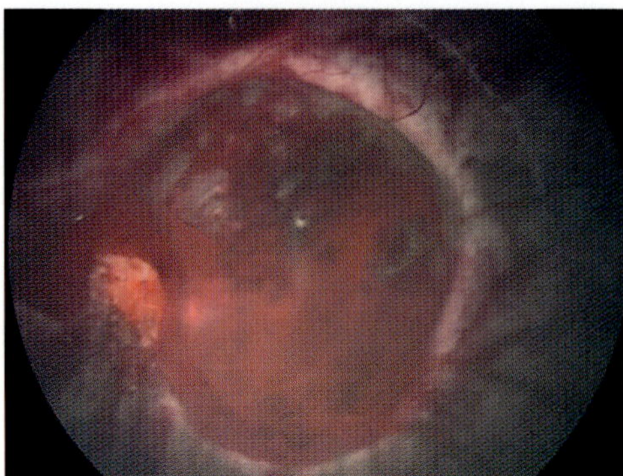

Fig. 14.4. Circinate elevated macular fold associated with traumatic retinoschisis in a shaken baby syndrome victim. The internal limiting membrane centrally has settled back against the retina

has a characteristic clinical presentation that is rarely of concern when considering SBS. Birth hemorrhage should be considered in the differential diagnosis for flame hemorrhage in the 1st week of life and dot/blot hemorrhage up to 4–6 weeks of age (with the exception of intrafoveal hemorrhage, which may last longer).

One form of hemorrhage seems to be particularly specific for SBS: traumatic macular retinoschisis. Although only present in up to one-third of patients [20], this characteristic finding is caused by traction applied to the macula by the tightly adherent vitreous as it is submitted to violent acceleration-deceleration forces. This entity has been confirmed by electroretinogram, ultrasound and histology [8, 16]. The latter often demonstrates the vitreous still attached to a retinal fold at the edge of the schisis cavity. Clinically, the schisis may be demarcated by a curvilinear fold, hemorrhagic line, or white line of depigmented retinal pigmented epithelium (Fig. 14.4). Most often the blood, which may fill the cavity in part or totally, is under the internal limiting membrane, although deeper cavities can also be seen. This may cause the ophthalmologist to confuse schisis with subhyaloid or preretinal blood. As paramacular folds in children have not previously been reported in any other entity except perhaps crush injury to the head [13], this finding has particular diagnostic significance. Blood may break through the cavity wall into the overlying subhyaloid or vitreous space (Fig. 14.4). Therefore, if the macula cannot be adequately viewed, it is wise to re-examine the child every 1–2 weeks until the underlying retina becomes visible to identify if schisis is present. Although many other entities may be associated with retinal hemorrhage, the presence of extensive hemorrhagic retinopathy, especially when macular retinoschisis is present, must raise strong suspicion that abusive head injury has occurred through a repetitive acceleration-deceleration mechanism.

Vitreoretinal traction and perhaps acceleration-deceleration injury to the orbital structures [16] appear to be the main mechanism by which retinal hemorrhage is generated in SBS [20]. Even with major accidental head injury such as motor vehicle accidents, retinal hemorrhage is uncommon, lending credence that there is something unique about the forces applied in inflicted neurotrauma [16, 32]. One author has suggested that short falls can very rarely result in significant retinal hemorrhage [23], but the study suffers from many flaws that make the reported case series difficult to interpret [17]. Other proposed mechanisms such as increased intracranial pressure, intracranial hemorrhage (Terson syndrome), and increased intrathoracic pressure (Purtscher retinopathy), seem to play little if any role [16, 20, 27]. The chest compressions of cardiopulmonary retinopathy rarely if ever cause retinal hemorrhage, and when they do, like most nonabusive causes of retinal hemorrhage other than birth, the findings would be confined to a small number of hemorrhages in the posterior pole [16]. The role of other factors such as mild coagulopathy secondary to brain injury, anemia, hypoxia, and autonomic dysregulation are worth further research but independently (i.e., in the absence of abusive head injury) do not cause severe hemorrhagic retinopathy. That retinal hemorrhages can occur with little or no apparent brain injury or hemorrhage on neuroimaging may support the isolated role of vitreoretinal traction, but some of these patients will exhibit intracranial pathology with alternative neuroimaging strategies or postmortem [21, 22].

When faced with an infant who has retinal hemorrhages, the examining ophthalmologist must begin by carefully documenting the findings. Detailed and well-labeled drawings are adequate, especially when accompanied by description of the number, type, pattern and extent of the retinal hemorrhages. Clinical photography is ideal but not required and even when obtained, may demonstrate artifacts brought on by the challenges of the moving eye, poorly dilated pupil, particular photographic technique and other technical factors. Postmortem photography, both gross and histologic, is also helpful. As we begin to realize the importance of orbital pathology, it is recommended that the orbital contents and globe be removed *en bloc* using a combined intracranial and transconjunctival approach and then fixated for 72 h followed by serial sections [16]. In the absence of other explanatory findings, if abuse is considered, skeletal radiographic examination, neuroimaging, blood studies and other tests where appropriate to rule out systemic disorders [16], consultation with a child abuse pediatrician and ultimately, reporting to child protective services are required.

Summary for the Clinician

- **Abusive head injury with an acceleration-deceleration component (Shaken baby syndrome) can result in potentially lethal brain injury, fractures, and retinal hemorrhage**
- **Children under 4 years old, and especially those less than 1 year old, are particularly susceptible**
- **The ophthalmologist must carefully characterize the types, distribution pattern, and number of retinal hemorrhages, as this will aid in differential diagnosis**
- **Whereas a few preretinal and intraretinal hemorrhages in the posterior pole are nonspecific, they may be due to inflicted neurotrauma**
- **Extensive hemorrhagic retinopathy with too numerous to count hemorrhages at all levels and extending to the ora serrata are rarely caused by systemic or ocular disease other than abuse**
- **Macular retinoschisis is a lesion highly suggestive of abusive head injury with acceleration-deceleration components**
- **The differential diagnosis of retinal hemorrhage can be refined based on the age of the child and the pattern of retinal hemorrhage**
- **Vitreoretinal traction plays a major role in the generation of eye injuries in Shaken baby syndrome**
- **Retinal hemorrhage can not be dated**

14.2.3 Munchausen Syndrome by Proxy (Factitious Illness by Proxy)

This uncommon and somewhat bizarre form of abuse involves the falsification or manipulation of medical data or physical findings such that the child has the appearance of having a medical disorder that is actually created by the perpetrator, usually the mother. For greater review of this entity, the reader is referred elsewhere [28]. Often, the mother may have secondary gains as a result of the attention the child's illness draws from a well-meaning medical team, that will often engage in numerous diagnostic interventions, even surgery, to solve the medical dilemma. These interventions may lead to prolongation of the time before the disorder is recognized and even iatrogenic injury. Reported ophthalmic manifestations include subconjunctival hemorrhages from covert suffocation, pupillary abnormalities or nystagmus from covert poisoning, recurrent periorbital cellulitis as a result of covert injections around the eye of foreign substances, corneal scarring secondary to covert instillation of noxious chemicals, and pupillary abnormalities due to indirect application of drops or even inhaler sprays (e.g., atropine) [15]. Ophthalmologists should expect Munchausen syndrome by proxy when they are faced with a child, usually preverbal, whose ocular illness does not fit into a known diagnosis, responds inconsistently to treatment, and has been presented by the parent to multiple ophthalmologists at different centers. The perpetrator will often appear as the "ideal" parent, often offering to help the nurses in the care of the child during inpatient stays and befriending hospital staff. The perpetrator may have a history of working in the health care field or having medical experience as a patient, perhaps even for Munchausen syndrome.

Summary for the Clinician

- **Munchausen syndrome by proxy is a disorder in which the caretaker, usually the mother, causes the child to appear to have an illness by the manipulation of samples from the patient, falsification of the history, or covert injury to the child**
- **Munchausen syndrome by proxy should be suspected when the eye condition does not make physiologic sense, responds inconsistently to treatment, and/or has been the subject of repeated visits to different physicians without satisfactory resolution. There may be a characteristic (although not necessarily required for diagnosis) profile to the family and victim**

14.3 Sexual Abuse

Sexual abuse of a child is very different from the violent isolated acts of adult rape. Rather, children become victims to chronic secretive abuse which may range from inappropriate touching to anal or vaginal penetration. Rarely, children may be victims of child pornography. Both victim and perpetrator may be either male or female although most commonly the victim is female and the perpetrator male. The perpetrator of child sexual abuse is often known to the child and in a position of authority which might be exploited through the use of threats to the child to maintain secrecy. Very young children may not even realize that the behavior of this trusted adult is abnormal. Over 90% of child abuse victims will show no physical evidence of the abuse. It may be years before sexual abuse is discovered or disclosed.

Although uncommon, sexual abuse may present as sexually transmitted ocular disease. Gonorrhea or chlamydial conjunctivitis, human papilloma virus of the conjunctiva, pubic lice of the eyelashes, periocular infection with molluscum or herpes simplex, or ocular involvement with HIV or syphilis may all occur in sexually abused children. However, there is evidence that some infections, such as gonorrhea [18], may be transmitted to the eye nonsexually. This is contrary to the well-documented exclusivity of sexual transmission for gonorrhea to the oropharynx, vagina, rectum and male urethra. There may be unique factors about the externalized conjunctival mucosa that allow for this nonsexual transmission to occur. Infections such as molluscum and herpes simplex are so frequently transmitted nonsexually that consideration of sexual abuse seems almost misdirected in the absence of other concerning findings. Nonsexual transmission of syphilis to children does not occur. But like virtually all sexually transmitted diseases, infection via the birth canal is an important consideration and some infections, particularly *Chlamydia*, may have very long latent periods. Consultation with child abuse and infectious disease specialists may be helpful. In teenagers, one must also consider the possibility of consensual sexual activity with peers as the source of infection. At the very least, sexually transmitted diseases with ocular manifestations should lead the ophthalmologist to place sexual abuse in the differential diagnosis, and communicate this concern to the child's primary care physician or a child abuse pediatrician, to consider further evaluation.

There is also important literature to suggest that covert sexual abuse, and perhaps other forms of abuse, may lead to functional visual loss in children [4, 30]. Although it would not be appropriate to question every child with functional visual loss regarding possible covert abuse, it is recommended that the evaluation of functional symptoms include consideration of possible stressors in the child's life.

Summary for the Clinician

- **Sexual abuse of a child is a chronic covert act that may escape detection or report by the child for years and is most often not associated with physical injury to the victim**
- **Ocular manifestations of sexually transmitted disease may be a sign of sexual abuse**
- **The ophthalmologist must consider the possibility of nonsexual transmission of sexually transmitted diseases to the conjunctiva, but when there is a suspicion of sexual abuse, the ophthalmologist should refer to expert professionals**

- Infection via the birth canal, and, in teenagers, via voluntary sexual activity, must be considered
- Functional visual loss and other symptoms may be a sign of covert abuse

14.4 Neglect and Noncompliance

Although this form of child abuse is perhaps the most common, it is also the most difficult to identify and manage. Although neglect may manifest as a more dramatic physical failure to thrive (psychosocial growth retardation), the ophthalmologist is more often confronted with parents and other caregivers who fail to attend scheduled appointments or adhere to prescribed treatment regimens such as occlusion therapy for amblyopia. Apparent noncompliance may result from confounding factors that significantly impair a parent's ability to comply: poverty leading to an inability to afford care, access to care (transportation, insurance coverage), lack of child care for siblings, inability to leave work, misunderstanding of the instructions or the seriousness of the eye disease, and others. When concerned about possible abusive neglect and noncompliance, the ophthalmologist should first explore such factors, perhaps with the help of a social worker or other support personnel. Absent such factors, the ophthalmologist can enter into written contracts with patients, documented in the chart and signed by the patient and a witness, that indicate the physician's expectations and the consequences (e.g., reporting to child protective services) should the behavior continue. This will empower the report once it is made, as otherwise, the agency receiving the report may blame misunderstanding and miscommunication rather than neglectful behavior.

Summary for the Clinician

- The ophthalmologist must ensure that explanatory factors (e.g., poverty) for noncompliance are identified and addressed
- Written contracts with parents/guardians can be helpful in managing non compliance

14.5 Emotional Abuse

Often it is the faces and affect of abused children that tell us the adverse emotional consequences of their abuse. Other times a physician may actually witness emotionally abusive interactions in the waiting room or examination room. Like all forms of abuse, it is sometimes difficult to draw a line between acceptable but harsh parental verbal discipline and emotional abuse, but clearly comments such as "You did not deserve to be born," "You are a good for nothing/stupid/evil child," and other forms of threat and intimidation cross the line into the realm of abuse. When such behavior is witnessed first hand, office staff should notify the ophthalmologist who can then approach the parent in a nonconfrontational, nonaccusatory way saying something like "Your child seems to be particularly challenging today" or "You seem to be feeling very angry with your child." The patient's entry into the examination room should be prioritized and the observed behaviors addressed in a fashion that explores the parental feelings rather than condemns them for their actions. Enlisting the support of social work or nursing services can be very helpful. Reporting to child protective services is indicated if emotional abuse is observed or suspected.

Summary for the Clinician

- Potentially abusive behavior by a child's caretaker that is observed by an ophthalmologist or their staff must be addressed

14.6 Conclusion

Every ophthalmologist who cares for children will be confronted with the challenges of child abuse. Every ophthalmologist is a mandated reporter. Yet we must carefully consider alternative explanations for the physical findings, and not rush to the conclusion that a child has been abused. Consideration of a broad differential diagnosis must also be balanced with the immediate protection needs of the child. Abuse should be reported when there is reasonable suspicion. One need not achieve complete medical certainty. By using an open and sensitive partnership with parents, they are more likely to understand the ophthalmologist's intentions and obligations to act on behalf of the child. The ophthalmologist must honor the responsibility to advocate for their child patients.

References

1. Adams G, Ainsworth J, Butler L et al (2004) Update from the Ophthalmology Child Abuse Working Party: Royal College Ophthalmologists. Eye 18:795–798
2. Bechtel K, Stoessel K, Leventhal J et al (2004) Characteristics that distinguish accidental from abusive injury in hospitalized young children with head trauma. Pediatrics 114:165–168
3. Brent RL (1982) The irresponsible expert witness: a failure of biomedical graduate education and professional accountability. Pediatrics 70:754–762
4. Catalano R, Simon J, Krohel G et al (1986) Functional visual loss in children. Ophthalmology 93:385–390
5. Cory CZ, Jones BM (2003) Can shaking alone cause fatal brain injury? A biomechanical assessment of the Duhaime shaken baby syndrome model. Med Sci Law 43:317–333
6. Duhaime A, Gennarelli T, Thibault L et al (1987) The shaken baby syndrome: a clinical, pathological, and biomechanical study. J Neurosurg 66:409–415
7. Geddes JF, Plunkett J (2004) The evidence base for shaken baby syndrome. BMJ 328(7442):719–720
8. Greenwald M, Weiss A, Oesterle C, Friendly D (1986) Traumatic retinoschisis in battered babies. Ophthalmology 93:618–625
9. Hampton R, Newberger E (1985) Child abuse and reporting by hospitals: significance of severity, class, and race. Am J Public Health 75:56–60
10. Kempe CH, Silverman FN, Steele BF, Droegemueller W, Silver HK (1962) The battered-child syndrome. JAMA 181:17–24
11. Kivlin J, Simons K, Lazoritz S, Ruttum M (2000) Shaken baby syndrome. Ophthalmology 107:1246–1254
12. Lane WG, Rubin DM, Monteith R, Christian CW (2002) Racial differences in the evaluation of pediatric fractures for physical abuse. JAMA 288:1603–1609
13. Lantz P, Sinal S (2002) Perimacular retinal folds in non-abusive head trauma. Fourth National Conference on Shaken Baby Syndrome, Salt Lake City, Utah
14. Lantz PE, Sinal SH, Stanton CA, Weaver RG Jr (2004) Perimacular retinal folds from childhood head trauma. BMJ 328(7442):754–756
15. Levin A (1995) Ophthalmic manifestations. In: Levin A, Sheridan M (eds) Munchausen syndrome by proxy; issues in diagnosis and treatment. Lexington, New York, pp 207–212
16. Levin A (2000) Retinal haemorrhage and child abuse. In: David T (ed) Recent advances in paediatrics, vol 18. Churchill Livingstone, London, pp 151–219
17. Levin A (2001) Fatal pediatric head injuries caused by short-distance falls. Am J Forensic Med Pathol 22:417–418
18. Lewis LS, Glauser TA, Joffe MD (1990) Gonococcal conjunctivitis in prepubertal children. Am J Dis Child. 144:546–548
19. Milunsky A (2003) Lies, damned lies, and medical experts: the abrogation of responsibility by specialty organizations and a call for action. J Child Neurol 18:413–419
20. Morad Y, Kim Y, Armstrong D, Huyer D, Mian M, Levin A (2002) Correlation between retinal abnormalities and intracranial abnormalities in the shaken baby syndrome. Am J Ophthalmol 134:354–359
21. Morad Y, Avni I, Benton S et al (2004) Normal computerized tomography of brain in children with shaken baby syndrome. J AAPOS8:445–450
22. Morad Y, Avni I, Capra L et al (2004) Shaken baby syndrome without intracranial hemorrhage on initial computed tomography. J AAPOS 8:521–527
23. Plunkett J (2001) Fatal pediatric head injuries caused by short-distance falls. Am J Forensic Med Pathol 22:1–12
24. Raghupathi R, Mehr MF, Helfaer MA, Margulies SS (2004) Traumatic axonal injury is exacerbated following repetitive closed head injury in the neonatal pig. J Neurotrauma 21:307–316
25. Reece R, Nicholson C (eds) (2003) Inflicted childhood neurotrauma. American Academy of Pediatrics, Chicago
26. Reece R, Alexander R, Dubowitz H et al (2004) The evidence base for shaken baby syndrome: response to editorial from 106 doctors. BMJ 328:1316–1317
27. Schloff S, Mullaney P, Armstrong D et al (2002) Retinal findings in children with intracranial hemorrhage. Ophthalmology 109:1472–1276
28. Sheridan M (2003) The deceit continues: an updated literature review of Munchausen syndrome by proxy. Child Abuse Negl 27:431–451
29. Starling S, Patel S, Burke B, Sirotnak A, Stronks S, Rosquist P (2004) Analysis of perpetrator admissions to inflicted traumatic brain injury in children. Arch Pediatr Adolesc Med 158:454–458

30. Taich A, Crowe S, Kosmorsky G, Traboulsi E (2004) Prevalence of psychosocial disturbances in children with nonorganic visual loss. J AAPOS 8:457–461
31. Taylor D et al (1999) The Ophthalmology Child Abuse Working Party: child abuse and the eye. Eye 13:3–10
32. Vinchon M, Noizet O, Defoort-Dhellemmes S, Soto-Ares G, Dhellemmes P (2002) Infantile subdural hematoma due to traffic accidents. Pediatr Neurosurg 37:245–253
33. Windham A, Rosenberg L, Fuddy L, McFarlane E, Sia C, Duggan A (2004) Risk of mother-reported child abuse in the first 3 years of life. Child Abuse Negl 28:645–667

Subject Index

A
Aberration 4
- chromatic 4, 11
- spherical 4
Ab-interno surgery 102
Acceleration-deceleration force 223
Accommodation 4
- lag of 8
Acetylcholine 6
Achromatopsia 158, 179
- complete 179
- incomplete 179
Acquired immune deficiency syndrome 115
Acyclovir 211
Age 26
- effect 26, 27, 32
- optimal 81
Ahmed valve 102
AIPL1 158, 164
Albinism 143
- ocular 145
- oculocutaneous 145
Alpha-2 agonist 101
Alstrom syndrome 158
Amblyogenic factor 21
Amblyopia 37, 151
- bilateral 21
- prevalence 22
- treatment 19, 21, 37, 46
Ametropia 151
Anemia 224
Anesthesia 84
- general 84, 97
- halothane 97
Animal model for myopia 1
Anisometropia 19, 21
Anophthalmia 210
Anterior segment 74
Antifibrotic agent 104
Antimetabolite 102
Anti-VEGF 53
Antiviral agent 215
Apnea, postoperative 84
Arden index 137
Arrestin 183
Arterial blood gas monitoring 64
A-scan sonography 96
- B-scan 98
Astigmatism 4, 22
Astrocytoma, juvenile pilocytic 127
Atropine 45
Autoimmune disease 95
Autorefraction 24
Avulsion of the vitreous base 221
Axial length 97

B
Baerveldt implant 102
Band keratopathy 106
Bardet-Biedl (BBS) 140, 158
Batten disease 145
- infantile 158
Battered child 219
Berson plates 185
Bestrophin 148
Beta-blocker, topical 101
Binocular correspondence, abnormal 43
Binocular input 15
Biomicroscopy 96
Bipolar cells 135
Birth weight 64
- extremely low see ELBW
Bleb 104
Blepharoptosis 116
Blepharospasm 96
Blindness 511
- childhood 63
- uniocular, cause 32
Blunt trauma 192
Blur sensitivity 15
Bone-spicule pigmentation 157
BPD (bronchopulmonary dysplasia) 56
Bradycardia 101
Brain contusion 223
Brimonidine 95, 101
Brinzolamide 101
Bronchopulmonary dysplasia (BPD) 56
Buphthalmia 95

C

CACA1F 182
CAM stimulator 46
Capillary hemangioma 111
Capsulotomy, posterior 89
Carbonic anhydrase inhibitor 101
- topical 101
Cataract 20, 81
- bilateral congenital 85
- infantile
- - management controversies 81
- simultaneous surgery 91
- surgery 81
- unilateral congenital 81
Central nervous system injury 222
Cerebral edema, secondary 223
Cerebral visual impairment 42
Chemoreduction 111, 121
Chemotherapy, systemic 111
Chick 2
- lens-reared 5
Chicken 3
Child abuse 219
Childhood 19
- amblyopia 27
- blindness 63, 157
Children 7
- full correction 7
- undercorrected 7
Chlamydial conjunctivitis 226
Chloral hydrate 97
Chloroidal detachment 106
Chloroma 128
Chorioretinal scar 206
Chorioretinitis 206, 210
Choristoma 117
- complex 117
- epibulbar osseous 117
Choroid 5
CHRPE (congenital hypertrophy of retinal pigment epithelium) 125
Ciliary process 107
CIMN see nystagmus
CLAMP study 9
Cleft palate 195
Clinical trial 64
$CNGA_3$ 145
$CNGB_3$ 145
Coagulopathy 224
Coat's disease 112, 202
COL (collagen)2 194
COL2A1 196
COL11A1 196
Coloboma 191
Colour vision testing 145
COMET 8
Commotio retinae 221
Complex malformation 95
Compliance 46, 85
Computer work 10
Cone 135
Cone dysfunction syndrome 145, 179
- XL, with dichromacy 179
Cone transducin, α-subunit 185
Congenital heart disease 212
Congenital hypertrophy of retinal pigment epithelium see CHRPE
Congenital myopia 191
Congenital nonattachment 191
Congenital stationary night blindness see CSNB
Congenital toxoplasmosis 206
Conjunctivitis 211
Contact-diode transscleral cyclophotocoagulation (TSCPC) 105
Contact lens 85
- compliance 83
Contrast adaptation 5, 12
Corectopia 86
Cornea, diameter 97
Corneal electrode 134
Corneal opacification, scarring 98, 225
Corneal opacity 39, 213
Cortical dysfunction 152
Cortical visual impairment (see also CVI) 223
Cost-effectiveness, benefit 19, 24
Cover testing 24
Craniopharyngioma 150
CRB1 (crumbs homologue 1 gene) 158, 167
Crowding 19, 41
Crumbs homologue 1 gene see CRB1
CRX 158, 162
- knockout mice 162
CRYO-ROP study 70
Cryotherapy 51
- prophylactic 200
CSNB (congenital stationary night blindness) 137, 140, 142, 180
- AD 180, 182
- AR 180, 182, 183
- complete 140, 182
- dominant 142
- incomplete 140, 182
- recessive 142
- XL 140, 180
Cup disc ratio 97
CVI (cortical visual impairment) 147
Cyclodestructive method 95
Cyclodestructive procedure 105
Cyclodialysis 102
Cyclopia 210
Cycloplegia 4, 21
Cytomegalovirus 205, 209

D

Deep sclerectomy 105
Defocus 2
– imposed 4
– negative 4
– positive 4
Dermoid 117
– conjunctival 117
– cyst 111, 126
Diffuse axonal injury 223
Digital imaging 76
Digital photography 75
Diopter 10
Diplopia 112
Disability 38
Disc pallor 143
Diurnal light rhythm 10
DOA (dominant optic atrophy) 149
Dopamine 6
Dorzolamide 101
Dystrophy 143
– cone 143
– dominant cone-rod 143
Dystrophy, macular 147
– Best vitelliform macular 148
– Stargardt macular 148

E

Early onset severe retinal dystrophy see EOSRD
Early Treatment of ROP Study Group see ETROP 68
Ecchymosis
– periorbital 221
– – differential diagnosis 222
Educational advice 188
Ehlers-Danlos syndrome 198
Ehlers-Danlos type VI 194
ELBW (extremely low birth weight) 69
Electronic monitor 46
Electro-oculogram see EOG
Electrophysiology 133
Electroretinogram see ERG
Electroretinography 133
Emmetropia 21
Emmetropization 11
Emotional abuse 227
Endophthalmitis 91, 104
Enhanced S-cone syndrome see ESCS
Enucleation 111
Environment
– extrauterine 54
– intrauterine 54
Environmental factor 1
EOG (electro-oculogram) 133
EOSRD (early onset severe retinal dystrophy) 157
Epigenetic variance 3
Epiphora 96
Episcleral plaque brachytherapy 121
Epstein-Barr virus 205, 214
ERG (electroretinogram) 133
– flicker 135
– full-field 134
– 30-Hz 137
– maturation 135
– maximal response 147
– negative 140
– OFF- 140
– ON- 140
– photopic 140
– rod-specific 183
– S-cone 140
– – specific 134
– scotopic 140
– single flash 135
– wave
– – ON-b- 148
– – OFF-d- 148
ESCS (enhanced S-cone syndrome) 142
Esotropia 39, 112
ETROP (Early Treatment of ROP Study Group) 68
EVR1, 2, 3 (Exsudative Vitreoretinopathy) 200
Excisional biopsy 113
Exotropia 39, 112
Extension patch 43
Extremely low birth weight see ELBW
Eye growth 1
– axial 1
– inhibitory effect on 9
– visual control 2
Eye injury
– nonaccidental 219
– physical 221
– unintended 222
Eyelashes, pubic lice of 226

F

Facial dysmorphia 147
FAF (fundus autofluorescence) 162
FBN1 198
FEVR see vitreoretinopathy 199
Fibrillin 198
Fine-needle aspiration biopsy see FNAB
Flash stimulation 136
Fluorescein angiography 121
5-fluorouracil 104
FNAB (fine-needle aspiration biopsy) 113
Focal length 2
Focal plane 5
Form vision 2
Form vision deprivation 21
Fracture 222
Fundus albipunctatus (FA) 142, 183
Fundus flavimaculatus 148
Fundus hypopigmentation 145
FZD4 (frizzled-4 gene) 200

G

Ganciclovir 210
Ganzfeld 134
Gene therapy 157, 170
General anesthesia 97
Genetic counselling 188
Genetic heterogeneity 185
Geniculate body, lateral 37
Genotype-phenotype correlation 160
Gestational age 64, 70
Glaucoma 105
- angle-closure 106
- aphakic 83, 95
- congenital 95
- episcleral venous pressure 105
- glaucomatous excavation 96
- implant 102, 104
- infantile 95
- - classification 95
- - prognosis 95
- inflammatory 95
- juvenile 96
- primary 96
- secondary 77, 96
- surgery 95
- - nonperforating 105
- uveitic 106
Glucagons 6
GNAT2 185
Goldenhar's syndrome 117
Gonioscopy 87, 96
Goniotomy 95
- endoscopic 102
Gonorrhea 226
Granuloma, pyogenic 119
Grating acuity 86
GRM6 183
Growth-controlling messenger 5
Growth factor 6
Growth rate 15
GUCY2D 158, 159
Guidelines for ROP see ROP

H

Haab striae 96
Hamartoma, astrocytic of retina 122
Hand-held tonometry 96
Harada's disease 202
Head trauma 222
- abusive 222
- blunt 223
Hearing difficulty 195
Hearing loss 208
Heart disease 208
Hemangioma 111
- capillary 111, 114, 127
- cavernous 111
- choroidal 111, 123
- racemose 111
- retinal 111
- - capillary 121
- - cavernous 121
- - racemose 122
- strawberry 114
Hemizygote 140
Hemorrhage 223
- birth 224
- subarachnoid 223
- subconjunctival 225
- subdural 223
- subretinal 223
Hepatosplenomegaly 212
Heritability 1
Herpes simplex virus (HSV) 205, 210
Heterozygote 137
- carrier 170
High arched palate 195
Hippel Lindau syndrome 121
HIV, congenital 214
Horner's syndrome 213
HSV (herpes simplex virus) 205, 210
- congenital 211
- transmission 210
Human immunodeficiency virus 205
Human papilloma virus
of the conjunctiva 226
Hydrocephalus 212
Hypermobile joint 195
Hyperopia 4, 14
Hyperoxia 52
Hyperplastic primary vitreous 106
Hyphema 102, 222
Hypomelanosis of Ito 201
Hypoplasia, foveal 145
Hypotony 104
Hypoxia 224
Hysteria 151

I

Iatrogenic injury 225
IATS (Infant Aphakia Treatment Study) 81, 89
IBIT (Interactive Binocular Treatment) 46
ICROP (International Classification
of ROP) 64, 65
- zones 64
- zone I disease 65
- zone II disease 65
IgA antibody 205
IGF (Insulin-like growth factor)1 51
IgM antibody 205, 208, 209
Illuminances 9
Immaturity 84
Immunofluorescent antibody (IFA) 212
Immunomodulative therapy 95

Implicit time 149
Incontinentia pigmenti 200, 201
Infant Aphakia Treatment Study see IATS
Infectious disease 202, 226
Inflammation, postoperative 90
Inflammatory disease 202
Inheritance
– autosomal dominant 158
– mode 179
Injection 225
– covert 225
Inner nuclear layer 160
Insulin-like growth factor-1 see IGF-1
Interactive Binocular Treatment see IBIT
Interocular difference 25
Intracranial calcification 211, 212
Intracranial misrouting 145
Intraocular lens see IOL
Intraocular pressure see IOP
Intraoperative complication 106
Intrauterine growth retardation 208
Intrauterine infection 205
– epidemiology 207
– prevention 207
– systemic manifestations 206
– transmission 207
– treatment 207
– – triple therapy 207
Intraventricular hemorrhage (IVH) 56
IOL (intraocular lens) 81, 85
– acrylic 90
– implantation 91
IOP (intraocular pressure) 87, 97
– control 95
Iridectomy 106
Iridociliary cyst 106
Iridocyclitis 211
Iridotrabeculodysgenesis, iridocorneotrabeculodysgenesis 96
Iris
– atrophy 211
– incarceration 107
– pigmentation 100
– transillumination 145
ISCEV standard 134
Isomerisation 160
IVH (intreventricular hemorrhage) 56

J

Joint mobility 195
Joubert syndrome 158

K

Kaposi's sarcoma 115, 119
Keratitis 211
Keratoconus 157
Keratoplasty 105
Ketamine 97
Kinetic manual perimetry 99
Kniest dysplasia 194
Kniest syndrome 197

L

Langerhans cell histiocytosis 129
Laser photocoagulation 51, 121
– cyclophotocoagulation 102
– diode- 69
Laser scanning optic disc morphometry 97
Latanoprost 100
Latent period 83
LCA (Leber's congenital amaurosis) 145
– autosomal recessive 157
LCA3 158, 169
LCA4 164
LCA5 158, 169
LCA6 165
LCA9 158, 169
LCMV (lymphocytic choriomeningitis virus) 212
Leber's congenital amaurosis see LCA
Leber hereditary optic neuropathy see LHON
Lecithin acyl transferase (LRAT) 158, 160
Lens
– contact 8
– power 4
– progressive addition 8
– reproliferation 84
– single vision 8
Lensectomy 83
Leukemia 126
Leukocoria 112
Leukodystrophy, neonatal adrenal 147
Lhermitte-Duclos syndrome 158
LHON (Leber hereditary optic neuropathy) 148
Light peak:dark trough ratio 137
LogMAR 19
Long-term safety 90
L-opsin gene 186
Low vision aid 188
Low-density lipoprotein receptor-related protein-5 see LRP5
LRP5 (low-density lipoprotein receptor-related protein-5) 200
Lymphangioma 114, 127
Lymphocytic choriomeningitis virus (LCMV) 205
Lymphoma 129

M

MAC-ELISA 214
Macrocephaly 212
Macroexcavation 98
Macular coloboma 157
Macular dysfunction 135
Maculopathy 142
– bull's eye 143

Mainzer-Saldino syndrome 158
Malingering 151
Marfan syndrome 194, 198
Maximal ERG response see ERG 147
Mechanical model 222
Media opacity 21
Medulloepithelioma, intraocular 111, 123
Megalocornea 96, 99
Melanocytoma, of the optic nerve 122
Melanocytosis, congenital ocular 118
Melanoma, choroidal 111
Melanoma, uveal 124
Mental retardation 208
MERTK 158
Messenger 5
- growth-controlling 5
- secondary 5
Metabolism 6
Microcephaly 208, 212
Microcornea 83, 206
Microphthalmia, microphthalmos 89, 206, 211
Microstrabismus 22
Miotics 100
Mitomycin C 104
Mizuo-Nakamua phenomenon 183
Molecular diagnostic testing 179
Molteno implant 102
Monitored Occlusion Treatment of Amblyopia Study see MOTAS
Monkey 2
- Rhesus- 3
Monochromatism 185
- blue cone 185
- rod 145
- S-cone 145
M-opsin gene 186
Morbidity 64
Mortality 64
MOTAS (Monitored Occlusion Treatment of Amblyopia Study) 26
Multisystem disorder 147
Munchausen syndrome 225
Myopia 1, 7
- development 1, 2
- deprivation 2
- management, treatment 7, 8
- progression 7
- regression of 15

N

Nanophthalmic eye 106
Nasolacrimal duct obstruction 92
NCL (neuronal ceroid lipofuscinosis) 147
Near work 8
NEC (necrotizing enterocolitis) 56
Necrotizing enterocolitis see NEC
Neglect 227
- abusive 227
NEMO 201
Neonatal adrenoleucodystrophy 158
Neonates 83
Nephronothisis, juvenile 158
Neurilemoma (Schwannoma) 116
Neuritis, optic 211
Neuroblastoma, metastatic 129
Neurodevelopmental defect 40
Neurofibroma 116
Neuroimaging 223
Neurological disorder 143
Neuromodulator 6
Neuronal ceroid lipofuscinosis see NCL
Neurotrauma 224
- inflicted 222
Nevus 111
- choroidal 111
- congenital 118
- eyelid 111
- flammeus, facial 115
- melanocytic 116
- uveal 124
Newborn 20
Nyctalopia 164
Night blindness 137
Night vision 183
Nonamblyopic eye 34
Norrie's disease 194, 200
NUB1 164
Nystagmus 21, 140, 225
- early onset 143
- idiopathic motor (CIMN) 143
- infantile 158
- sensory 143
NYX 182

O

Objective refraction 99
Occlusion therapy 26
Occlusion, unilateral 21
OCT (optical coherence tomography) 113, 148
Ocular coloboma 201
Ocular disease, sexually transmitted 226
Ocular involvement with HIV 226
Ocular oncology 111
Ocular trauma, penetrating 193
Oculodigital sign 145
Oguchi disease 179
Oligocone trichromacy 179, 186
OPA_1 149
Ophthalmitis 104
Ophthalmoscopy, binocular indirect 73
Optic atrophy 149, 206
- dominant see DOA, familial 150

Optic disc
- cupping 97
- pits 201
Optic nerve 3
- abnormalities 143
- coloboma 210
- disease 89
- dysfunction 135
- glioma 149
- hypoplasia 210
Optical coherence tomography see OCT
Optical correction 24
Ora serrata 73
Oral levodopa 46
Orbital cellulitis 126
Orbital haemangioma 39
Orthoptic examination 24
Orthoptist 24
Osteoma, choroidal 123
Oxygen 51, 64, 70
- supplemental 54

P

Papillary abnormality 225
Papilloma 117
Papillomavirus 117
Paramacular fold 224
Patching 43, 83
- full-time 44
Pattern electroretinogram see PERG
Pattern offset 136
PaVEP see VEP
PEDIG (US Pediatric Eye Disease Investigator Group) 43
PERG (pattern electroretinogram) 133
- P50 component 151
Periocular infection with molluscum 226
Periorbital cellulitis, recurrent 225
Peripheral refraction 8
Peripheral schisis 148
Peroxisomal disorder 147, 158
Perpetrator 225
Persistent fetal vasculature 83
Peters' anomaly 96
Phenotyping 133
Photocoagulation 201
Photography 225
- clinical 225
- postmortem 225
Photophobia 96, 145
Photoreceptor specific guanylate cyclase 160
Photoreceptor transplantation 171
Photo-ROP study 76
Phthisis 106, 206
Pilocarpine 100
Plus disease 64
PMA (postmenstrual age) 67
PMMA (polymethylmerthacrylate) lens 90
Poisoning 225
- covert 225
Polymethylmerthacrylate see PMMA
Postmenstrual age (PMA) 67
Predictive value, positive 23
Pregnancy 55, 207
Prematurity 51
Previtelliform stage 148
Prophylactic treatment 191
Proptosis 112, 128, 149
Prostaglandin 101
Pseudophakic eye 83, 86
Psychomotor retardation 147
Psychosocial distress 27
Ptosis 21
Pupil 157
Pupillary block 106
Pupillary membrane 83
Purtscher retinopathy 224

Q

Quality of life 38

R

Radiotherapy, orbital 111
RAMSES (Rotterdam Amblyopia Screening Effectiveness Study) 30
Randomised treatment 25
RDH12 158, 169
RDH5 183
Reading distance 10
Reading glasses 8
Referral criteria 25
- over- 24
- under- 24
Refraction 5
Refractive adaptation 43
Refractive correction 46
Refractive development 1
Refractive error 19, 43
Refractive growth 91
Refsum disease, infantile 147, 158
Retina 2
- deprivation 2
- primate 7
Retinal astrocytic hamartoma 111
Retinal dehydrogenase, 11-cis 183
Retinal detachment 77, 191, 194
- familial 194
- dominant rhegmatogenous 198
- exudative 202
Retinal dialysis 191
- nontraumatic 193
Retinal dysfunction 135
- syndrome, stationary 179
Retinal dystrophy, early onset severe see EOSRD

Retinal dystrophy, progressive 137
Retinal ganglion cells 135
Retinal hemorrhage 222
Retinal hypoxia 53
Retinal image 3, 4
- brightness 9
- degradation 4
- processing 3
- sharpness 4, 7
Retinal molecular genetics 179
Retinal neovascularization 51
Retinal pigment epithelium 5, 157
Retinal telangiectasia, congenital 112
Retinal thickness 167
Retinal transplantation 171
Retinal vascular growth 51
Retinal wide-field imaging 75
Retinal 11-cis 171
Retinal 9-cis 171
Retinitis 210
- pigmentosa (rod-cone dystrophy) 137
- punctata albescens 142
Retinoblastoma 20, 111, 119
- genetics of 121
Retinopathy
- hemorrhagic 224
- of prematurity see ROP
- pigmentary 147
- Purtscher see Purtscher retinopathy
- salt and pepper 208
Retinoschisis
- traumatic macular 224
- X-linked (XLRS) 148, 149, 199
Retrolental fibroplasia 63
Rhabdomyosarcoma 111, 128
Rhesus monkey see monkey
Rhodopsin kinase 183
Rieger's syndrome 96
RM-ROP 68
RM-ROP2 68
Rod dysfunction syndrome 179
Rod-cone dystrophy 137
ROP (retinopathy of prematurity, see also RM-ROP) 3, 20, 51
- CRYO- 70
- epidemiology 69
- incidence 63, 70
- international classification see ICROP
- mouse model 52
- national guidelines 73
- phase II 52
- referral-warranted 76
- treatment-requiring 76
- threshold 69
- type 1 68, type 2 68
Rotterdam Amblyopia Screening Effectiveness Study see RAMSES
RPE transplantation 171
RPE65 157, 158
- knockout mice 160, 162
RPGR interacting protein see RPGRIP
RPGRIP1 158, 165
- knockout mice 165
Rubella 205
Ruptured globe 221

S

Sarcoma, granulocytic (chloroma) 128
SBS (shaken baby syndrome) 222
Schwannoma 116
Sclera 5
Scleritis, posterior 202
Screening see vision screening
SEDC (spondyloepiphyseal displasia congenita) 197
Seizure 147, 212
Senior-Loken syndrome 158
Sensitive period of visual development 37
Sensitivity 19
- contrast 41
Sensory deprivation 39
Sexual abuse 226
- covert 226
S-FFM 148
Shaken baby syndrome (SBS) 222
Shaken impact syndrome 222
Skiascopy 96
Smith-Magenis 194
Snellen-based acuity measurement see visual acuity
Spatial frequency 5
Spatial information 2
Spectacle correction, appropriate 188
Spectacles 8
Spectral sensitivity measurement 145
Spherophakia 106
Spoke wheel 148
Spondyloepimetaphyseal dysplasia (Strudwick type) 194, 198
Spondyloepiphyseal dyplasia congenita (SEDC) 194, 197
Stargardt fundus flavimaculatus 145
Stargardt macular dystrophy see dystrophy
Stem cell therapy 171
Stereo test 2
Stereoacuity 39
Steroid 111
Stickler syndrome 191
- type 1 194
- type 2 196
Strabismus 19
- cyclovertical 39
Strudwick type of spondyloepiphyseal displasia congenita see spondyloepiphyseal displasia congenita

Sturge-Weber-Krabbe syndrome 105
Suffocation 225
- covert 225
Surface electrode 134
Synechiae, posterior 211
Synechiolysis, posterior 87
Syphilis 226
- congenital 213
Systemic immunomodulation 106

T

Telemedicine 76
Teratogenic effect 210
Teratoma 127
Terson syndrome 224
Thermotherapy 111, 121
Timolol 101
Tonometer 97
- Perkins- 97
- Schiötz- 97
- Tonopen- 97
Tonometry 96, 97
- hand-held 96
Topical antiviral 211
TORCH 205
Toxoplasma gondii 205
Trabeculectomy 95
Trabeculodysgenesis 96
Trabeculotomy 95
- 360° 103
Trabeculotomy-trabeculectomy, combined 103
Transmitter 6
Transscleral illumination 105
Trauma 191
Tree shrew 3
Treponema pallidum 205
TSCPC (contact-diode transscleral cyclophotocoagulation), contact-diode 105
Tubby like protein see TULP
Tube implant 95
TULP1 (Tubby like protein) 158, 166
Tumor 111
- benign 111
- conjunctival 111
- cutaneous 114
- intraocular 111
- malignant 111
- orbital 111
- vasoproliferative 111
Tunica vasculosa lentis 74

U

Ultrasound biomicroscopy 96
Uniocular blindness see blindness
US Pediatric Eye Disease Investigator Group see PEDIG
Usher syndrome 140
Uveitis 89
- chronic 95

V

Vaccine RA-27 209
Varicella-zoster virus 205
Vascular development 51
Vascular endothelial growth factor see VEGF
Vasoconstriction 65, 74
Vasoobliteration 65
VEGF (vascular endothelial growth factor) 51
- Anti- 53
VEP (visual evoked potential) 41, 133
- appearance (PaVEP) 151
- flash 136, 145
- onset-offset 145
- pattern 143
- - reversal 151
Viscocanalostomy 105
Vision loss, lifetime risk 41
Vision screening 19
- defects 19
- false-negative 20, 24
- false-positive 20
- in childhood 19
- methodology 23
- photorefractive 24
- population-based 20
- preschool 19
- programs 20
- selective 22
- tests 19
Visual acuity 42, 135
- binocular 40
- monocular 24
- Snellen-based measurement 42
- testing 19
Visual chart 23
- age-appropriate 23
- crowded 23
Visual cortex, primary 37
Visual cues 2
Visual cycle 160
Visual evoked potential see VEP
Visual experience 13
Visual feedback 3, 13
Visual field testing 97
Visual handicap 63
Visual loss
- functional 226
- nonorganic 147, 151
Visual maturation, delayed 162
Visual outcome 51, 83
Visual pathway evaluation 133
Visual rehabilitation 84, 92
Visual stimulation 2, 46

Vitelliruptive stage 148
Vitrectomy 69, 83
- anterior 89
- lens-sparing 69
Vitreoretinal displasia 191
Vitreoretinal traction 224
Vitreoretinopathy
- associated with phalangeal epiphyseal dysplasia 198
- familial exudative (FEVR) 194
- hereditary 191
- Wagner 194, 199
Vitreous detachment, posterior 191
Vitreous haemorrhage 39
VMD_2 148
Vogt-Koyanagi-Harada 202
VPED 194

W

Wagner vitreoretinopathy see vitreoretinopathy
Weill-Marchesani syndrome 106
West Nile virus (WNV) 205, 214
Western blot assay 212

X

X-linked carrier 137
XLRS see retinoschisis

Y

YAG laser 83

Z

Zellweger disease, syndrome 147, 158